T0298319

Management of lameness causes in sport horses

Management of lameness causes in sport horses

Muscle, tendon, joint and bone disorders

edited by:
Arno Lindner

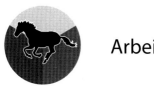 Arbeitsgruppe Pferd

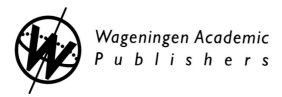 *Wageningen Academic*
P u b l i s h e r s

ISBN-10: 90-8686-004-4
ISBN-13: 978-90-8686-004-3

ISBN-10: 3-00-019187-9
ISBN-13: 978-3-00-019187-9

First published, 2006

Wageningen Academic Publishers
The Netherlands, 2006

All rights reserved.
Nothing from this publication may be
reproduced, stored in a computerised system
or published in any form or in any manner,
including electronic, mechanical, reprographic
or photographic, without prior written
permission from the publisher, Wageningen
Academic Publishers, P.O. Box 220, NL-6700 AE
Wageningen, The Netherlands.

The individual contributions in this publication
and any liabilities arising from them remain the
responsibility of the authors.

The publisher is not responsible for possible
damages, which could be a result of content
derived from this publication.

Foreword

This time the book is available because of CESMAS taking place in Cambridge, England! Many factors have contributed to make it easy to run the conference at this site. First of all the support of Sue Dyson, Pat Harris and their partners. Because of them over the years I have had so many opportunities to be in the area that I knew that nothing could go wrong. Second, the city hosts such a large number of conferences every year that also the logistics of organisation could not fail. And third, many industrial partners were willing from early on to sponsor the meeting.

The contents of this book complement very well the information presented at the CESMAS meeting in Oslo (2004) published in the book „The Elite Race and Endurance Horse". That book focussed on how to have a healthy sport horse and maintain that status, while this one gives more information on how to manage an injured horse and how to rehabilitate it.

I would like to wish readers pleasure reading the book.

Arno Lindner

Scientific Committee
Warwick M. Bayly, USA
Hilary Clayton, USA
Anne Courouché-Malblanc, France
Jean-Marie Denoix, France
Sue Dyson, United Kingdom
Adriana Ferlazzo, Italy
Arne Holm, Norway
Arne Lindholm, Sweden
Arno Lindner, Germany
José Luis López Rivero, Spain
Marianne Sloet van Oldruitenborgh-Oosterbaan, Netherlands
Steven Wickler, USA

Partners
Boehringer Ingelheim Vetmedica
Equine Veterinary Journal
Innovative Technologies & Systems / IDEXX
Vetray

Electro Medical Systems
Intervet
Life Data Labs
Videomed

Table of contents

Articles

Deep digital flexor tendon lesions in the fetlock region: A retrospective study of 108 tenoscopies of digital flexor tendon sheaths suspected of deep digital flexor tendon laceration

Hans Wilderjans and Bernard Boussauw
Equine Hospital De Bosdreef, Spelonckvaart 46, 9180 Moerbeke-Waas, Belgium

The superficial digital flexor tendon (SDFT) and suspensory ligament are more commonly injured in performance horses in comparison to the deep digital flexor tendon (DDFT). Lesions in one of the lobes of the DDFT are a common diagnosis following MRI examination of the front foot (Dyson *et al.*, 2005; personal observations).

DDFT lesions are associated with chronic (non-infected) tenosynovitis of the digital flexor tendon sheath (DFTS) in the fetlock area. The most common presentation of DDFT lesions within the DFTS is longitudinal tears in the lateral border of the DDFT (Wright and McMahon, 1999; Wilderjans *et al.*, 2003; Smith and Wright, 2006). Central core lesions, dorsal or palmar/plantar lesion in the DDFT are seen but are less common. Manica flexoria (MF) tears, longitudinal and branch tears of the SDFT, desmitis of the palmar annular ligament (PAL) and tears in the DFTS itself can also result in a chronic tenosynovitis of the DFTS.

Anatomy of the digital flexor tendon sheath and its content

The DFTS surrounds the SDFT and DDFT palmar or plantar to the fetlock joint. The DFTS begins 4 to 7 cm proximal to the proximal sesamoid bones and extends distally to the middle third of the middle phalanx. At this level a thin wall separates the DFTS from the proximal recess of the podotrochlear bursa and the proximopalmar recess of the distal interphalangeal joint (Denoix, 1994). The DFTS is surrounded by the PAL and the proximal and distal digital annular ligament. The PAL attaches on the palmar/plantar aspect of the sesamoid bones and creates an inelastic canal between the sesamoid bones, intersesamoidean ligament and the PAL. The proximal digital annular ligament is a thinner quadrilateral sheet located over the palmar/plantar aspect of the proximal phalanx. This ligament is mostly adherent to, and very difficult to differentiate from, the DFTS in normal limbs. The distal digital annular ligament is located distally in the pastern and is adherent to the palmar/plantar surface of the distal part of the DFTS (Denoix, 1994). Just proximal to the proximal sesamoid bones the SDFT encircles the DDFT forming a ring called the MF. The distal aspect of the MF is located underneath the PAL (personal observation). Proximal to the MF the DDFT is attached to the DFTS by a medial and lateral band. This band is called the mesotendon. It can easily be recognised on a transverse ultrasound image especially if the tendon sheath is distended (Dik *et al.*, 1995). On the palmar aspect of the fetlock, the SDFT is also attached sagittally with a mesotendon to the DFTS (Dik et al, 1995; Nixon, 1990). This band can clearly be visualised on an ultrasound image of a distended DFTS when there is no important constriction of the PAL (personal observation). The mesotendon of the SDFT, both medial and lateral mesotendon of the DDFT and the MF can also clearly be visualised by tenoscopy of the DFTS (Wright and McMahon, 1999; Wilderjans *et al.*, 2003).

Material and methods

The medical records of 108 cases with non-infected tenosynovitis of the DFTS that had a diagnostic tenoscopy were reviewed between 1999 and 2005 with a follow-up period of minimum 6 months. Seventy-one horses (66%) were diagnosed with a longitudinal tear in a digital flexor tendon, 37 (34%) horses did not have flexor tendon lesions. From those 71 horses with flexor tendon lesions in the DFTS the case history, clinical, ultrasonographic and tenoscopic finding, surgical treatment and post-operative treatment were reviewed. Follow-up information was obtained from the owner, the referring veterinary surgeons or from follow-up examinations performed at the hospital.

We were interested in the final outcome of horses suffering from longitudinal tears in one or more flexor tendons, aiming to compare those horses performing at equal or better level than before the onset of the problem with those performing at a reduced level of performance or with permanent lameness. To this end, average convalescence period, cosmetic end result (reduced, similar or worse distensions of the DFTS than before surgery), limb prevalence, the ultrasonographic accuracy to predict longitudinal tears in the border of the flexor tendons, was measured. The associations between the length and the depth of the tear and final outcome, association between duration of the clinical signs and final outcome, and comparison of the final outcome between tenoscopic treatment with and without PAL desmotomy and the final outcome between treatment with shaver versus treatment with shaver and coblation (ArthroCare) were also measured.

Results

In the 71 horses suffering from LT's, 73 DFTS were examined tenoscopically, 2 horses had bilateral problems; 35 mares, 29 geldings and 7 stallions. They ranged in age between 5 and 18 years with a mean of 12 years. Thirty-four were show-jumpers, 23 dressage horses, 5 standardbreds, 5 general-purpose riding and 4 eventers. Fifty-five horses were warmblood horses, 7 standardbreds, 4 ponies, 2 thoroughbreds, 3 unknown.

The right front limb was affected in 39 cases (55%), the left front in 18 (25%) cases, the right hind limb in 8 (11%) cases and the left hind limb in 6 cases (8%) (Figure 1).

Presence of clinical signs before referral to the hospital varied from 2 days to 4 years with an average of 21 months. Fourteen cases (24%) were presented within the 4 weeks of onset of clinical signs, 14 (24%) between 5 and 15 weeks and 31 (52%) at greater than 15 weeks. In 12 horses this information was unknown. Distension of the DFTS was noticed

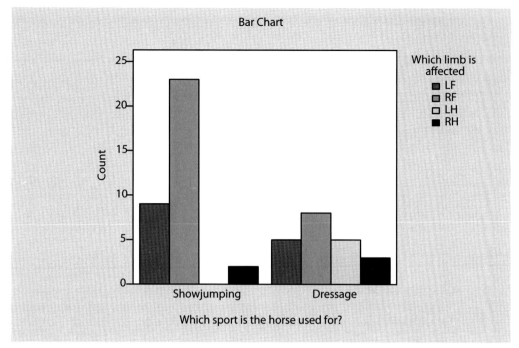

Figure 1. Show jumping horses and the right front fore limb seems to be the most commonly affected.

before referral in 58 cases (98%), 1 (2%) had no obvious distension of the DFTS and in 12 horses this information was unknown. Lameness was present before referral in 43 cases (81%), absent in 10 (19%) and not recorded in 18 horses. Fifty-one horses were treated before referral; 19 (37%) with rest only, 29 (57%) with rest and medical treatment and 3 (6%) had previous surgery, which consisted of PAL desmotomy.

In the 71 horses all DFTS's demonstrated effusion. Forty-two horses (64%) were still lame at the time of examination at the referral hospital, 24 (36%) were sound and in 5 horses this information was not available not recorded. A positive flexion test was present in 40 cases (61%), negative in 26 (39%) and not recorded in 5 cases. A clear "notching" was visible in 20 (30%) horses, absent in 46 (70%) and in 5 horses this information was not recorded.

Local anaesthesia

Intrathecal anaesthesia was performed in 6 of the 71 horses (8%). In 4 horses this abolished the lameness completely and in 2 horses partially.

Radiography

In 15 horses the fetlock was radiographed (21%). In one case there was irregular new bone formation and bone remodelling over the palmar aspect of the sesamoid bones.

One horse had several calcification foci in the DFTS. The remaining 13 horses had no bony abnormalities related to the clinical problem.

Ultrasonography

Ultrasonographic examination was performed with a 7.5 MHz linear transducer with detachable standoff (Toshiba Sonolayer SSH-140A) and from 2005 with a 10 and 12 MHz linear transducer (ESAOTE).

Ultrasonographic information was available on 67 DFTS's. Distension of the DFTS was present on ultrasound in 63 (94%) DFTS's, 4 (6%) showed no abnormal increase in synovial fluid. Obvious thickening of the synovium/tendon sheath wall was present in 39 (58%) of the cases, in 28 (42%) no abnormal thickening was recorded. Thickening of the lateral mesotendon of the DDFT was present in 22 (33%) of the cases, thickening of the lateral and medial mesotendon of the DDFT in 10 (15%) and no obvious thickening in 35 (52%) of the cases. Thickening of the soft tissue palmar/plantar to the SDFT was visible in 37 (55%) cases and considered normal in 30 (45%) cases. This soft tissue thickening included synovium, fibrous part of the DFTS, PAL and subcutaneous tissue. A clear differentiation between those structures is not always possible and for this reason they were grouped together as thickening palmar/plantar to SDFT.

In 36 (54%) cases the DDFT showed ultrasonographic changes indicative of LT's (irregular border of the DDFT, hypoechoic foci, echogenic mass continuous with DDFT border), in 31 (46%) cases the borders of the DDFT were normal on ultrasound. Three horses had an irregular border of the SDFT. One horse had a thickened MF. Additional changes on ultrasound examination included free-floating fibrin (n = 5), obvious synovio-synovial adhesions (n = 1) and intra synovial echodens material (n = 15).

Surgery

All tenoscopies were performed under general anaesthesia: horses were placed in lateral recumbency with the affected site of the limb placed uppermost. An Esmarch bandage and tourniquet at the proximal metacarpus/metatarsus were used in all cases.

Tenoscopy was performed with a 4 mm 25° forward oblique arthroscope with the limb in extension. The technique for tenoscopy of the digital flexor tendon sheath and desmotomy of the PAL as described by Nixon (1990; Nixon *et al.*, 1993) was slightly modified for the treatment of this case series. The tendon sheath was distended in the pastern, between the proximal and distal digital annular ligament, to facilitate entrance of the arthroscopic sleeve using a blunt trocar. The arthroscope was inserted just distal to the PAL almost halfway between the digital neurovascular bundle and the ergot. The lateral or medial entrance portal was positioned lateral or medial to the respective edge of the SDFT. This position allowed both easy passage between the SDFT and the PAL and between SDFT and DDFT. A complete inspection of the tendon sheath and it contents was performed. The instrument portal was made 5 to 10 mm proximal to the PAL almost lateral to the SDFT. A hook probe or curette was introduced through the instrument portal to palpate the flexor tendons. The LT's were not always easy recognised by only viewing the tendons. Palpation of the edge of the flexor tendons is absolutely necessary to appreciate the full depth and extend of the LT's. In all cases torn tendon fibrils protruding from the edge of the DDFT or SDFT indicated the presence of a LT. Palpating the edge of the DDFT within the MF, using the above described instrument portal just proximal to the PAL, is only possible if a small stab incision is made through the MF. At this level the MF still surrounds the DDFT. This precludes visualisation and free passage of instruments to the lateral edge of the DDFT. To gain access to the most proximal part of the LT, a third instrument portal was made as proximal as possible in the tendon sheath between the deep and superficial flexor tendon. This portal allowed full access to the LT not only within but also distal to the MF. For long tears extending further distal to the sesamoidean canal, arthroscope and instrument portals were switched to gain better access to the most distal part of the LT. The MF was never cut to gain access to the most proximal part of the tear.

Desmotomy of the PAL was performed standard from 1999 to 2003 using a hook meniscetomy knife. From 2003, PAL desmotomies was only performed if there was an obvious thickening of the PAL. The PAL was easily transected in a distoproximal direction. Complete division of the PAL often resulted in an important separation of both edges of the cut ligament. Because the most distal part of the PAL is located close to the arthroscope portal, switching portals is recommended to check for complete division of the most distal aspect of the PAL.

Results of tenoscopic inspection

Seventy-nine LT's were detected in 73 DFTS. Sixty-eight (86%) LT's were identified in the DDFT involving 58 fore- and 10 hindlimbs, 9 (11%) in the SDFT involving 5 fore- and 4 hindlimbs and 2 (3%) in the distal margin of the MF of forelimb. Six horses had 2 LT's per DFTS involving DDFT and MF in 2 horses and DDFT and SDFT in 4 horses. The length of the tear was classified as long or a short tears. Long tears (n = 26) (39%) extended from the level of the mesotendon of the DDFT (proximal in the DFTS) to distal to the sesamoidean canal. Short tears (n = 41) (61%) extended from distal to the MF to mid P1 level or from proximal in the DFTS to somewhere in the sesamoidean canal. In 12 cases the length of the tear was not recorded. In 29 cases (62%) the tear was classified as superficial (< 5 mm) in 18 cases (38%) as deep (> 5 mm). In 32 cases this information was not available. LT's in the DDFT were located in the lateral edge in 60 cases (88%), medial edge in 4 cases (6%), plantar in 3 cases (4.5%) and lateropalmar in 1 case (1.5%).

LT's in the SDFT were located lateral in 6 cases (67%), medial in 1 case (11%) and dorsal in 2 cases (22%). In 2 cases the laterodistal free border of the MF was partially torn. In 12 cases there was a mild fibrillation of the free border of the MF without a tear. In 7 cases of lateral LT's of the DDFT, large masses of torn tendon bundles where curled up in the distal part of the tear where they formed a mass of tissue often adhered to the surrounding synovium distal to the sesamoidean canal.

Synovio-synovial adhesions were present in 21 cases. Other less common findings were free floating collagen fibrils (n = 14), fibrin clots, hypertrophic synovium, rough or fibrillated palmar/plantar surface of the SDFT or intersesamoidean ligament, calcifications in the DFTS (n =1), thickened MF (n = 1) and in 1 horse the MF was absent.

Treatment

In 27 LT's (37%) the torn fibrils were resected using a motorised synovial resector (Dyonics-Smith&Nephew-PS3500EP), in 46 LT's (63%) the bulk of torn tendon tissue was removed with a motorised synovial resector followed by further microdebridement and smoothing of the remaining smaller tendon fibres using coblation wands (ArthroCare). Arthroscopic Ferris-Smith rongeurs were used to remove the larger masses of torn tendon fibres, fibrin and to remove the synovio-synovial adhesions. Fibrillation of the palmar/plantar surface of the SDFT was smoothened with coblation.

Forty-six cases (63%) had the PAL transacted and 27 cases (37%) had no transection. From 2003 routine sectioning of the PAL was discontinued. In the following 24 tenoscopies for treatment of LT's only 2 PAL desmotomies were performed because of obvious thickening.

Skin portals were closed with single interrupted vertical mattress suture of 3 metric polydioxanone (PDS). A padded bandage was applied to the lower limb. In 2 horses that had previous unsuccessful tenoscopic treatment of a LT in the DDFT, a follow up tenoscopic evaluation was converted into an open approach because the LT's were too deep and too long. The DDFT was opened through a vertical incision from proximal to distal to the PAL as described by Wright and McMahon (1999). The MF was divided to gain full access to the tear. In one case the previously sectioned edge of the PAL was adhered over its entire length with the SDFT. Those adhesions were removed. The LT's were debrided and the torn edges were removed with a scalpel n°11. Flexion of the fetlock joint improved access to the tear. In both cases the LT was sutured with a 2 metric polydioxanone (PDS). Wound closure consisted of suturing the MF, PAL and DFTS with a polyglactin 910 (vicryl) 3 metric, subcutaneous layer was closed with monocryl 3 metric and the skin was closed with stainless skin staples (Ethicon). A double layer padded bandage was applied to the operated leg for recovery. All recoveries were rope-assisted recoveries (Wilderjans, 2000).

Drug therapy

All horses received preoperative procaine penicillin G (22,000 iu/kg bwt i.m., B.I.D.) and phenylbutazone (2.2 mg/kg bwt i.v., S.I.D.). Penicillin treatment was continued post operatively for 3 days. Phenylbutazone (equipalazone) was continued for 8 days after surgery.

Post operative care

The bandage was changed 4-6 days after surgery and maintained for 2 weeks post operatively. Skin sutures were removed 2 weeks after surgery. There were no post-operative complications. Horses were box rested for the first 3 months after surgery but a controlled ascending walking exercise program was started 10 days after surgery. Ridden walking exercise was allowed 4 weeks after surgery. Walking-time was gradually increased from 15 minutes to 45-60 minutes per day. At the end of this period, owners were asked to present their horse for clinical and ultrasonographical re-evaluation. Horses, which were sound received 3 months walking, trot and light canter work for the next 3 months. After this period the horses were re-evaluated and if sound they gradually returned to normal work. Owners were asked not to resume the normal work level until 8 months post surgery.

Follow up results

Follow-up information of > 6 months (6-78; mean 41) was available for 71 DFTS (69 horses). Twenty-six horses (38%) returned to a level of work equal or higher than before the onset of the lameness. Twenty-six horses (38%) returned to a lower level of work than before the onset of clinical signs and 17 horses (24%) remained lame. Some horses could return to the previous level of competition but at reduced frequency and with intrathecal hyaluronan and corticosteroid treatment. Others competed initially at equal or higher level but had recurrence of the clinical signs after several months. Those horses were classified in the "lower level of work" or "lame" group.

Distension of the DFTS was completely resolved in 5 cases (7%), reduced and mild in 43 cases (62%), similar compared to the pre-operative situation in 15 cases (22%) and worse compared to the pre-operative situation in 6 cases (9%). The relation between final outcome and return to previous level of work is summarised in Table 1.

On 27 horses re-examined at 6 months post-operative we had some ultrasonographic data. In 11 cases a mild irregularity was still visible. Three (27%) were in the equal/ higher level group, 6 (55%) in the lower level group and 2 (18%) in the "lame" group. We had insufficient consistent ultrasonographic data to draw conclusions on the long-term outcome versus ultrasonographic appearance of the DFTS and its contents. However we observed on ultrasound examination that the majority of cases which had thickening of the soft tissue palmar/plantar to the SDFT, reduced in size but never returned to normal thickness. Thickened mesotendons reduced to normal or almost normal size in the majority of the horses. Synovial fluid and echodens material decreased.

The relation between final outcome and treatment with synovial resector, coblation, PAL resection, length of the tear, presence of post operative distension and duration of clinical signs are summarized in Table 1.

Table 1. Relation between final outcome and treatment with synovial resector, coblation, PAL resection, length of the tear, presence of post operative distension and duration of clinical signs.

Performance group	Equal or higher	Lower	Lame	Unknown
Tenoscopic treatment	26 (38%)	26 (38%)	17 (24%)	2
PAL desmotomy n = 46	18 (41%)	16 (36%)	10 (23%)	2
No PAL desmotomy n = 27	7 (26%)	13 (48%)	7 (26%)	
Synovial resector n = 27	14 (52%)	7 (26%)	6 (22%)	
Synovial resector and coblation n = 46	11 (25%)	22 (50%)	11 (25%)	2
Synovial resector + PAL desmotomy n = 23	12 (52%)	6 (26%)	5 (21%)	
Synovial resector + no PAL desmotomy n = 4	2 (50%)	1 (25%)	1 (25%)	
Synovial resector + Coblation + PAL desmotomy n = 21	6 (23%)	8 (42%)	5 (26%)	2
Synovial resector + Coblation + no PAL desmotomy n = 23	5 (22%)	12 (52%)	6 (26%)	
Long tear n = 25	6 (24%)	14 (56%)	5 (20%)	
Short tear n = 38	15 (42%)	12 (33%)	9 (25%)	8
< 5 w before referral n = 14	6 (43%)	6 (43%)	2 (13%)	
5-15 w before referral n = 14	6 (43%)	3 (21%)	5 (36%)	
> 15 w before referral n = 31	8 (26%)	17 (55%)	6 (19%)	12
DFTS distension resolved n = 5	1 (20%)	4 (80%)	0 (0%)	
DFTS distension reduced n = 43	15 (35%)	16 (37%)	12 (28%)	
DFTS distension similar n = 15	8 (53%)	5 (33%)	2 (13%)	
DFTS distension increased n = 6	1 (17%)	2 (33%)	3 (50%)	2

Discussion and conclusions

Statistic analyses of the results are not available yet.

There was no gender predisposition and warmblood horses were over-represented, but this reflects the hospital's caseload. Non-infected tenosynovitis caused by LTs is more common in the older (11-15 years old) warmblood show jumper. Longitudinal tears affect the forelimb more frequently than the hindlimb and the right forelimb is significant more affected than the other limbs (see Figure 1). The reason for this is unclear. Smith and Wright (2006) also identified more marginal tears of the DDFT in the forelimb. The precise aetiology of those LTs is unknown but stress or trauma is very likely to be the cause.

Longitudinal tears will mainly affect the lateral border of the DDFT. The proportion of LTs affecting the lateral border was much greater than as reported by Smith and Wright

(2006). One of the reasons is probably the type of work and the higher presence of show jumping horses in our case study. Conversely, tears of the MF were more common in Smith and Wright (2006) series but were very uncommon in our study.

Distension of the DFTS is almost always present but can disappear temporarily in acute cases with some rest. Lameness and a positive flexion of the Mc/Mt phalangeal joint are often present. More than 80% of the horses where lame at referral or had a history of lameness. More than 50% of the horses had distension of the DFTS for more than 15 weeks, unresponsive to rest and medical treatment.

Ultrasound examination is the best non-invasive diagnostic tool to identify longitudinal tears in the border of the DDFT. Ultrasonography predicted the lesions identified at tenoscopy in 36 (54%) of the cases. With growing experience and based on case history, clinical and ultrasound examination, the examiners where able to suspect LT's as the underlying cause of tenosynovitis in 50 (70%) of the cases. Smith and Wright (2006) predicted marginal tears of the DDFT with a sensitivity of 71%, specificity of 71%, a positive predictive value of 71% and a negative predictive value of 55%. Typical but non specific changes on ultrasonographic examination of distended DFTS's are thickening of the tendon sheath wall, increased synovial fluid, thickening of the PAL, thickening of the mesotendons of the DDFT and thickening the soft tissue palmar/plantar to the SDFT (synovium, PAL, subcutaneous tissue).
Irregular outlining, hypoechoic lesions and echogenic masses at the margin of the DDFT are strongly indicative for longitudinal marginal tears. These changes are often best visible just proximal to the proximal border of the PAL. At this level the DDFT is still surrounded by the MF. Slightly oblique views can help identifying the LT's. Unilateral distension of a DFTS especially in a forelimb, with a history of lameness and non-responding to rest, are strongly suspected of LT's of a flexor tendon even if only non specific changes are visible on ultrasound examination.

Constriction of the PAL was present in 24 (37%) of the cases and is mainly a problem in chronic long-standing tenosynovitis of the DFTS. Constriction of the PAL is in most cases of tenosynovitis a secondary problem with LT's in the DDFT being the primary problem. If synovial fluid is present between the SDFT and the PAL we consider the PAL not to cause constriction of the sesamoidean canal. Only low pressure should be applied on the ultrasound probe to allow visualisation of this fluid and to avoid pushing the PAL against the SDFT.

Tenoscopy of the DFTS is the only way to confirm and accurately describe the morphology of the longitudinal tears. The length of the LT appears to affect the outcome (Table 1). Long tears have less chance to return to previous level of work. This is in agreement with the findings of Smith and Wright (2006). Torn tendon fibrils, protruding from the edge of the flexor tendons, always indicates the presence of a LT. However the tenoscopic appearance can vary from subtle fraying of the margin of the tendon to large pieces of torn tendon bundles floating in the irrigation fluid. In some cases a large mass of tissue is sitting in the distal or proximal end of the tear representing retracted and curled up tendon bundles often adhered to the surrounding synovial membrane. Palpation of the tendon border and placing the arthroscope in the tear is necessary to appreciate the depth of the tear.

Disrupted collagen fibrils protruding from the tendon are the most likely cause of chronic irritation of the DFTS, creating distension of the sheath, thickening of the sheath wall, synovial hypertrophy and annular ligament constriction syndrome (ALCS) in chronic cases. Within a tendon sheath there are no mechanisms available that can remove disrupted collagen fibres (Wright and McMahon, 1999). The results after suturing the tear with an open approach were inferior to tenoscopic debridement and second intention healing (Wright and McMahon, 1999). In our case series all the longitudinal tears were treated by tenoscopic debridement with or without PAL desmotomy and smoothing of the fibres with coblation. Suturing the LTs, as described by Wright and McMahon (1999), was only performed on 2 cases with LT's of the lateral edge of the DDFT unresponsive to tenoscopic debridement. One horse returned to previous level of work, the other one to a lower level of work.

Initially, PAL desmotomy was performed on all cases in combination with tenoscopic debridement of the LT. Later we considered that this was not contributing a lot to the case management and PAL desmotomy was only performed in 2 of 24 cases where ALCS was obviously present on ultrasound and tenoscopy. We noted extensive adhesions between the sectioned PAL edge and the SDFT during tenoscopy of 2 cases that had PAL desmotomy surgery before referral. This indicates that PAL desmotomy is not free of complication and should be restricted to those cases showing clear signs of ALCS.

We introduced coblation in combination with resection of the torn tendon fibres to further minimise the exposure of torn collagen tissue. Motorised synovial resectors are not capable to create a smooth surface and careful use of radiofrequency energy in saline is capable of gently dissolving the remaining fibres. Coblation wands were used in no contact mode after first debriding the bulk of fibres with a motorised synovial resector.

The relation between final outcome and treatment with synovial resector, with and without coblation and with and without PAL resection are summarized in Table 1.

The long-term prognosis for horses following tenoscopic treatment of longitudinal tears is guarded. Twenty-six horses (38%) returned to an equal or higher level of work, 26 (38%) to a lower level of work and 17 (24%) remained lame. This is in accordance with the findings of Smith and Wright (2006) who reported 14 of 33 horses (42%) with marginal tears of the DDFT returning to previous level of work. Longer tears and horses operated after 15 weeks seemed to carry a worse prognosis. Early diagnosis and treatment seems to improve the final outcome. Those findings are in accordance with the case series described by Smith and Wright (2006). Persistence of post-operative distension of the DFTS is normal but marked distension after surgery indicates incomplete healing and increased chance of permanent lameness. Those findings are comparable with Smith and

Wright (2006). Desmotomy of the PAL and the use of coblation do not seem to affect the final outcome (Table1).

A long and controlled postoperative program was considered to be important in the final outcome of the cases. Controlled exercise was started 10 days after the surgery but return to normal work was postponed until 8 months after surgery. In most cases clinical symptoms improved quickly after surgery but a final evaluation is only possible after resuming the intended work level.

It is important to note that even after a successful surgery the cosmetic result is seldom completely perfect. In most cases a firm non-painful distension will remain visible and palpable. The typical non-specific ultrasonographic changes will improve but never disappear completely.

The results of this study indicate that the majority of unilateral tenosynovitis of the DFTS, especially in forelimbs, is caused by longitudinal tears in the DDFT. Ultrasonography is the most reliable non-invasive diagnostic tool but tenoscopy is the only accurate way to identify the location and morphology of those longitudinal tears. Until now, tenoscopic debridement with a motorised synovial resector was the best treatment option but long-term results are guarded. New treatment options to improve the healing of the tears should be investigated and further methods to prevent this type of injury especially in middle-aged show-jumpers should be sought.

References

Denoix, J.M., 1994. Functional anatomy of tendons and ligaments in the distal limbs (manus and pes). Vet. Clin. N. Am. Equine Pract. 10: 273-322.

Dik, K.J., S.J. Dyson and T.B. Vail, 1995. Aseptic tenosynovitis of the digital flexor tendon sheath, fetlock and pastern annular ligament constriction. Vet. Clin. N. Am. Equine Pract. 11: 151-162.

Dyson, S.J., R. Murray and M.C. Schramme, 2005. Lameness associated with foot pain: results of magnetic resonance imaging in 199 horses (January 2001-December 2003) and response to treatment. Equine Vet. J. 37: 113-121.

Nixon, A.J., 1990. Endoscopy of the digital flexor tendon sheath in horses. Vet. Surg. 19: 266-271.

Nixon, A.J., A.E. Sacus and N.G. Ducharme, 1993. Endoscopically assisted annular ligament release in horses. Vet. Surg. 22: 501-507.

Smith, M.R.W. and I.M. Wright, 2006. Noninfected tenosynovitis of the digital flexor tendons: A retrospective analysis of 76 cases. Equine Vet. J. 38: 134-141.

Wilderjans, H., 2000. BEVA Equine Specialist Meeting, Royal college of Physicians, London: Advances in assisted recovery from anaesthesia of horses with fractures.

Wilderjans, H., B. Boussauw, K. Madder and O. Simon, 2003. Tenosynovitis of the digital flexor tendon sheath and annular constriction syndrome caused by longitudinal tears in the deep digital flexor tendon: a clinical and surgical report of 17 cases in Warmblood horses. Equine Vet. J. 35: 270-275.

Wright, I.M. and P.J. McMahon, 1999. Tenosynovitis associated with longitudinal tears of the digital flexor tendons in horses: A report of 20 cases. Equine Vet. J. 31: 12-18.

Treatment results for the causes of digital flexor tendon sheath distension

Matthew R.W. Smith

Reynolds House Referrals, Greenwood Ellis & Partners, 166 High Street, Newmarket, United Kingdom

This paper describes the causes and results of treatment of 125 cases of non-infected tenosynovitis of the DFTS. The animals were all working adults used for a variety of purposes but racehorses were under-represented. The duration of clinical signs prior to surgery ranged from 1-104 (mean 16) weeks. The DFTSs were affected in 58 forelimbs and 65 hindlimbs (including 3 animals affected bilaterally). One hundred and twenty-four animals were lame at presentation with the severity ranging from 1 to 8/10. All sheaths were distended. Radiological abnormalities were detected in 4 animals; 2 cases had irregular new bone formation on the abaxial margins of the proximal sesamoid bones and 2 cases had foci of dystrophic mineralisation (one in the PAL and one the DDFT).

Ultrasonography confirmed fluid distension in all cases, and frequently demonstrated non-specific findings including thickening of the sheath wall, thickened DDFT plicae and intra-thecal echogenic material. In 52 cases ultrasonographic features were consistent with the presence of tearing of the DDFT (43) or SDFT (9) and in 23 animals tearing of the manica flexoria. Other ultrasonographic features included thickening of the PAL (13), disruption of the insertion of the SDFT (3), disruption of the straight distal sesamoidean ligament (2), mineralisation of the SDFT (1) or DDFT (1), and sheath rupture and/or synovioceole formation (6).

Ninety-seven animals underwent tenoscopy in lateral recumbency and 28 in dorsal recumbency. All limbs were exsanguinated with an Esmarch bandage and proximal tourniquets applied. Initial arthroscopic evaluation was performed through a portal between the PAL and proximal digital annular ligament (Nixon, 1990). The tenoscopic diagnoses are recorded in Table 1.

Ultrasonography accurately predicted the lesions identified at tenoscopy in 54% of cases.

In DFTSs with torn tissue, treatment aimed to reduce exposure of disrupted tissue to the synovial environment. In 110 cases treatment was performed using tenoscopic techniques only, with instrument portals sited according to lesion location. Large masses of torn tendon tissue and granulomata were dissected free with arthroscopic scissors or meniscectomy knives before removal with Ferris-Smith arthroscopic rongeurs. Tendonous defects were also debrided with a motorised synovial resector in an oscillating mode with suction applied. When necessary, arthroscope and instrument portals were

Table 1. Tenoscopic diagnoses in 128 digital flexor tendon sheaths.

Diagnosis	Number
Marginal tear DDFT	66
Marginal tear DDFT only	50
Marginal tear DDFT + other	16
Torn manica flexoria	41
Torn manica flexoria only	28
Torn manica flexoria + other	13
Marginal tear SDFT	13
Marginal tear SDFT only	5
Marginal tear SDFT + other	4
Torn medial branch only	3
Torn medial branch SDFT + other	1
Sheath tear	12
Sheath tear only	1
Sheath tear + other	11
Adhesions/fibrosis	14
Adhesions only	1
Adhesions + other	13
Torn digital manica	3
Torn digital manica only	2
Torn digital manica + other	1
Torn lateral plica DDFT	3
Torn lateral plica DDFT only	2
Torn lateral plica DDFT + other	1

interchanged to optimise accessibility of lesions for assessment and treatment. Access to tears of the DDFT which commenced beneath the MF was optimised by creation of an instrument portal at the proximal DFTS reflection which permits instruments to pass between the MF and DDFT. Partial tears of the MF (12) were debrided, and the MF was removed in its entirety when one margin was disrupted completely (29). In 4 latter cases, partially torn MF were removed in their entirety. Removal was effected by division of the intact margin opposite the tear from the SDFT, and subsequently its attachments to the proximal sheath reflection, using arthroscopic scissors and / or meniscectomy knives. Occasionally a second instrument was utilised concurrently to grasp and to stabilise the torn MF in order to aid division. Following tenoscopic evaluation 15 DFTSs were treated with open surgical techniques. This included repair (7) or debridement (1) of marginal tears of the DDFT, repair (1) or removal (4) of torn manica flexoria, repair of tears of the sheath wall (4) and repair (1) or debridement (2) of marginal tears of the SDFT.

Medical management consisted of peri-operative systemic antimicrobial and non-steroidal anti-inflammatory drugs only. A controlled, ascending exercise program commenced immediately following surgery and the horses returned to normal work between 3 and 18 (mean 7) months post-operatively.

Follow-up information of between 4 and 64 (mean 17 months) post-operatively was available for 99 horses. Seventy animals (70%) were sound and 54/94 (57%) returned to a level of work equal or better than obtained pre-operatively. Distension of the DFTS resolved in 30/87 (35%) horses and was considered improved in a further 36 (41%) animals.

For tears of the DDFT, 30/55 (55%) animals became sound following surgery, and 20/50 (40%) returned to previous levels of performance. Distension resolved in 13/48 (27%) sheaths, and was improved in a further 17 (35%). Compared to all other diagnoses, marginal tears of DDFT were associated with reduced post-operative soundness and performance, and no improvement in distension post-operatively. Further to this, long tears were associated with reduced post-operative performance when compared to short tears (18% and 68% respectively returned to work at their previous levels). Treatment with tenoscopic debridement alone resulted in a higher rate of return to pre-injury levels of performance than open surgical repair of DDFT lesions.

Manica flexoria tears had a better rate of return to soundness (81%) and previous levels of performance (73%), and reduction in post-operative distension (90%) than seen with marginal tears of the DDFT. Favourable outcomes were seen following both complete excision of the MF (84% sound, 76% return to previous performance), and debridement of tears (60% sound, 50% return to previous performance).

Horses without tearing of a tendon or the MF had excellent outcomes, with 9/11 (81%) becoming sound and returning to previous levels of performance. DFTS distension resolved in 7/10 (70%) and reduced in 9/10 (90%).

Increasing duration of clinical signs was associated with reduced post-operative soundness and performance, and a lack of improvement in distension post-operatively. Marked pre-operative distension was associated with both reduced levels of post-operative performance and no improvement in post-operative distension.

The nature and distribution of lesions seen in this series differs from reported experiences in the United States (Fortier *et al.*, 1999; Nixon, 2003), but is similar to other European series (Smith and Wright, 2006; Wilderjans *et al.*, 2003; Wright and McMahon, 1999). It has been hypothesised that the pathogenesis of complex tenosynovitis involves inflammation and subsequent fibrous thickening of the sheath and PAL resulting in pressure, irritation of the tendons within the DFTS and ultimately formation of teno-synovial masses (Fortier *et al.*, 1999; Nixon, 2003). Desmotomy of the PAL has therefore been considered to have therapeutic benefit. In this series the PAL was considered contributory only when thickened, and therefore transected in the minority of cases. The surgeons treating the cases in this series hypothesised that the intra-thecal lesions identified are primary, and these have been treated without desmotomy of the PAL.

The results of this series indicate tenoscopic debridement offers a reasonable prognosis for the majority of animals with non-infected tenosynovitis of the DFTS. The prognosis for long tears of the DDFT remains guarded, even following tenoscopic debridement, and alternative or adjunctive therapeutic interventions need considering.

Acknowledgements

The author would like to thank Ian Wright for the contribution of 100 cases for which he was primary surgeon.

References

Fortier, L.A., A.J. Nixon, N.G. Ducharme, H.O. Mohammed and A. Yeager, 1999. Tenoscopic examination and proximal annular ligament desmotomy for treatment of equine "complex" digital sheath tenosynovitis. Vet. Surg. 28: 429-435.

Nixon, A.J., 1990. Endoscopy of the digital flexor tendon sheath in horses. Vet. Surg. 19: 266-271.

Nixon, A.J., 2003. Arthroscopic surgery of the carpal and digital tendon sheaths. Clin. Tech. Equine Pract. 1: 245-256.

Smith, M.R.W. and I.M. Wright, 2006. Noninfected tenosynovitis of the digital flexor tendons: A retrospective analysis of 76 cases. Equine Vet. J. 38: 134-141.

Wilderjans, H., B. Boussauw, K. Madder and O. Simon, 2003. Tenosynovitis of the digital flexor tendon sheath and annular constriction syndrome caused by longitudinal tears in the deep digital flexor tendon: a clinical and surgical report of 17 cases in Warmblood horses. Equine Vet. J. 35: 270-275.

Wright, I.M. and P.J. McMahon, 1999. Tenosynovitis associated with longitudinal tears of the digital flexor tendons in horses: A report of 20 cases. Equine Vet. J. 31: 12-18.

Diagnosis of superficial digital flexor tendonitis and paratendonitis

Eddy Cauvin
Le Sanmoranth, 3314 Route des Serres, F-06570 Saint-Paul, France

Introduction

Tendonitis is one of the most common conditions affecting horses. The diagnosis has been revolutionised by the advent of ultrasonography. Thanks to improving technology, we are able to detect increasingly subtle, even subclinical disease, and provide an accurate prognosis at an early stage. This has changed the way we can follow-up cases and gear the management.

Clinical presentation

The initial presentation may be quite variable. Sudden onset lameness may occur during or immediately after exercise, but in some cases the horse slows down or only shows pain and swelling the day after the injury. The lesions are most often spontaneous and there are rarely prodromal signs. However, some horses will tend to present mild swelling or filling of the 'tendon' area with no apparent lameness on several occasions before overt tendonitis. With typical tendonitis, there is heat and swelling over the palmar aspect of the metacarpus (less commonly plantar metatarsus) particularly marked 24 hours after injury. There may be palpable pain. This gradually recedes over 4 to 10 days, leaving a firm, bow-shaped swelling over the 'tendon' area ('bowed tendon'). There may be associated distension of the carpal and / or digital sheath(s), depending on the site of lameness. The latter may be moderate to severe initially and usually recedes after 7 to 20 days. The severity of the swelling and lameness do not correlate well with the severity of the tear and it is not unusual to see severe lesions in the absence of lameness after only a few days of rest. Early return to exercise may then cause a more severe strain.

Paratendonitis relates to inflammation or trauma to the paratenon, most often from direct trauma (interference, hitting solid objects, rub from bandages, *etc.*). The paratenon is a thin layer of loose connective tissue surrounding the tendon in unsheathed areas. This is increasingly recognised with the use of high frequency transducers. This condition has long been recognised in man but lacks recognition in horses. Although this does not affect the tendon per se, this condition may be very painful and is often indistinguishable from tendonitis clinically, at least in the first 5 to 20 days where there is subcutaneous oedema, peritendinous swelling, lameness and pain on palpation.

Clinical examination

Suspicion is usually based on lameness associated with swelling, heat and pain over the palmar metacarpal or plantar metatarsal area. These signs are not pathognomonic as there may be marked oedema in that region with a number of other conditions. In the acute stage, swelling is usually very diffuse and it may be difficult to detect tendon thickening. One should be cautious of not overinterpreting pain on deep palpation over the tendon as many horses tend to respond to that test in the absence of significant lesion.

In subacute and chronic cases, thickening is usually easy to palpate, although there may be a lot of peritendinous thickening and fibrosis, which may be difficult to differentiate from intratendinous thickening. There is actually little correlation between clinical presentation, palpation and the severity of the lesions as based on ultrasonographic appearance.

Ultrasonography

Ultrasonography is the diagnostic method of choice and should be performed whenever there is suspicion of soft tissue injury in the palmar metacarpus / plantar metatarsus. However, it is best carried out at 7 to 10 days, as the lesions may initially continue to increase in size and the ultrasonographic appearance may be confusing before that subacute stage. In fact, in the initial, acute stage, the intratendinous haematoma may look echogenic and may be indistinguishable from the surrounding, normal tendon tissue. Longitudinal scans should show some loss of fibre alignment but in any case, proteolytic enzymes, oedema and cell infiltration systematically cause enlargement of the lesion. In case of suspicion of tendonitis, an initial scan may be performed rapidly after the onset of swelling, but the owners / trainers should be warned that it may be difficult to give them an accurate prognosis and that lesions may only become evident after 7 to 10 days. In that case, it is probably best to rest the horse, start treatment and rescan after a week.

High definition ultrasound systems, using 7.5 to 12 MHz linear array transducers, are most adequate. A systematic approach must be used and comparison with the opposite limb is often valuable. The limb should be clipped. It is possible to scan horses without clipping, but this will significantly decrease image quality, create artefacts, especially with high frequency probes, and it may impair the detection of subtle lesions. The whole area should be assessed, including the suspensory ligament and the pastern in case of low bows or in the presence of digital sheath effusion.

Typical lesions in the SDFT appear as discrete, well defined hypo (= dark grey)- or an-echogenic (black) areas in cross (transverse) sections. These are most often located near the centre of the tendon but it may also occur at the periphery. The size of the defect should be measured and its ratio to the whole cross sectional area of the tendon calculated (most scanners make it possible).

Associated swelling of the tendon due to oedema, haemorrhage and cell infiltration causes an increased cross-sectional surface area, although this should be differentiated from peritendinous swelling. Some lesions may be more diffused and less well defined and some may show a heterogeneous pattern. This is particularly obvious in recurring cases where there may be small foci of decreased echogenicity associated with hyperechogenic areas. Longitudinal scans should always be performed as they will show the proximodistal extent of the lesion and degree of loss of the normal fibre pattern, typical of type I collagen fibres.

In completely ruptured tendons, the fibrous tissue is replaced by amorphous, hypoechogenic tissue containing anechogenic foci (haematoma formation). This tissue is gradually replaced by homogeneous, hypoechogenic granulation tissue. No normal tendon tissue is visible at the level of the rupture. The frayed ruptured ends are hypoechogenic and heterogeneous.

In all cases, with time, the echogenicity of the lesion tends to increase because of decreased infiltration and increased collagen deposition. Scar tissue is iso- to hyperechogenic to normal tendon tissue but lacks a normal fibrillar pattern on longitudinal scans. Mineralisation may be present in chronic cases, causing hyperechogenic interfaces casting an acoustic shadow. Lesions most often occur in the metacarpal, unsheathed area. They may also occur, though much less commonly, either within the carpal flexor tendon sheath or the digital sheath.

Distal SDFT branch injuries are increasingly recognised. The branch will appear enlarged, hypoechogenic and heterogeneous. The lesion may be defined or, more frequently, diffuse. One or both branches may be affected but the medial branch appears to be most commonly involved. There is usually associated digital sheath effusion. In the author's experience, this is very rare, except in trotters. The initial examination will confirm the diagnosis, and determine the localisation, size, extent and severity of the lesion.

Ultrasonography should then be used regularly (every 8 to 12 weeks) to monitor the progress and quality of healing. Ideally, there should be an increase in echogenicity (fibrous tissue formation) and fibre alignment on longitudinal scans. Adequate healing is characterised by isoechogenicity of the damaged portion with normal tendon tissue and near-longitudinal alignment of the replacement fibres. In many cases, however, immature or poorly organised fibrous tissue will replace the damaged tendon. This will give an echogenic, often heterogeneous tissue on cross sections, but longitudinal scans will show poor to absent fibre alignment.

In cases of recurrence, peritendinous thickening, decreased echogenicity and multiple hypoechogenic foci are visible. Full size lesions may occur and tend to be worse than the initial injury. Most recurring lesions occur proximal or distal to the original site of injury.

The diagnosis of paratendonitis may be more subtle. In most cases, there is focal, hypoechogenic thickening of the paratenon, which normally forms a thin layer of moderately echogenic tissue around the tendon. The lesion is most often encountered over the palmar/plantar aspect of the tendon at any level in the metacarpus or metatarsus. It is probably as common in the hind as fore limb. In acute cases, there may be extensive peritendinous and subcutaneous oedema. Within a few days, this recedes leaving a variably sized, hypoechogenic area just palmar/plantar to the tendon. The lesion may extend as a notch into the substance of the tendon. These lesions can persist for several weeks. Obvious haematomas may form in some cases. After a few weeks, the echogenicity increases and the lesion size decreases although some fibrous tissue thickening may remain. This may occasionally interfere mechanically with the function of the tendon. Adhesions can also develop abaxially, especially with the accessory ligament of the deep digital flexor tendon. Paratendonitis is often present in combination with tendonitis.

There is some controversy as to the ability to detect subclinical or pre-clinical lesions with ultrasound. Certainly, gradual degeneration as observed biochemically or histologically most often goes undetected. However, with increasing use of ultrasound as a preventive means, slightly hypoechogenic foci are occasionally encountered in the SDFT of race horses without obvious signs of tendonitis. This has been suggested to represent subclinical tears or degeneration (R.K. Smith, personal communication).

Prognosis

Early publications suggested that the greater the ratio of lesion size over total tendon cross section, the poorer the prognosis. However, many factors will have to be taken in consideration.

The prognosis can be based on increased cross sectional area of the tendon, and decrease of echogenicity, cross sectional surface area (relative to that of the tendon) and proximo-distal length of the lesion. Diffuse lesions carry a worse prognosis than central core lesions.

The prognosis for soundness is always good, even with severe tears. Even very severe lesions will heal eventually. However, the prognosis for return to the same level of activity and performance is often moderate to guarded, depending on the severity of the lesion. Up to 50% of affected racehorses never return to racing, while recurrence occurs in up to 80% of cases. In other athletic activities, the prognosis is probably better but the risk of recurrence remains high. A more useful parameter to take into account is the quality of the repair tissue, *i.e.* primarily the quality of the fibre alignment in repair tissue.

Further references

Crass, J.R., R.L. Genovese, J.A. Render and E.M. Bellon, 1992. Magnetic resonance, ultrasound and histopathologic correlation of acute and healing equine tendon injuries. Vet. Radiol. and Ultrasound 33: 206-216.

Denoix, J.M., M. Mialot, I. Levy, et al., 1990. Etude anatomo-pathologique des lesions associees aux images echographiques anormales des tendons et ligaments chez le cheval. Recueil de Medecine Veterinaire 166: 45-55.

Dyson, S., 1992. Ultrasonographic examination of the metacarpal and metatarsal regions in the horse. Equine Vet. Educ. 4: 139-144.

Genovese, R.L., N.W. Rantanen, M.L. Hauser, et al., 1986. Diagnostic ultrasonography of equine limbs. Vet. Clin. North Am. [Equine Pract.] 2: 145-226.

Genovese, R.L., N.W. Rantanen, B.S. Simpson and D.M. Simpson, 1990. Clinical experience with quantitative analysis of superficial digital flexor tendon injuries in Thoroughbred and Standardbred racehorses. Vet. Clin. North Am. [Equine Pract.] 6: 129-145.

Genovese, R.L., V.B. Reef, K.L. Longo, J.W. Byrd and W.M. Davis, 1996. Superficial digital flexor tendonitis: Long term sonographic and clinical study of racehorses. In: Proceedings Dubai International Equine Symposium 1, pp. 187-205.

Gillis, C.L., D.M. Meagher, R.R. Pool, S.M. Stover, T.J. Craychee, N. Willits, 1993. Ultrasonographically detected changes in equine superficial digital flexor tendons during the first months of race training. Am. J. Vet. Res. 54: 1797-1802.

Gillis, C., D.M. Meagher, A. Cloninger, L. Locatelli and N. Willits, 1995. Ultrasonographic cross-sectional area and mean echogenicity of the superficial and deep digital flexor tendons in 50 trained Thoroughbred racehorses. Am. J. Vet. Res. 56: 1265-1269.

Marr, C.M., I. McMillan, J.S. Boyd, N.G. Wright and M. Murray, 1993. Ultrasonographic and histopathological findings in equine superficial digital flexor tendon injury. Equine Vet. J. 25: 23-29.

Rantanen, N.W., R.L. Genovese and R. Gaines, 1983. The use of diagnostic ultrasound to detect structural damage to the soft tissues of the extremities of horses. J. Equine Vet. Sci. 3: 134-135.

Reef, V.B., B.B. Martin and K. Stebbins, 1989. Comparison of ultrasonographic, gross and histologic appearance of tendon injuries in performance horses. In: Proceedings 35th Annu. Conv. Am. Assoc. Equine Pract., pp. 279.

Smith, R.K.W., R. Jones and P.M. Webbon, 1994. The cross-sectional areas of normal equine digital flexor tendons determined ultrasonographically. Equine Vet. J. 26: 460-465.

Spurlock, G.H., S.L. Spurlock and G.A. Parker, 1989. Ultrasonographic, gross and histologic evaluation of a tendinitis disease model in a horse. Vet. Radiol. 30: 184-188.

Yovich, J.V., H. Sawdon, T. Booth, et al., 1995. Correlation of ultrasonographic findings and long term outcome in racehorses with superficial digital flexor tendon injury. Aust. Equine Pract. 13: 89-92.

Management of superficial digital flexor tendonitis

Lisa A. Fortier
Cornell University, Ithaca, NY, USA

Management of superficial digital flexor tendonitis (SDFT tendonitis) should encompass medical, surgical, rehabilitation and prevention therapies. Proper management requires an accurate diagnosis, including ultrasound examination of tendons within the carpal and digital sheaths. This is important since tendon lesions within either sheath may require surgical attention. The majority of medical treatments for equine tendonitis have centered on delivery of a single or multiple growth factors to the site of injury. Growth factors are protein signaling molecules that regulate cellular metabolism. They enhance tendon and ligament healing by stimulating cell proliferation, increasing extracellular matrix synthesis and promoting vascular ingrowth. In addition to their anabolic effects, growth factors down regulate catabolic, matrix degrading cytokines such as interleukins and matrix metalloproteinases. Due to their broad beneficial effects, growth factor-enhanced tendon/ligament healing holds tremendous promise for the future and is an active area of research.

The growth factors most widely studied in tendon and ligament healing include platelet derived growth factor (PDGF), insulin-like growth factor-I (IGF-I), transforming growth factor-B (TGF-B), vascular endothelial growth factor (VEGF), growth/differentiation factor (GDF), basic fibroblast growth factor (bFGF) and bone morphogenetic protein-12 (BMP-12). Growth factors are available as recombinant, purified proteins, or within a less defined slurry of bone marrow aspirate or platelet rich plasma. Clinical data, animal studies and tissue culture studies strongly support the use of IGF-I for the treatment of equine SDFT tendonitits; however, the benefits of IGF-I will be reported in a subsequent presentation by Britton and therefore, our results will not be presented herein. The disadvantage of such an approach is the lack of additional growth factors to compliment the effects of IGF-I and potentially the lack of transplanted cells (a requirement for cells in tendon regeneration has not yet been conclusively determined).

Bone marrow aspirate

The beneficial effects of bone marrow aspirate injections are theoretically twofold; delivery of mesenchymal stem cells (MSCs) and growth factors. MSCs injected into an area of damaged tendon could differentiate into mature tendon (or ligament) fibroblasts under the signaling influences of the tissue and produce the appropriate matrix products for repair. And bone marrow contains high concentrations of several of the growth factors listed above, which have been shown to improve the healing of tendons and ligaments in a variety of models.

Peer-reviewed literature on the efficacy of MSCs in tendon regeneration is sparse. With the exception of a few rabbit studies, there is little scientific evidence to support the use of bone marrow aspirate for enhanced tendon/ligament healing. Herthel (2002) reported the largest case series (123 horses) of bone marrow injections for suspensory desmitis. He reported that without treatment, 15% returned to soundness within 12 months, compared to 84% return to soundness within 6 months in the bone marrow injection group. Our clinical experience would suggest more variable results than Herthel (2002) experienced.

Laboratory data suggests that the growth factors TGF-B and PDGF are present in high concentrations in bone marrow aspirate, while IGF-I is less abundant (Figure 1). Presumably, other growth factors are also present in high concentrations; however our testing has been limited to these peptides. Figure 1 also demonstrates the increased growth factor concentration obtained by making a platelet rich plasma concentrate from venous blood (PRP; discussed further below).

Our data also suggests that 1-2 x 10^5 putative stem cells (defined as those cells that adhere to tissue culture plates) can be obtained from 10mls of sternal bone marrow aspirate from horses 2-5 years of age. We are developing a method by which the bone

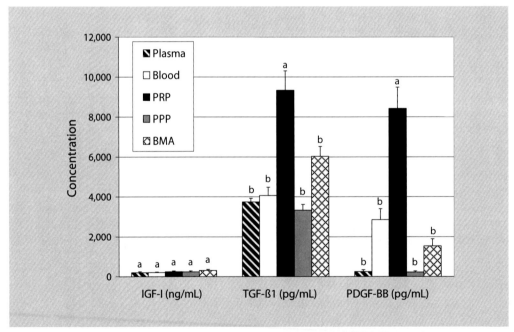

Figure 1. IGF-I (ng/mL), TGF-ß1(pg/mL), and PDGF-BB (pg/mL) concentrations in plasma, whole blood, platelet rich plasma (PRP), platelet poor plasma (PPP), and bone marrow aspirate (BMA). TGF-ß1 and PDGF-BB concentrations were significantly higher in PRP compared to all other blood products (p=0.0003 and p=0.0000 respectively). No significant differences in IGF-I concentration were observed between blood products (p=0.5320). Bars represent mean n=6 +/-SE; superscript letters indicate significant differences between the blood products (ANOVA with Tukey's post-hoc test). Source: Schnabel et al., 2006.

Management of lameness causes in sport horses

marrow stem cells and platelets can be concentrated from bone marrow aspirates (bone marrow aspirate concentrate; BMAC). In conjunction, a molecular marker profile is being generated to identify those cells in bone marrow which are stem cells based on cell surface antigen expression. Establishing a marker profile to definitely identify MSCs will be important for evaluation of research and clinical study outcomes.

Platelet rich plasma

Platelets are known for their role in homeostasis. Platelets also release substances that promote tissue repair and influence the reactivity of vascular and other blood cells in angiogenesis and inflammation. They contain a storage pool of growth factors including PDGF, TGF-B and VEGF. Several companies are marketing specialized centrifuges designed to create platelet rich plasma (PRP) which can be combined, if desired, with thrombin to create a moldable fibrin clot (Figure 2).

We performed an *in vitro* study to examine gene expression patterns and DNA content of equine SDFT explants cultured in media consisting of PRP and other blood products. (Schnabel *et al.*, 2006) Blood and bone marrow aspirate (BMA) were collected from horses and processed to obtain plasma, PRP, and platelet poor plasma (PPP). IGF-I, TGF-ß1, and PDGF-BB were quantified in all blood products using ELISAs. SDFT tensile regions were cultured in explant fashion with blood, plasma, PRP, PPP, or BMA at concentrations of 100%, 50%, or 10% in serum-free DMEM with amino acids. Quantitative RT-PCR for expression of collagen types I and III, cartilage oligomeric matrix protein (COMP), and matrix metalloproteinase-13 (MMP-13) were performed as well as DNA and total soluble collagen assays. TGF-ß1 and PDGF-BB concentrations were higher in PRP compared to all other blood products tested (Figure 1). Tendons cultured in 100% PRP showed enhanced gene expression of all anabolic tendon matrix

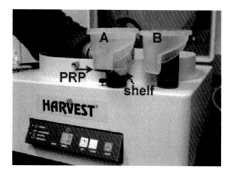

Figure 2. Equine platelet rich plasma (PRP) generated from 60mls of venous blood using a commercially available centrifuge and disposable chambers from Harvest Technologies. Chamber A has been processed (centrifuged) to generate PRP with platelet poor plasma in the supernatant. Red blood cells are retained in the central compartment by a shelf which moves during centrifugation. For comparison, chamber B contains unprocessed blood.

molecules examined and no increase in the catabolic molecule MMP-13. These findings support further *in vivo* and clinical investigation of PRP as an autogenous, patient-side treatment for tendonitis.

When applied to tendonitis/desmitis, the advantages of using PRP compared to the other modalities mentioned include ease of availability and application, use of autologous materials, and delivery of a combination of growth factors. The disadvantage is the cost associated with the purchase of a dedicated centrifuge and disposable supplies necessary for making PRP. We have used PRP in 18 clinical cases of SDFT tendonitis with no adverse effects such as heat, swelling, pain or infection after injection. However, return to athletic function data is not currently available for assessment.

Bone marrow aspirate concentrate (BMAC)

The same machine as depicted in Figure 2 can be used to concentrate platelets and putative MSCs from bone marrow aspirates.

Our preliminary data suggests that MSCs are concentrated approximately 8-fold (based on flow cytometry using cell surface markers, tissue culture, and total nucleated cell counts) and platelets are concentrated an average of 6 fold after centrifugation. Although the same machine can be used, the floating shelf in the disposable chamber must be more dense when generating BMAC compared to PRP; at least when using the Harvest Technologies system. The creation of BMAC could allow for a patient-side method that would immediately deliver MSCs and growth factors without the need for manipulation of the biological product in the laboratory.

Tenoscopy

Tenoscopy of the carpal sheath with desmotomy of the accessory ligament of the superficial digital flexor tendon (proximal check ligament) should be considered for animals with SDFT lesions (Southwood *et al.*, 1999). Transection of the check ligament lengthens the musculo-tendinous unit which should help compensate for the loss of elasticity associated with tendon scar formation, thereby diminishing the incidence of re-bowing. There is conflicting clinical data about the utility of a proximal check desmotomy, and large retrospective or prospective studies are still required to determine their effectiveness in the prevention of recurrence of tendonitis. Carpal or tarsal sheath tenoscopy should also be performed in those cases where ultrasonographic examination indicates tendon pathology within the sheath. Exploration may suggest the need for tendon debridement or release of the carpal canal or tarsal sheath.

The most commonly operated tendon sheath is the digital sheath. The surgical approach and pathologies of the digital sheath have been described (Nixon, 1990; Fortier *et al.*, 1999). When operated, an annular ligament transection is always performed. Removal of masses and adhesions is also required for return to athletic performance. Masses and adhesions may be present on the sheath, tendon, or between the tendons, necessitating a thorough examination of the digital sheath. The use of a synovial resector is essential for efficient surgical time although thin adhesions may be removed with the use of a biopsy punch. Potential intraoperative complications include lack of maneuverability and bleeding. When digital sheath fibrosis prevents surgical maneuvers, it is beneficial to transect the annular ligament prior to mass/adhesion removal. The use of a specialized endoscope (reverse viewing) will also aid in surgical manipulations. These scopes have their viewing angle oriented 180° compared to standard arthroscopes. In this way, interference between the light cable and foot is eliminated.

Post-operatively prevention of adhesion and mass re-formation are paramount to a successful outcome. Methods which should be employed include intraoperative and frequent (every 2 weeks for 3-4 treatments) post-operative use of intrathecal (not IV) high molecular weight hyaluronan (40 mg). It is generally believed, and increasingly well documented, that high molecular weight hyaluronan is more beneficial than a less expensive, lower molecular weight product. Also important are immediate post-operative exercise consisting of frequent walking (every 4 hours), range of motion exercises, and aggressive pain management so the patient is willing to use the operated limb.

Rehabilitation

Regardless of the medical or surgical therapy applied, a controlled exercise program with regular ultrasonographic recheck examinations is required. One example of a post-therapy exercise protocol is listed below and the clients are clearly informed that any stage might be prolonged based on the outcome of recheck examinations.

- Day 0-30: Stall rest, surgery, PRP/BMAC/IGF injection.
- Day 30-60: Stall rest with walking. Recheck ultrasound at day 60.
- Day 60-90: Ponying, swimming or extra walking.
- Day 90-120: Walk under saddle; 1 or 2 trot periods weekly. Recheck ultrasound at day 120.
- Day 120-150: Add periods of canter every week.
- Day 150-180: Increase periods of canter; add slow gallop. Recheck ultrasound at day 180.
- Day 180- 240: Conditioning gallops.

During and after rehabilitation, regular shoeing to ease break-over and maintain a balanced foot is also required. The prognosis for return to athletic function for horses with SDFT tendonitis is variable and depends primarily on the degree of tendon pathology present, but also on the age, conformation, and intended use of the horse.

References

Herthel, D.J., 2002 Suspensory desmitis therapies. In: ACVS, Equine Orthopedics Proceedings, 2002.

Fortier, L.A., A.J. Nixon, N.G. Ducharme, H.O. Mohammed and A. Yeager, 1999. Tenoscopic examination and proximal annular ligament desmotomy for treatment of equine "complex" digital sheath tenosynovitis. Vet. Surg. 28: 429-435.

Nixon, A.J., 1990. Endoscopy of the digital flexor tendon sheath in horses. Vet. Surg. 19: 266-271.

Schnabel, L.V., H.O. Mohammed, B.J. Miller, W.G. McDermott, M.S. Jacobson, K.S. Santangelo and L.A. Fortier, 2006. Platelet rich plasma (PRP) enhances anabolic gene expression patterns in flexor digitorum superficialis tendons. J. Orthop. Res. (in press).

Southwood, L.L., T.S. Stashak, R.A. Kainer and R.H. Wrigley, 1999. Desmotomy of the Accessory Ligament of the Superficial Digital Flexor Tendon in the Horse with Use of a Tenoscopic Approach to the Carpal Sheath. Vet. Surg. 28: 99-105.

Diagnosis of proximal suspensory desmitis in the forelimb and hindlimb

Sue Dyson

Centre for Equine Studies, Animal Health Trust, Lanwades Park, Kentford, Newmarket, Suffolk CB8 7UU, United Kingdom

Anatomy

The suspensory ligament (SL) (third interosseous muscle) can be divided into 3 separate regions which are subject to injury, the proximal part, the body and the branches. For clinical purposes the proximal part extends from approximately 8 to 14 cm distal to the accessory carpal bone and 2 to 10 cm distal to the tarsometatarsal (TMT) joint. In the forelimb the SL originates from 2 heads which rapidly fuse. In the hindlimb this division is less obvious. The SL contains a variable amount of muscular tissue (2 - 11%), which tends to be bilaterally symmetrical. In the forelimb the SL originates from the palmar carpal ligament and the proximal aspect of the third metacarpal bone (Mc III), whereas in the hindlimb the SL originates principally from the proximoplantar aspect of the third metatarsal bone (Mt III). The SL in the forelimb is approximately rectangular in cross-section, but is more rounded in the hindlimb. The body of the SL descends between the second (Mc/Mt II) and fourth (Mc/Mt IV) metacarpal/metatarsal bones and divides into 2 branches at a variable site in the mid metatarsal region. The level of division is usually bilaterally symmetrical. Each branch inserts on the abaxial surface of the corresponding proximal sesamoid bone (PSB). Each branch detaches a thin extensor branch dorsodistally, that courses obliquely across the pastern to join the dorsal digital extensor tendon just above the proximal interphalangeal (PIP) joint. Each extensor branch also blends with the corresponding collateral sesamoidean ligament. Proximally there is a distinct fascial band in close apposition to the plantar aspect of the SL, with horizontally orientated fibres extending between Mc/Mt II and Mc/Mt IV.

In the forelimb the SL is innervated by the palmar metacarpal nerves, derived from the lateral palmar nerve, which receives fibres from both the ulnar and median nerves. The hindlimb SL is innervated by the plantar metatarsal nerves, branches from the deep branch of the lateral plantar nerve, which is derived from the tibial nerve. The proximal SL is closely related to the palmar outpouching of the carpometacarpal joint capsule in the forelimb and the plantar outpouching of the TMT joint capsule in the hindlimb.

The principal function of the SL is to prevent excessive extension of the fetlock joint. During weight bearing the relative tension in the SL and flexor tendons regulates the stresses applied to different aspects of the Mt III. When a limb is fully load bearing the distal part of the SL branches are closely apposed to the abaxial aspects of the metatarsal condyles and then move to the plantar aspect as the fetlock drops. During hyperextension, the PSBs move distally and dorsally, so the branches of the SL act as articular surfaces to balance the position of the Mt III. If the limb is loaded asymmetrically, so there is torque on the fetlock, the SL branches contribute to joint stability on the side opposite compression of the joint.

In the forelimb there is some evidence that training increases the strength of the SL; the mean absolute load to failure in a single load to failure compression test was significantly higher in horses that had been in racehorse training compared to those that had been confined to box or paddock rest (Bramlage *et al.*, 1989). In the trained group failure was most likely to be by fracture of a PSB, whereas in the untrained group, the SL failed. However when six 2 year old Thoroughbred fillies underwent an 18 month controlled exercise programme including galloping, and were compared to 6 fillies which were restricted to walking exercise, there were no differences in the collagen fibril mass-average diameter (MAD) in the body of the SL (Patterson-Kane *et al.*, 1998). MAD is correlated with ligament strength. Similar studies have not been conducted in hindlimbs.

Proximal suspensory desmitis in the forelimb

Proximal suspensory desmitis (PSD) results in sudden onset lameness, which can be remarkably transient, resolving within 24 hours unless the horse is worked hard. In horses with more chronic injury lameness may be persistent. PSD in forelimbs occurs in horses of all ages and from all disciplines. Extravagantly moving young dressage horses and older upper level competition horses are particularly at risk of injury. Lameness varies from mild to moderate and is rarely severe, unless the lesion is extensive. Lameness in Standardbred racehorses may only be apparent at high speeds. Bilateral PSD may result in loss of action rather than overt lameness. This occurs more commonly in flat racehorses, probably due to failure of recognition of earlier, subtle unilateral lameness. Lameness is usually worse on soft ground, especially with the affected limb on the outside of a circle and, when subtle, may be more easily felt by a rider than seen by an observer. Occasionally lameness is only apparent ridden, sometimes with the limb on the inside of a circle. Lameness may not be apparent at the working trot, but may be detectable at the medium or extended trot. Recognition of these features in the history may be important, since acute lameness often resolves rapidly and it may be undesirable to work the horse hard to reproduce lameness, with the inherent risk of worsening the injury. Lameness is often transiently accentuated by distal limb flexion. In the acute phase there may be slight oedema in the proximal metacarpal region, localised heat and distension of the medial palmar vein, but these features may be transient or absent. Pressure applied to the SL against the palmar aspect of the Mc III may elicit pain. Forced extension and protraction of the limb may elicit pain.

The feet should be evaluated carefully since frequently foot imbalance is a predisposing factor. Back at the knee and tied in below the knee conformation may also be predisposing factors. PSD is a common compensatory injury, therefore the horse should be evaluated as a whole to insure that other causes of lameness are not missed.

Proximal suspensory desmitis in the hindlimb

The diagnosis of proximal suspensory desmitis (PSD) in the hindlimb has increased in recent years unquestionably due to improved recognition, but possibly also due to increased frequency of occurrence. This may relate to a change in both training methods and training surfaces and the increasing athletic demands placed on upper level competition horses. It results in either an insidious onset, or sudden onset lameness, which may be mild or severe, either unilateral or bilateral. However, some horses present with poor performance, rather than a recognised lameness. Complaints include loss of hindlimb impulsion; unwillingness to go forward freely; stiffness; resistant behaviour; lack of power when jumping; refusing jumps uncharacteristically; difficulties in performing specific dressage movements, *e.g.* canter pirouette; poor performance at high speed in racehorses; evasive behaviour such as bolting. In contrast to PSD in the forelimb, lameness may persist and remain severe, despite restriction to box rest. This is probably due to a compartment-like syndrome and pressure on the adjacent plantar metatarsal nerves (Dyson, 1995b). In view of the chronicity of some lesions when first identified, and the finding of secondary radiological changes in sound horses, it is likely that some lesions exist sub-clinically, or are associated with a low grade lameness that goes unrecognised. The prevalence of bilateral lesions is higher than in forelimbs.

PSD in the hindlimb occurs in horses in all athletic disciplines and of all ages. It is a particular problem in dressage horses working at advanced level. Horses with either straight hock conformation, and or hyperextension of the metatarsophalangeal (MTP) joint, appear predisposed to injury. Such conformational abnormalities were identified in 9 of 42 horses (21%) with hindlimb PSD, but in only 4 of 50 (8%) horses examined consecutively with hindlimb lameness unrelated to the suspensory apparatus (Dyson, 1994, 1995a) Hyperextension of the MTP joint may develop as a sequel to PSD. A long toe and low heel conformation may also be a predisposing factor, especially if associated with abnormal orientation of the distal phalanx, with the plantar aspect lower than the toe (Dyson and Genovese, 2003).

Clinical features

In horses with acute hindlimb PSD there may be localised heat and swelling and pain on pressure applied to the SL, but frequently there are no localising clinical features. At the walk there may be reduced extension of the MTP joint of the lame limb, unless the integrity of the SL is severely compromised resulting in hyperextension of the joint. Lameness is often characterised by a reduced height of arc of foot flight, with or without intermittent catching of the toe. The cranial phase of the stride may be shortened. Lameness may be accentuated by either proximal or distal limb flexion. Bilateral lesions may result in poor hindlimb action, with poor hindlimb impulsion and engagement, rather than obvious hindlimb lameness, and may compromise the movement of the entire horse. Lameness may be more obvious on a circle on the lunge, but unlike forelimb PSD, the lameness is not necessarily worse with the lamer limb on the outside. Like many hindlimb lamenesses, lameness is usually more obvious when the horse is ridden, especially when the rider sits on the diagonal of the lame or lamer limb, and in some horses gait abnormalities are only evident when ridden.

Diagnosis

Local analgesic techniques

Forelimb lameness is often worse after palmar (abaxial sesamoid) nerve blocks. Perineural analgesia of the palmar/plantar nerves (at the junction of the proximal ⅔ – ¾ and distal ⅓ - ¼ of the metacarpal/ metatarsal region) and palmar metacarpal/ plantar metatarsal nerves may result in slight improvement in lameness, due to proximal diffusion of the local anaesthetic solution, and if a '4 point' or '6 point' block is done more proximally the risk of false positive results increases.

Forelimb PSD

Perineural analgesia of either the lateral palmar nerve (2 ml mepivacaine) or the medial and lateral palmar metacarpal nerves (2 ml per site) should result in substantial improvement in, or alleviation of, lameness within 10 minutes, assuming PSD is the only cause of lameness. However neither technique is necessarily specific. Blockade of the lateral palmar nerve also has the potential to alleviate pain associated with a lateral source of pain in the more distal limb (*e.g.* a 'splint'). The risks of influencing middle carpal (MC) joint pain are less than using the sub-carpal approach, but local anaesthetic solution may diffuse and result in improvement in lameness associated with the MC joint or with the carpal canal using a lateral approach (Ford *et al.*, 1989). However, a medial approach to the lateral palmar nerve eliminates these risks (Castro *et al.*, 2005). Perineural analgesia of the palmar metacarpal nerves may alleviate pain associated with either the MC or carpometacarpal (CMC) joints, due to local diffusion or inadvertent deposition of local anaesthetic solution into the distopalmar outpouchings of the CMC joint capsule. A false negative result may be achieved either due to inadvertent injection into the carpal sheath, or failure of the local anaesthetic solution to diffuse proximally to the most proximal extent of a lesion. Although the SL receives innervation from fibres from both the median and ulnar nerves, perineural analgesia of the ulnar nerve usually resolves, or substantially improves, lameness associated with PSD.

Intra-articular analgesia of the MC joint may result in either partial improvement, or complete alleviation, of pain associated with the proximal suspensory ligament in some horses (15/25 horses, 60%). Using a dorsal approach to the MC joint, rather than a palmarolateral approach, should theoretically reduce the risks of diffusion of local anaesthetic solution to the proximal SL and palmar metacarpal nerves, however in practice there appears to be little difference. Comparison of the relative responses to MC joint analgesia (6 ml mepivacaine; assessed 10 minutes after injection) and perineural analgesia of the lateral palmar nerve or the palmar metacarpal nerves is potentially useful, but it can be highly misleading. Generally a horse with lameness due to PSD shows a better response to perineural analgesia than intra-articular analgesia, but this is not universal. Similarly primary MC joint pain is usually best improved by intra-articular analgesia, but this is not always the case. Middle carpal joint pain and PSD may occur concurrently, especially in Standardbred racehorses. The clinician should evaluate the response to these local analgesic techniques in the light of:

- the use of the horse and thus the likelihood of the site of injury, and other clinical signs;
- other clinical signs *e.g.* distension of the MC joint capsule, pain on passive manipulation of the carpus;
- the degree and character of the lameness.

Hindlimb PSD

Lameness is usually substantially improved by perineural analgesia of either the deep branch of the lateral plantar nerve distal to the tarsus (3 – 5 ml mepivacaine 2%), or by local infiltration axial to the second and fourth metatarsal bones, but may not be alleviated fully. Improvement is usually seen within 10 minutes of injection. In some horses it may be difficult to deposit the local anaesthetic solution as proximal as ideal, due to the shape of the base of Mt IV. This may result in only partial improvement in lameness. False negative results may also be obtained due to inadvertent injection into either the tarsal sheath, or the TMT joint capsule (Dyson and Romero, 1993). In a horse presenting with poor hindlimb impulsion it might theoretically be expected that if pain was alleviated from one limb the horse should then show overt lameness on the other. Although this sometimes happens, it does not always and this can result in false negative results. In such horses a much more dramatic improvement in gait may be seen if perineural analgesia of the deep branch of the lateral plantar nerve is performed bilaterally. This technique should theoretically only remove ligamentous pain and not osseous pain at the ligament's origin. Osseous pain is more likely to be abolished by directing the needle in a dorsal direction and infiltrating as deeply as possible. However, diffusion of local anaesthetic solution from the site for perineural analgesia of the deep branch of the lateral planar nerve may produce some confusing results and nuclear scintigraphy may be a more reliable means of establishing whether there is active concurrent bony pathology at the SL's origin.

Sub-tarsal analgesia can influence TMT joint pain, and occasionally (2/24 horses, 8%; Dyson, 1994) intra-articular analgesia of the TMT joint alleviates pain associated with PSD. If a horse which had lameness abolished by intra-articular analgesia of the TMT joint, but with only minor radiological change of the TMT and centrodistal joints, fails to respond adequately to treatment consideration should be given to the presence of PSD. Therefore a comparison of the responses to intra-articular analgesia and subtarsal analgesia can be useful. Perineural analgesia of the tibial nerve alone alleviates pain associated with PSD, without significantly influencing tarsal pain. However this is a larger nerve, therefore it may take 20 minutes before analgesia is effectively achieved. This is an extremely useful block to perform to differentiate between distal hock joint pain and PSD, especially in horses in which false negative results to subtarsal analgesia have been obtained. Occasionally PSD occurs together with pain associated with osteoarthritis of the TMT joint.

Diagnostic ultrasonography

High quality ultrasonographic images, in both transverse and sagittal planes, are essential for accurate diagnosis. Transverse images are best acquired from the palmar aspect in the forelimb, but the plantaromedial aspect of the metatarsal region (Dyson, 1998). Large vessels plantarolateral to the SL may result in broad linear anechogenic artefacts within the SL in hindlimbs. Air artefacts after local analgesia may also be a problem, especially in hindlimbs. In large Warmblood horses in particular, the SL is situated deeply and the ultrasound transducer must be focused accordingly so that a clear image of the plantar cortex of Mt III is obtained. In both transverse and longitudinal images the most proximal part of the SL in hindlimb of a normal horse may appear slightly less echogenic than the DDFT. Detection of subtle abnormalities requires careful comparison with the contralateral limb and measurement of cross-sectional area.

Abnormalities associated with forelimb PSD include:
- Enlargement of the cross sectional area. This may result in reduction of space between the SL and the palmar cortex of the Mc III, or reduced space between the SL and the ALDDFT.
- Poor demarcation of the margins of the SL, especially the dorsal margin.
- Focal or diffuse areas of reduced echogenicity. These may extend less than 1 cm proximodistally and occupy from less than 10%, to up to the entire cross-sectional area of the ligament.
- Focal anechogenic core lesions.
- Reduced strength of fibre pattern.
- Focal mineralisation (rare in acute cases).

In a horse with bilateral PSD an obvious lesion may be detectable in the lamer limb, but abnormalities may be much more subtle, and occasionally not apparent in the less lame limb. In a 3 year old Thoroughbred that had sustained PSD at 2 years of age, there may be recurrent mild lameness and it may not be possible to discern any structural abnormality other than enlargement of the SL.

The degree of ultrasonographic abnormality (cross sectional area involved and proximodistal extent of the lesion) usually reflects the severity of the lameness. In horses with acute PSD the ultrasonographic abnormalities may be very subtle, although if lameness is unilateral, slight enlargement of cross-sectional area may be detectable. Care should be taken to compare measurements in the contralateral limb at the same distance distal to the accessory carpal bone. Ultrasonographic abnormalities may deteriorate over the next 10 to 14 days and re-evaluation may be useful to confirm the diagnosis. In very chronic cases the SL may be diffusely hyperechogenic due to fibrosis and lesions are easily missed.

In hindlimb PSD focal anechogenic areas are relatively unusual, except in the Standardbred racehorse. More commonly there is enlargement of the SL, with poor demarcation of its borders, especially the dorsal border and a diffuse reduction in echogenicity of part, or all, of the cross sectional area of the ligament. Ectopic fibrosis or mineralisation occurs more often in hindlimbs compared with forelimbs. Lesions are easily missed unless the most proximal aspect of the SL is examined. Familiarity with the normal ultrasonographic appearance is crucial for recognition of mild lesions. An irregular contour of the plantar aspect of the Mt III may reflect entheseophyte formation. In the author's experience, in the vast majority of horses with a positive response to subtarsal analgesia, ultrasonographic abnormalities are detectable, unless it is a very acute lesion (days), or fibrosis is the predominant change in a chronic injury, or in the less lame limb of a bilaterally lame horse.

In some horses, especially those with abnormal conformation, the lesions may progress despite box rest.

Radiography

Radiological changes occur more commonly in hindlimbs than in forelimbs. Diagnosis should never be based on radiography alone, since some sound horse have some sclerosis of the proximal aspect of the McIII or Mt III. In horses with chronic active PSD this may be more extensive. In the dorsoplantar view there is increased opacity of the proximal aspect of the Mt III, often more obvious laterally. In a lateromedial projection there may be sub-cortical sclerosis and alteration of the trabecular pattern of the proximoplantar aspect of the MT III due to endosteal new bone, extending up to 4cm proximodistally. The plantar cortex may itself be thickened and in addition there may be entheseophyte formation on the plantar aspect. However in many horses no radiological abnormality is detectable.

Nuclear scintigraphy

Recognition of normal patterns of radiopharmaceutical uptake (RU) is crucial for accurate image interpretation. In normal horses, it is normal in plantar images of hindlimbs to see relatively greater RU in the proximoplantar lateral aspect of Mt III compared with medially or dorsally (Murray *et al.*, 2005; Weekes *et al.*, 2005). Nuclear scintigraphy is not a sensitive means of detecting PSD in forelimbs or hindlimbs. Pool phase images were positive in only 25% of 20 horses with ultrasonographic evidence of PSD (Dyson and Genovese 2003). Approximately 12% of 126 horses with forelimb or hindlimb PSD had increased RU (IRU) in bone phase images (Dyson *et al.*, 2006). IRU associated with PSD should be differentiated from those horses with primary bony pathology, with no detectable ultrasonographic abnormality of the SL and no radiographic change associated with enthesopathy.

Magnetic resonance imaging

The interpretation of magnetic resonance (MR) images is complicated by the high signal intensity of muscle within the ligamentous structure; however, lesions are characterised by enlargement of the affected lobe and increased (intermediate) signal intensity. MR imaging is also useful for explaining concurrent bony pathology in horses in which the degree of ultrasonographic abnormality is not commensurate with the degree of lameness. In most of these horses there is IRU in the region of origin of the SL or slightly distal to this. This has been associated with endosteal mineralisation and fluid accumulation in T1 and T2 weighted MR images and increased signal intensity in fat suppressed images. MRI may also enable diagnosis of concurrent syndesmopathy of Mc/Mt II & III or Mc/Mt IV & III.

Differential diagnosis

PSD should be differentiated from pain associated with the MC or CMC joint or the TMT joint, an avulsion fracture of the McIII/Mt III at the origin of the SL, and primary stress reactions in the McIII/Mt III.

Gross pathology and histopathology

Post mortem examinations have been performed on both hindlimbs of 14 horses, 8 with unilateral lameness and 6 with bilateral lameness (Dyson, 1995, 2003). Abnormalities of the SLs were confined to the lame limbs. There was gross enlargement of the SLs, with thickening of surrounding fascia and periligamentous tissues, especially on the plantar aspect. Histological changes in the SL included hypercellularity and acellular areas, haemosiderin deposition, fibrosis, hyalinisation of collagen, an increased number of fibrous septae, some with blood vessels, neovascularisation and chondroid metaplasia. Although chondroid metaplasia was seen at the ligament bone interface in both lame and sound limbs, intra-ligamentous chondroid metaplasia was only seem in the lame limbs. There was evidence of compression of adjacent peripheral nerves in the lame limb of 12 horses. Abnormalities of the plantar metatarsal nerves included thickening of the perineurium, perineural fibrosis, reduction or absence of nerve fibres and Renaut bodies. These changes support the theory of PSD in the hindlimb resulting in a compartment syndrome.

Concurrent injuries

Forelimb PSD often occurs together with foot pain. Hindlimb PSD may also be accompanied by injury of the lateral or, less commonly, the medial branch of the SL. This may be unapparent at the time of initial clinical examination, unless there is gross swelling. However, ultrasonographic examination may reveal evidence of damage. Several horses had been successfully treated surgically only to incur recurrent lameness due to desmitis of the lateral or, less commonly, the medial branch of the SL that was not recognised at the time of initial examination (unpublished data). One horse with acute PSD was managed successfully conservatively and 1 year later had recurrent lameness due to desmitis of the proximal aspect of the lateral oblique sesamoidean ligament. Chronic PSD has also been seen in association with sacroiliac joint region pain.

References

Bramlage, L., C. Buckowiecki and A. Gabel, 1989. The effect of training on the suspensory apparatus of the horse. Proc. Amer. Assoc. Equine Pract. 35: 245–247.

Castro, F., J. Schumacher, F. Pauwels and J. Blackford, 2005. A new approach for perineural injection of the lateral palmar nerve in the horse. Vet. Surg. 34: 539–542.

Dyson, S., 1994. Proximal suspensory desmitis in the hindlimb: 42 cases. British Vet. J. 150: 279–291.

Dyson, S., 1995a. Proximal suspensory desmitis in the hindlimb. Equine Vet. Educ. 7: 275–278.

Dyson, S., 1995b. Problems encountered in equine lameness diagnosis with special reference to local analgesic techniques, radiology and ultrasonography. R. & W. Publications Ltd, Newmarket, pp. 31-54.

Dyson, S., 1998. The suspensory apparatus. In: N. Rantanen and A. McKinnon. Equine Diagnostic Ultrasonography. 1st ed. Baltimore, Williams & Wilkins, pp. 447-474.

Dyson, S. and R. Genovese, 2003. The suspensory apparatus. In: M. Ross and S. Dyson. Diagnosis and management of lameness in the horse. 1st ed. St. Louis, Saunders, pp. 654–672.

Dyson, S. and J. Romero, 1993. An investigation of injection techniques for local analgesia of the equine distal tarsus and proximal metatarsus. Equine vet. J. 25: 30 – 35.

Dyson, S., J. Weekes and R. Murray, 2006. Scintigraphic evaluation of the proximal metacarpal and metatarsal regions of horses with proximal suspensory desmitis. Vet. Radiol & Ultrasound (In press).

Ford, T., M. Ross and P. Orsini, 1989. A comparison of methods for proximal palmar metacarpal analgesia in horses. Vet. Surg. 18: 146 – 150.

Murray, R., S. Dyson, J. Weekes, C. Short and M. Branch, 2005. Nuclear scintigraphic examination of the distal tarsal region in normal horses. Vet. Radiol. and Ultrasound 46: 171–178.

Patterson-Kane, J., E. Firth, D. Parry, et al., 1998.: Effects of training on collagen fibril populations in the suspensory ligament and deep digital flexor tendon of young Thoroughbreds. Am. J. Vet. Res. 59: 64–68.

Weekes, J., R. Murray and S. Dyson, 2006. Scintigraphic evaluation of the proximal metacarpal and metatarsal region in clinically sound horses. Vet. Radiol. and Ultrasound (In press).

Management of proximal suspensory desmitis

Andrew P. Bathe
Rossdales Equine Hospital, Cotton End Road, Exning, Newmarket Suffolk, CB8 7NN, United Kingdom

Introduction

As in any orthopaedic condition, an accurate diagnosis is a prerequisite for optimal treatment but proximal suspensory desmitis (PSD) has a complex clinical picture. Many cases present as acute onset lameness, whereas more and more cases of chronic, active PSD – especially in the hindlimb, are being recognised. Forelimb PSD tends to respond well to conservative treatment, whereas in the hindlimb there is s much poorer prognosis with rest alone. These cases often stay lame despite protracted periods of convalescence and apparent healing of the ligament. It has been hypothesised that this is due to the development of a local compartment syndrome. Figure 1 demonstrates the enclosed

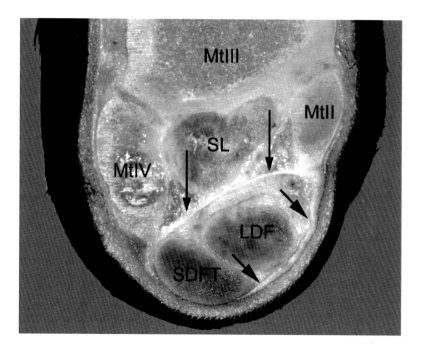

Figure 1. Cross section of the right proximal metatarsus, 3 cm distal to the tarsometatarsal joint. The origin of the suspensory ligament (SL) is bordered by the second (Mt II), third (Mt III) and fourth (Mt IV) metatarsal bones and the deep laminar plantar metatarsal fascia (long arrows). The deep plantar metatarsal fascia (short arrows) also encloses the superficial deep flexor tendon (SDFT) and lateral digital flexor tendon (LDF).

surroundings of the proximal suspensory ligament in the hindleg. It is surrounded by the metatarsal bones on three sides and is overlain on its plantar border by the deep laminar plantar metatarsal fascia, creating a tight compartment. Enlargement of the ligament in this region can cause chronic pain due to swelling within this compartment. There may also be a component of neuritis of the deep branch of the lateral plantar nerve, and even the development of abnormal innervation following injury – which can lead to chronic pain. There also appears to be a spectrum of disease. Some horses have a true desmitis with very clear cut ultrasonographic changes. Other cases which have blocked to this region appear to have more of an enthesiopathy at the actual origin on the proximal plantar third metatarsal bone and may have minimal ultrasonographic changes but positive bone phase scintigraphic changes in this region. Other cases may have pain and inflammation from both these regions. Optimal treatment requires an understanding of the specific pathology in the individual, as one treatment does not fit all.

Conservative and medical management

Management of acute injuries should involve rest, anti-inflammatory therapy and controlled exercise under serial ultrasound monitoring. Intra-lesional medication with products such as hyaluronan or polysulphated glycosaminoglycans does not appear to offer any clinical benefits. I do not consider that systemic medication with PSGAGs or nutraceuticals has been shown to improve the outcome. Intravenous infusion of bisphosphonates has been useful in some cases of enthesis-related pain.

One-off regional infiltration with corticosteroids (*e.g.* 10 mg triamcinolone in 3 ml of local anaesthetic) can be beneficial in decreasing the inflammation in acute cases. It can also be useful in managing low-grade chronic/active cases in the short term. This is often the most appropriate form of treating flat racing Thoroughbreds, as there is not time in their short careers for the lay-off associated with surgery.

Bone marrow injections have been employed in a large number of cases of suspensory disease, especially in the United States (Herthel, 2001). This is a simple but crude technique for injecting a combination of growth factors and stem cells, although only a low number of the latter are present. Bone marrow is normally harvested from the sternebrae. The author has treated a number of horses in this way. This has tended to give a good improvement on apparent healing, as assessed ultrasonographically, but there has been no significant abolition of lameness in hindlimb PSD. I have since treated horses with xenogenic extracellular matrix (ACell) instead, but the results have not been as satisfactory as with the bone marrow. I do not feel that the additional expense and complication of using stem cells is necessary in the suspensory ligament.

Extracorporeal Shockwave Therapy (ESWT)

ESWT has now been employed for a number of years in the treatment of proximal suspensory desmitis. In my experience it has been extremely helpful in the management of chronic active cases of proximal suspensory desmitis in the forelimb. Crowe *et al.*

(2004) reported on a series of cases of hindlimb PSD treated with radial ESWT, and improved the prognosis to around 41%. This is significantly better than with conservative treatment, but still poorer than the surgical treatments that will be described. In the hindlimb I tend to use it in either mild, acute cases or for the management of low-grade, chronic cases, and continued treatments may be necessary. Clinically there does not seem to be any difference between radial and focused machines in the outcome following treatment. I now use higher settings for the hindlimb than the forelimb: with the EMS Swiss Dolorclast Vet 2,500 pulses at 3.5 bar with a 10 mm applicator versus 2,000 pulses at 3 bar (Figure 2).

Surgery

Ligament splitting (desmoplasty)

Ligament splitting has been performed for many years, without ever gaining full acceptance for regular use. There is a rationale for its use in decompressing an acute

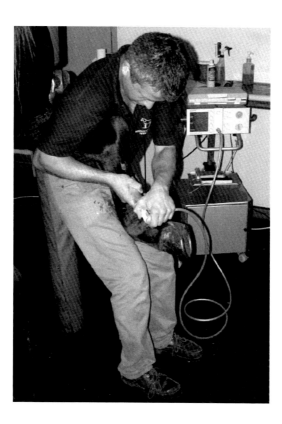

Figure 2. Swiss Dolorclast Vet radial shockwave machine being used to treat a hindlimb proximal suspensory ligament injury.

core lesion. White (2003) has described ultrasound guided percutaneous ligament splitting under general anaesthesia for the management of chronic hindlimb PSD, with encouraging results. However, there is less decompression than can be achieved with the open surgical technique which I will describe later.

Osteostixis

The drilling of multiple holes into the region of the origin of the suspensory ligament was originally described for the treatment of non-healing fractures in this region but has also been employed for the management of proximal suspensory desmitis (Launois *et al.*, 2000). This is a relative crude technique however, and there must be questions over its benefits in a true case of desmitis, although there is logical application in the management of non-responsive bone-related pain. I use it in combination with plantar metatarsal neurectomy and fasciotomy for treating hindlimb PSD with a component of bone or enthesis related pain, as diagnosed by the response to local analgesia being better to local infiltration than to blocking the deep branch of the lateral plantar nerve.

Plantar metatarsal neurectomy and fasciotomy

This treatment was developed as the surgical option for the management of proximal suspensory ligament desmitis in the hindlimb. This procedure combines decompressive fasciotomy of the deep laminar plantar metatarsal fascia with neurectomy of the deep branch of the lateral plantar nerve. This nerve branch is the common origin of the medial and lateral plantar metatarsal nerves, which apply sensory innervation to the origin of the suspensory ligament. Surgery has been restricted to those cases that have had a very good response to a block of the deep branch of the lateral plantar nerve. Over 250 horses have been operated on by the author to date, and long term follow-up has yielded a long term success rate of 79% returning to normal function. Approximately 4-5 cm of nerve is removed through a 3.5 cm incision (Figure 3). The same procedure has also been used successfully in a smaller number of forelimb cases.

Conclusions

My current treatment regime involves a combination of the techniques described above. Extracorporeal shockwave therapy is used in persistent lameness due to proximal suspensory desmitis in the forelimb and low-grade cases of hindlimb proximal suspensory desmitis. In hindlimb proximal suspensory desmitis a plantar metatarsal neurectomy and fasciotomy is employed if the block pattern is appropriate. In cases with marked hypoechogenicity this is combined with a bone marrow injection. In cases with significant bone involvement osteostixis is also performed. With aggressive surgical management I would consider that the prognosis is dramatically improved in a large number of cases. Follow-up of these cases during the rehabilitation period is important in optimising the outcome.

Management of lameness causes in sport horses

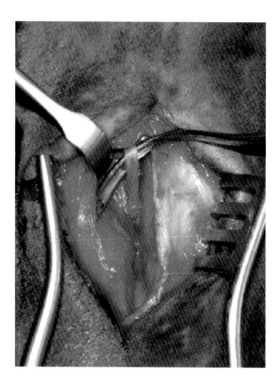

Figure 3. Intra-operative view of plantar metatarsal neurectomy and fasciotomy, with nerve branch elevated. Proximal to top, lateral to right.

References

Crowe, O.M., S.J. Dyson, I.M. Wright, M.C. Schramme and R.K. Smith, 2004. Treatment of chronic or recurrent proximal suspensory desmitis using radial pressure wave therapy in the horse. Equine Vet. J. 36: 313-316.

Herthel, D.J., 2001. Enhanced suspensory ligament healing in 100 horses by stem cells and other bone marrow components. AAEP Proceedings, pp. 319-321.

Launois, T., F. Desbrosse and R. Perrin, 2000. Osteostyxis, a new surgical technique in the treatment of tendinous injuries at the proximal insertion of the 3rd interosseous muscle (suspensory ligament) with bone lesions of the proximal palmar (plantar) cortical metacarpus (metatarsus). ECVS Proceedings, pp. 69-70.

White, N.A., 2003. Surgical treatment of suspensory desmitis. ACVS Symposium Equine and Small Animal Proceedings, October 9, 2003.

A system for monitoring of training and disease of Thoroughbreds in the UK

Anthony Stirk
Horseracing Regulatory Authority, 151 Shaftesbury Avenue, London WC2H 8AL, United Kingdom

Racecourse injuries, whilst rare, carry welfare and economic implications which the racing industry must recognize and approach. There is likely to be further public interest in the subject as a result of increased worldwide television coverage and the activities of 'animal rights' organizations.

English language reports describing the incidence of racecourse injuries first began to appear in the scientific press in the mid 1970's. Results have since been published from a variety of countries, including Australia, Canada, Japan, New Zealand, Scandinavia, South Africa, UK, USA and detailing a variety of race types and surfaces (Bourke, 1995; Johnson *et al.*, 1994; McKee, 1995; Parkin *et al.*, 2004a; Vaughan and Mason, 1975; Williams *et al.*, 2001). Data sources have included published race results, course, trainer and veterinarian questionnaires, and official regulatory records. The research has been conducted by a variety of groups, most usually university based, but also encompassing individual research bodies and regulatory authorities. The emphasis has moved from mere descriptive studies of incidence to identification of risk factors for individual injury types, and the recommendation of preventive strategies.

Experimental randomized controlled trials and observational cohort and case-control studies have been utilised and described (Bailey *et al.*, 1998; Cohen *et al.*, 2000; Estberg *et al.*, 1998; Kane *et al.*, 1996; Mohammed *et al.*, 1998; Parkin *et al.*, 2004b, 2004c, 2005; Perkins *et al.*, 2005; Verheyen *et al.*, 2005; Wood *et al.*, 2005). Statistically validated epidemiological studies will remain the 'gold standard' in the investigation and analysis of risk factors for fatalities, injuries and medical events in the racing and training thoroughbred. However, data capture, validation, and analyses are time-consuming. The capacity to produce up to date results, whilst not necessarily statistically validated, can also benefit the industry as a monitoring process, and can indicate areas of potential research interest. There is also a need for an internationally agreed simplified uniform terminology.

Whilst there is now a substantial volume of data on racecourse injuries, the incidence of in-training injuries has received less attention. Increasingly, training methodology is being cited as a risk factor in injuries both on and off the track. Trainers have been traditionally reluctant to divulge their training methods, or their injury incidence, and vary greatly in their use of records. Data recording can be encouraged by emphasising the potential improvement in their own performance, the longer term contribution to equine welfare, and by the provision of attractive features such as vaccination reminders and medical records. Confidentiality must be stressed at all times.

In 1990 a custom-designed Windows-based system for the collection of veterinary data on the racecourse was introduced in the UK by the (then) Jockey Club Veterinary Department. In conjunction with a racing industry performance database it allows an up to the minute descriptive monitoring facility, and the ability to investigate some two hundred potential risk factors.

A voluntary confidential website (accessed via the BHB/Weatherbys Administration site) has also recently been made available for trainers to record details of work schedules, injuries, medical events, physical and medical treatments, routine medication and vaccination, and general health monitoring (including weight, temperature, blood and respiratory fluid sample results). A daily task list is generated. A variety of listing procedures are available, including daily customisable worksheets detailing horses by 'lot', exercise description and jockey. Reports comparing workloads and incidence of physical and medical problems with previous time periods, or with the average for (unidentified) contributing trainers can be presented in tabular or graphical format.

As well as helping trainers to objectively measure their own performance, it is hoped that over time the system will enable significant studies and analyses in the 'in training' area. Standardised exercise descriptions (intensity, duration, frequency, incline, total workload) which would benefit the international collection and analysis of data, especially that obtained under field conditions, are proposed. Both systems would be readily customisable for use in other racing jurisdictions.

References

Bailey, C.J., S.W.J. Reid, D.R. Hodgson, J.M. Bourke and R.J. Rose, 1998. Flat, hurdle and steeple racing: risk factors for musculoskeletal injury. Equine Veterinary Journal 30: 498-503.

Bourke, J.M., 1995. Wastage in Thoroughbreds. Proceedings of the Annual Seminar of the Equine Branch of the New Zealand Veterinary Association, pp. 107-119.

Cohen, N.D., S.M. Berry, J.G. Peloso, G.D. Mundy and I.C. Howard, 2000. Association of high-speed exercise with racing injury in thoroughbreds. Journal of the American Veterinary Medical Association 216: 1273-1278.

Estberg, L., S.M. Stover, L.A. Gardner, B.J. Johnson, R.A. Jack, J.T. Case, A. Ardans, D.H. Read, M.L. Anderson, B.C. Barr, B.M. Daft, H. Kinde, J. Moore, J. Stoltz and L.W. Woods, 1998. Relationship between race start characteristics and risk of catastrophic injury in thoroughbreds: 78 cases (1992). Journal of the American Veterinary Medical Association 212: 544-549.

Johnson, B.J., S.M. Stover, B.M. Daft, H. Kinde, D.H. Read, B.C. Barr, M.L. Anderson, J. Moore, L.W. Woods, J. Stoltz and P. Blanchard, 1994. Causes of death in racehorses over a 2 year period. Equine Veterinary Journal 26: 327-330.

Kane, A.J., S.M. Stover, I.A. Gardner, J.T. Case, B.J. Johnson, D.H. Read and A.A. Ardans, 1996. Horseshoe characteristics as possible risk factors for fatal musculoskeletal injury of thoroughbred racehorses. American Journal of Veterinary Research 57: 1147-1152.

McKee, S.L., 1995. An update on racing fatalities in the UK. Equine Veterinary Education 7: 202-204.

Mohammed, H.O., T. Hill and J. Lowe, 1991. Risk factors associated with injuries in thoroughbred horses. Equine Veterinary Journal 23: 445-448.

Parkin, T.D.H., P.D. Clegg, N.P. French, C.J. Proudman, C.M. Riggs, E.R. Singer, P.M. Webbon and K.L. Morgan, 2004a. Risk of fatal distal limb fractures among thoroughbreds involved in the five types of racing in the United Kingdom. Veterinary Record 154: 493-497.

Parkin, T.D.H., P.D. Clegg, N.P. French, C.J. Proudman, C.M. Riggs, E.R. Singer, P.M. Webbon and K.L. Morgan, 2004b. Horse level risk factors for fatal distal limb fracture in racing Thoroughbreds in the UK. Equine Veterinary Journal 36:513-519.

Parkin, T.D.H., P.D. Clegg, N.P. French, C.J. Proudman, C.M. Riggs, E.R. Singer, P.M. Webbon and K.L. Morgan, 2004c. Race and course level risk factors for fatal distal limb fracture in racing Thoroughbreds. Equine Veterinary Journal 36:521-526

Parkin, T.D.H., P.D. Clegg, N.P. French, C.J. Proudman, C.M. Riggs, E.R. Singer, P.M. Webbon and K.L. Morgan, 2005. Risk factors for fatal lateral condylar fracture of the third metacarpus/metatarsus in UK racing. Equine Veterinary Journal 37:192-199.

Perkins, N.R., S.W.J. Reid and R.S. Morris, 2005. Risk factors for musculoskeletal injuries of the lower limbs in Thoroughbred racehorses in New Zealand. New Zealand Veterinary Journal 53: 171-183.

Vaughan, L.C. and B.J.E. Mason, 1975. A Clinico-pathological Study of Racing Accidents in Horses. A report of a study on Equine Fatal Accidents on Racecourses. London: Horserace Betting Levy Board.

Verheyen, K.L., W.E. Henley, J.S. Price and J.L.N. Wood, 2005. Training-related factors associated with dorsometacarpal disease in young Thoroughbred racehorses in the UK. Equine Veterinary Journal 37: 442-448.

Williams, R.B., L.S. Harkins, C.J. Hammond and J.L.N. Wood, 2001. Racehorse injuries, clinical problems and fatalities recorded on British racecourses from flat racing and National Hunt racing during 1996, 1997 and 1998. Equine Veterinary Journal 33: 478-486.

Wood, J.L.N., L.S. Harkins and K. Rogers, 2000. A retrospective study of factors associated with racehorse fatality on British racecourses from 1990-1999. Proceedings of the International Conference of Racing Analysts and Veterinarians 13: 274-277.

How are chronic tendon injuries tackled in humans?

Håkan Alfredson
Sports Medicine Unit, University Hospital, S-901 87 Umeå, Sweden

The chronic painful human tendon is well known to be difficult to treat, and the source of pain has not been scientifically clarified. The condition has for many years been treated as an inflammatory condition, secondary to overuse of the tendon (Schepsis *et al.*, 1987; Nelen *et al.*, 1989; Kvist, 1994; Leadbetter *et al.*, 1992; Myerson and McGarvey, 1998). Even the terminology used, tendinitis, implies involvement of an inflammation. This has not been based on scientific knowledge, on the contrary, histological examinations of tendon tissue specimens has repeatedly shown the absence of inflammatory cell-infiltrates (Movin *et al.*, 1997; Khan *et al.*, 1999). Still, cortico-steroidal injections, and tons of anti-inflammatory tablets, have been used in the treatment (Weiler, 1992; Leadbetter, 1995; Schrier *et al.*, 1996). Fortunately, during the recent years, researchers have started to question this treatment, and studied the background to pain in the chronic painful tendon (Khan et al, 2000; Alfredson *et al.*, 1999, 2000a, 2001).

Based on the absence of inflammatory cell-infiltrates in biopsies, the terminology has recently been changed to tendinopathy (pain and impaired function of the affected tendon) and tendinosis (where ultrasound, MRI, or biopsies, show specific changes in the affected tendon) (Movin *et al.*, 1997; Maffuli *et al.*, 1998).

Research on basic biology

Microdialysis

Microdialysis is a method to study concentrations of certain substances, in certain tissues, over a period of time (Darimont *et al.*, 1994; Thorsen *et al.* 1996). Intra-tendinous microdialysis was first done in 1999, and showed normal prostaglandin E_2 (PGE_2) levels in chronic painful Achilles tendinosis (Alfredson *et al.*, 2000a). The same findings, normal PGE_2 levels, were found when microdialysis was performed in chronic painful patellar tendinosis (Jumper´s knee) (Alfredson *et al.*, 2001). In those studies, for the first time, the neurotransmitter glutamate that is well known to be an important and potent modulator of pain in the central nervous system (Dickenson *et al.*, 1997), was found in it´s free form outside the central nervous system in humans. Interestingly, the glutamate concentrations were found to be significantly higher in the painful tendinosis tendons, compared to pain-free normal control tendons. A parallell study showed glutamate NMDAR-1 receptors localised in close relation to nerve structures in biopsies from Achilles tendinosis tissue (Alfredson *et al.*, 2000b). To try to evaluate the possible importance glutamate had for tendon pain, in a prospective study using microdialysis in chronic painful Achilles tendinosis, it was found that there were no differences in the intra-tendinous glutamate concentrations after succesful treatment with eccentric training (Alfredson and Lorentzon, 2003). The importance of the glutamate findings in the chronic painful tendons is still under scientific evaluation. Also using microdialysis, significantly higher lactate levels were found in chronic painful Achilles tendinosis tendons, compared to pain-free normal tendons, implying possibly hypoxic conditions, or maybe a high metabolic rate, in tendinosis (Alfredson *et al.*, 2002). If there is hypoxia, the hypoxia could either be preceeding tendinosis, or a result of tendinosis.

Gene technological analyses

Using cDNA-arrays and PCR techniques, it was demonstrated that there was no up-regulation of multiple so-called pro-inflammatory cytokines in chronic pain Achilles tendinosis tissue compared with normal pain-free Achilles tendon tissue (Alfredson *et al.*, 2003a). This finding, again, indicates that there is no intra-tendinous inflammation involved in this condition.

Grey-scale ultrasonography (US) and colour Doppler (CD)

US is an established reliable method to examine tendons (Åström *et al.*, 1996; Paavola *et al.*, 1998). The structure of the tendon can be accurately evaluated. CD is a method to study flows, and direction of flows, like blood flow (Terslev *et al.*, 2001; Weinberg *et al.*, 1998). The normal blood flow in tendons has a low flow rate and cannot be visualised, but vessels with high flows, like neovessels, can be detected. Using US and CD together, a neovascularisation was found inside and outside the area with structural tendon changes in chronic painful Achilles tendinosis tendons, but not in pain-free normal Achilles tendons, suggesting a relationship between neovascularisation and pain (Öhberg *et al.*, 2001). To further analyse the possible relationship between neovascularisation and pain, small amounts of a local anaesthetic was injected under US and CD-guidance towards the neovessels outside the tendon (Alfredson *et al.*, 2003b). This resulted in temporarily pain-free tendons, and indicated that the area with neovessels was of importance for the tendon pain.

Immunohistochemical analyses of tendon tissue specimens

Biopsies from the area with tendinosis and neovascularisation showed nerve structures in close relation to the vessels (Alfredson *et al.*, 2003b), and following studies have shown Substance-P (SP) nerves in the vascular wall, and Calcitonin Gene Related Peptide (CGRP) close to the vascular wall (Bjur *et al.*, 2005; Ljung *et al.*, 2004, 1999). Also, the Neurokinin-1-receptor (NK-1R), that is known to have a high affinity for SP, has been found in the vascular wall(Forsgren *et al.*, 2005). The findings of neuropeptides indicate that there still might be an inflammation in the tendon, however, not a so-called chemical inflammation via PGE_2, but instead a so-called neurogenic inflammation mediated via neuropeptides like SP.

Clinical research

About 10 years ago we designed a special type of eccentric calf muscle training to be used on patients with chronic painful mid-portion Achilles tendinosis (Alfredson et al., 1998). The results of that treatment have been shown to be very good, with more than 80% satisfied patients (Alfredson et al., 1998; Mafi et al., 2001; Fahlström et al., 2003). Also, US follow-ups have shown that the tendon thickness was significantly decreased and the structure looked ultrasongraphically "more normal" in the successfully treated cases (Öhberg et al., 2004a). We have not been able to explain the background to why this treatment works so well, but the follow-ups using US and CD together, showed that the neovascularisation was gone in the cases with a good clinical result, but remained in the cases with a poor clinical result, indicating a possible effect of this treatment on the area with neovascularisation (Öhberg et al., 2004b). By performing dynamic US+CD examinations, it was possible to demonstrate that the flow in the neovessels stopped during dorsiflexion of the ankle joint, and came back in the neutral ankle joint position (Öhberg et al., 2004b). During the eccentric training regimen, the ankle joint is in loaded dorsiflexion 180 repetitions/day, and possibly, in this position the vessels and nerves could be injured/destroyed? This is the only mechanism we have been able to objectively visualise, that possibly could explain how the eccentric training regimen works.

Coming back to the findings that US and CD-guided injections of small amounts of a local anaesthetic targeting the neovessels outside the tendon, temporarily cured the tendon pain. This raised the hypothesis that destroying the area with neovessels and nerves outside the tendon would affect the tendon pain. In a pilot study, US and CD-guided injections of a sclerosing substance, targeting the area with neovessels outside the tendon, was given to patients with chronic painful Achilles tendinosis (Öhberg et al., 2002). Polidocanol (an aliphatic non-ionised nitrogen-free substance with a sclerosing and anaesthetic effect) was used as a sclerosing agent. This substance has been in use for many years primarily with the purpose to treat varicose veins and tele-angiectasies (Guex, 1993), and has been demonstrated to have very few side-effects (Conrad et al., 1995). In the pilot study, the majority of the patients were pain-free after a mean of 2 treatments, with 6-8 weeks in between (Öhberg et al., 2002). Two-year follow-ups of these patients have shown a reduced tendon thickness, no remaining neovessels, and a ultrasonographically "normalised" structure in the successfully treated patients (non published material). In additional pilot studies using the same type of treatment on patients with similar findings in the Achilles tendon insertion (Öhberg et al., 2003), and in the patellar tendon (Alfredson and Öhberg, 2005a) the good short term results have been reproduced. Recently, in a randomized double-blind study, the effects of injecting Polidocanol was compared with the effects of injecting lidocaine+Adrenaline. The results clearly demonstrated good clinical effects using Polidocanol, but not when using lidocaine+Adrenaline (Alfredson and Öhberg, 2005b). This type of treatment has been extended in our clinic, and we have now treated more than 500 tendons. The group of patients is a mixture, ranging from relatively non-active individuals to Olympic level athletes. All types of complications possibly related to the treatment, are carefully noticed. We have only had three complications, two total and one partial Achilles tendon ruptures. All patients having had this treatment are routinely followed-up, clinically, and by US and CD, to be able to identify side-effects, and to present the results of mid- and long-term follow-ups in the future. Altogether, based on the short- and mid-term results of these studies, it seems that there is a potential to cure the pain, and also to decrease the thickness and ultrasonographically "normalise" the structure (non-published material) of the tendon, by "destroying" the area with neovessels and nerves outside the tendon with Polidocanol injections.

Conclusions

There is no scientific proof for an on-going prostaglandin-mediated inflammation inside the chronic painful Achilles-, patellar-, and ECRB-tendon. However, there might well be a neurogenic inflammation, mediated via neuropeptides like SP and CGRP. The area with neovascularisation (vessels and nerves) that can be visualised (vessels) in the chronic painful tendons using US and CD, is most likely the source of pain. Treatment focusing on destroying this area by US and CD-guided injections of the sclerosing substance polidocanol, targeting the neovessels, has in short-term studies been demonstrated to have a potential to cure the pain in the majority of patients.

Twelve weeks of painful eccentric calf-muscle training has been demonstrated to be a good treatment model for patients with chronic painful mid-portion Achilles tendinosis, but not for the chronic painful Achilles insertion.

References

Alfredson, H. and R. Lorentzon, 2003. Intra-tendinous glutamate levels and eccentric training in chronic Achilles tendinosis-a prospective study using microdialysis technique. Knee Surg, Sports Traumatol, Arthrosc 11: 196-199.

Alfredson, H. and L. Öhberg, 2005a. Neovascularisation in chronic painful patellar tendinosis-promising results after sclerosing neovessels outside the tendon challenges the need for surgery. Knee Surg, Sports Traumatol, Arthrosc 13: 74-80.

Alfredson, H. and L. Öhberg, 2005b. Sclerosing injections to areas of neovascularisation reduce pain in chronic Achilles tendinopathy: A double-blind randomized controlled trial. Accepted Knee Surg, Sports Traumatol, Arthrosc 13: 338-244.

Alfredson, H., D. Bjur, K. Thorsen and R. Lorentzon, 2002. High intratendinous lactate levels in painful chronic Achilles tendinosis. An investigation using microdialysis technique. J. Orthop. Res. 20: 934-938.

Alfredson, H., S. Forsgren, K. Thorsen, M. Fahlström, H. Johansson and R. Lorentzon, 2000b. Glutamate NMDAR1 receptors localised to nerves in human Achilles tendons. Implications for treatment? Knee Surg Sports Traumatol, Arthrosc 9: 123-126.

Alfredson, H., S. Forsgren, K. Thorsen and R. Lorentzon, 2001. In vivo microdialysis and immunohistochemical analyses of tendon tissue demonstrated high amounts of free glutamate and glutamate NMDAR1 receptors, but no signs of inflammation, in Jumper´s knee. J. Orthop. Res. 19: 881-886.

Alfredson, H., B.O. Ljung, K. Thorsen and R. Lorentzon, 2000a. In vivo investigation of ECRB tendons with microdialysis technique: no signs of inflammation but high amounts of glutamate in tennis elbow. Acta Orthop. Scand. 71: 475-479.

Alfredson, H., M. Lorentzon, S. Bäckman, A. Bäckman and U. Lerner, 2003a. cDNA-Arrays and Real-Time Quantitative PCR Techniques in the investigation of chronic Achilles tendinosis. J. Orthop. Res. 21: 970-975.

Alfredson, H., L. Öhberg and S. Forsgren, 2003b. Is vasculo-neural ingrowth the cause of pain in chronic Achilles tendinosis?-An investigation using ultrasonography and colour doppler, immunohistochemistry, and diagnostic injections. Knee Surg, Sports Traumatol, Arthrosc 11:334-338.

Alfredson, H., T. Pietilä, P. Jonsson and R. Lorentzon, 1998. Heavy-loaded eccentric calf-muscle training for the treatment of chronic Achilles tendinosis. Am. J. Sports Med. 26: 360-366.

Alfredson, H., K. Thorsen and R. Lorentzon, 1999. *In situ* microdialysis in tendon tissue: high levels of glutamate, but not prostaglandin E_2 in chronic Achilles tendon pain. Knee Surg, Sports Traumatol Arthrosc 7: 378-381.

Åström, M., C.F. Gentz, P. Nilsson, A. Rausing, S. Sjoberg and N. Westlin, 1996. Imaging in chronic Achilles tendinopathy: a comparison of ultrasonography, magnetic resonance imaging and surgical findings in 27 histologically verified cases. Skeletal Radiol. 25: 615-620.

Bjur, D., H. Alfredson and S. Forsgren, 2005. The innervation pattern of the human Achilles tendon -Studies on the normal and tendinosis tendon using markers for general, sensory and sympathetic innervations. Cell Tiss. Res. 320: 201-206.

Conrad, P., G.M. Malouf, M.C. Stacey, 1995. The Australian polidocanol (aethoxysklerol) study. Results at 2 years. Dermatol. Surg. 21: 334-336.

Darimont, C., G. Vassaux, D. Gaillard, G. Ailhaud and R. Négrel, 1994. *In situ* microdialysis of prostaglandins in adipose tissue: stimulation of prostacyclin release by angiotensin II. Int. J. Obesity 18: 783-788.

Dickenson, A.H., V. Chapman and G.M. Green, 1997. The pharmacology of excitatory and inhibitory amino acid-mediated events in the transmission and modulation of pain in the spinal cord. A Review. Gen. Pharmac. 28: 633-638.

Fahlström, M., P. Jonsson, R. Lorentzon and H. Alfredson, 2003. Chronic Achilles tendon pain treated with eccentric calf-muscle training. Knee Surg, Sports Traumatol, Arthrosc 11: 327-333.

Forsgren, S., P. Danielsson and H. Alfredson, 2005. Vascular NK-1R receptor occurrence in normal and chronic painful Achilles and patellar tendons. Studies on chemically unfixed as well as fixed specimens. Regul. Pept. 126: 173-181.

Guex, J.J., 1993. Indications for the sclerosing agent polidocanol. J. Dermatol. Surg. Oncol. 19: 959-961.

Khan, K.M., J.L. Cook, F. Bonar, P. Harcourt and M. Åström, 1999. Histopathology of common tendinopathies. Update and implications for clinical management. Sports Med. 27: 393-408.

Khan, K.M., J.L. Cook, N. Maffuli and P. Kannus, 2000. Where is the pain coming from in tendinopathy? It may be biochemical, not only structural, in origin. Br. J. Sports Med. 34: 81-83.

Kvist, M., 1994. Achilles tendon injuries in athletes. Sports Med. 18: 173-201.

Leadbetter, W.B., 1995. Anti-inflammatory therapy and sports injury: The role of non-steroidal drugs and corticosteroid injection. Clin. Sports Med. 14: 353-410.

Leadbetter, W.B., P.A. Mooar and G.J. Lane, 1992. The surgical treatment of tendinitis. Clinical rationale and biologic basis. Clin. Sports Med. 11: 679-712.

Ljung, B.O., H. Alfredson and S. Forsgren, 2004. Neurokinin 1-receptors and sensor neuropeptides in tendon insertions at the medial and lateral epicondyles of the humerus. Studies on tennis elbow and medial epicodylalgia. J. Orthop. Res.22: 321-327.

Ljung, B.O., S. Forsgren and J. Fridén, 1999. Substance-P and calcitonin gene-related peptide expression at the extensor carpi radialis brevis muscle origin: implications for the etiology of tennis elbow? J. Orthop. Res. 17: 554-559.

Maffulli, N., K.M. Khan and G. Puddu, 1998. Overuse tendon conditions: time to change a confusing terminology. Arthroscopy 14: 840-843.

Mafi, N., R. Lorentzon and H. Alfredson, 2001. Superior results with eccentric calf-muscle training compared to concentric training in a randomized prospective multi-center study on patients with chronic Achilles tendinosis. Knee Surg, Sports Traumatol, Arthrosc 9: 42-47.

Movin, T., A. Gad and F.P. Reinholt, 1997. Tendon pathology in long-standing Achillodynia. Biopsy findings in 40 patients. Acta Orthop. Scand. 68: 170-175.

Myerson, M.S. and W. McGarvey, 1998. Disorders of the insertion of the Achilles tendon and Achilles tendinitis. J. Bone and Joint Surg. 80-A: 1814-1824.

Nelen, G., M. Martens and A. Burssens, 1989. Surgical treatment of chronic Achilles tendinitis. Am. J. Sports Med. 17: 754-759.

Öhberg, L. and H. Alfredson, 2002. Ultrasound guided sclerosis of neovessels in painful chronic Achilles tendinosis: pilot study of a new treatment. Br. J. Sports Med. 36: 173-177.

Öhberg, L. and H. Alfredson, 2003. Sclerosing therapy in chronic Achilles tendon insertional pain-results of a pilot study. Knee Surg, Sports Traumatol, Arthrosc 11:339-343.

Öhberg, L. and H. Alfredson, 2004. Effect on neovascularisation behind the good results with eccentric training in chronic mid-portion Achilles tendinosis. Knee Surg, Sports Traumatol, Arthrosc 12: 465-470.

Öhberg, L., R. Lorentzon and H. Alfredson, 2001. Neovascularisation in Achilles tendons with painful tendinosis but not in normal tendons: an ultrasonographic investigation. Knee Surg. Sports Traumatol, Arthrosc 9: 233-238.

Öhberg, L., R. Lorentzon and H. Alfredson, 2004. Eccentric training in patients with chronic Achilles tendinosis-normalized tendon structure and decreased thickness at follow-up. Br. J. Sports Med. 38: 8-11.

Paavola, M., T. Paakkala, P. Kannus and M. Jarvinen, 1998. Ultrasonography in the differential diagnosis of Achilles tendon injuries and related disorders. Acta Radiol. 39: 612-619.

Schepsis, A.A. and R.E. Leach, 1987. Surgical treatment of Achilles tendinitis. Am. J. Sports Med. 15: 308-315.

Schrier, I., G.O. Matheson, and H.W. Kohl III, 1996. Achilles tendonitis: Are corticosteroid injections useful or harmful? Clin. J. Sport Med. 6: 245-250.

Terslev, L., E. Qvistgaard, S. Torp- Pedersen, J. Laetgaard, B. Danneskiold- Samsøe and H. Bliddal, 2001. Ultrasound and Power Doppler findings in jumper's knee - preliminary observations. European Journal of Ultrasound 13: 183-189.

Thorsen, K., A.O. Kristoffersson, U.H. Lerner and R.P. Lorentzon, 1996. *In situ* microdialysis in bone tissue. Stimulation of prostaglandin E_2 release by weight-bearing mechanical loading. J. Clin. Invest. 98: 2446-2449.

Weiler, J.M., 1992. Medical modifiers of sports injury. The use of nonsteroidal anti-inflammatory drugs (NSAIDs) in sports soft-tissue injury. Clin. Sports Med. 11: 625-644.

Weinberg, E.P., M.J. Adams and G.M. Hollenberg, 1998. Color Doppler sonography of patellar tendinosis. A.J.R. 171:743-744.

A scientific approach to training Thoroughbred horses

Allan J. Davie
School of Exercise Science & Sport Management, Southern Cross University, P.O. Box 157, 2480 Lismore, Australia

This review will discuss the literature in relation to key factors influencing training adaptations in the horse. The major emphasis will be on the equine discipline, however, in areas where equine literature is lacking, directly relevant literature from the studies in the human area will be discussed.

The review will focus on peripheral and central adaptations to training, the level of stimuli required to trigger these adaptations and finally some recommendations relating the requirements for adaptation to the design of training programs will be offered.

Introduction

The goal of any conditioning program is to stimulate adaptations within the animal's body in order to bring about improvements in efficiency of performance. These adaptations both central and peripheral that enhance performance occur mainly at a cellular level and are controlled by DNA. A number of biochemical processes take place that enable the nucleotide sequence in the DNA to be translated into proteins for an adaptation to occur. This process incorporates two key steps: transcription, copying of the gene sequence on DNA to RNA forming mRNA and translation in which the gene sequence on the mRNA is use to produce new proteins.

The controlling mechanisms underlying this process are not well understood, although the physiological signalling pathways that regulate transcription such as mechanical loading, intra-cellular calcium, hypoxia and cellular redox state, each of which is a response to mechanical loading, have been established.

Baar *et al.* (1999) reported that the adaptations to training are highly specific to the type and duration of exercise with the mechanisms and factors that regulate the transcriptional process limited. Available evidence indicates cellular adaptations arise from the cumulative effects of changes in gene transcription occurring during the recovery period (Pilegaard *et al.*, 2000). Pilegaard *et al.* (2000) reported that activation of transcription occurs for several hours post exercise and that this process was transient as all genes had returned to control levels by 22 hours post exercise. The mRNA content of genes however was still elevated at 22 hours post exercise indicating the transient increases in transcription from consecutive bouts results in accumulation of mRNA which they suggest may represent the basis for adaptation. It seems probable then that the accumulative effect of several training sessions or weeks of transient increases in transcription is likely to produce sufficient changes in mRNA to promote protein growth (Pilegaard *et al.*, 2000).

Adaptations occur in both aerobic and anaerobic energy systems. Long slow aerobic work stimulates increases in plasma volume and hemoglobin levels thus improving oxygen carrying capacity and at the cellular level, increases in myoglobin, number of mitochondria and activity levels of enzymes involved in energy production, increases the capacity to produce energy aerobically.

The increased anaerobic energy changes come principally in the form of an increased capacity of the ATP-CP system, CP levels in muscle, activity of creatine kinase and an increased glycolytic capacity.

Some physiological components responsible for performance

In this paper the major physiological components responsible for performance, cardiac output, maximal oxygen consumption ($VO_{2\,max}$), lactate threshold and efficiency will be discussed in relation to the level of stimuli and type of training most appropriate for promoting adaptation. Further key areas such as bone and tendon development will be briefly discussed in relation to impact of training on their development.

Maximum cardiac output and VO_{2max} determine the upper limits for a high performance potential (MacDougall *et al.*. 1991). It is well established that a high level of aerobic power (maximum oxygen consumption, VO_{2max}) provides the physiological foundation for elite performance in both humans and horses. VO_{2max} is mainly determined by two factors, cardiac output or the capacity of delivering oxygen to muscles and the capacity of muscles to utilize oxygen for energy production which is very much dependent on mitochondrial density and function. In humans VO_{2max} has been used as an indicator for potential success. However, this same relationship has not been demonstrated in horses, although the volume of research investigating this relationship in the horse has not been as extensive as it has in humans (Gauvreau *et al.*, 1995). Although these factors may provide a gauge for potential success they alone do not guarantee success. Further, VO_{2max} changes with training do not always provide the best foundation to monitor and design training programs. In contrast, the lactate threshold, or the lactate responses to exercise, can provide valuable information in relation to how much of the cardiovascular capacity can be taken advantage of in a sustained gallop. Both VO_{2max} and lactate threshold are affected by genetic factors and training status.

Cardiac output

Cardiac output is the product of heart rate and stroke volume and as maximal heart rate does not change with training, cardiac performance at sub-maximal levels is largely dependant on the determinants of stroke volume, including preload, afterload and contractility. Preload is the end-diastolic pressure which is the result of the heart chamber being stretched with increased venous return (Brooks *et al.*, 2005). An increased preload (volume overload) results in an increased end diastolic volume and increased stroke volume (Frank-Starling Law). In contrast an increased afterload (pressure overload) increases the resistance to blood leaving the heart, resulting in a decreased stroke volume.

Cardiac output is a function of the effectiveness of the heart, the performance of which is measured in several ways. Cardiac function has been evaluated in the horse with the quantitative two-dimensional echocardiograph being introduced in the early 1990's (Voros, 1997). Standardised techniques have now been established for quantification of cardiac size and assessing flow (Long et al., 1992; Lord and Croft, 1990; Reef, 1991). In addition echocardiology has been used to examine the correlation between heart score and maximal oxygen uptake (Young et al., 2002) to examine cardiac dimensions in Standardbreds (Bakos et al., 2002) and recording changes in cardiac dimensions during reconditioning in horses (Kriz et al., 2000).

Cardiac adaptations have been shown to respond to both preload and afterload training stimuli. However, the nature of cardiac hypertrophy differs in response to a volume versus a pressure overload. The implications of afterload from a training perspective are an increased left ventricular mass and wall thickness. In human studies of athletes that are involved in training modes that create high afterloads (weight training) there have been reported increases in left ventricular wall thickness and left ventricular mass (Morganroth et al., 1975) and interventricular septum thickness (Menapace et al., 1982). These changes increase cardiac oxygen requirements, however generally without concomitant increases in capillary density.

Preload training in contrast results in an increase in myocardial muscle mass, chamber size and increased capillary density. This increase (hypertrophy) results in an increased heart capacity (endurance), which in turn results in an increased volume of blood being pumped per heart beat (stroke volume). A higher stroke volume means that for a specific blood flow rate the heart rate can be lower, as more blood is being pumped per beat. This response is the major adaptation that we see with training. Recovery of heart rate following exercise is also improved with training (Evans, 1994) with the time period for heart rate to return to within a designated range (100-110 bpm) being directly related to the relative fitness of the horse.

Maximal oxygen uptake

The maximum oxygen uptake of Thoroughbred horses can vary from approximately 100 to 160ml.kg^{-1} min $^{-1}$ (Evans and Rose, 1987; Lund and Guthrie, 1995; Tyler et al., 1996a, b). VO_{2max} has been shown to continuously increase with training for several weeks to months, with the capacity for improvement in VO_{2max} in an untrained horse being up to 20 percent. The initial improvements in VO_{2max} are rapid and appear not to be effected by the relative intensity of the training. Further change in VO_{2max} depends on the level of training stimulus (intensity/duration), with increases in intensity having been shown to elicit only small further increases. This is supported in the human literature which has shown that the training intensity is of greater importance than duration to stimulate further improvements in VO_{2max}.

In stimulating an adaptation within the cardiovascular system we need to understand the level of stimuli required. Von Wittke et al. (1994) in examining the training programs of several training establishments, showed that the number of days of gallop workouts showed a significant correlation with performance, and that the number of gallop workouts and total time of training correlated with the changes in V4. Most gallops were done at speeds of less than 10 m/s (9.6 to 12.5 m/s) and at distances of 1600-1850 m. Evans *et al.* (1995) compared the effects of high versus low intensity treadmill training for 9 weeks at lactate concentrations of 4-8 mmol/l with the slow group training at half the speed of the fast group. Training intensities ranged from 49-84% to 53 to 97% VO_{2max} for the two groups from weeks 1 to 9 respectively. VO_2 increased by 20% in both groups indicating that intensity is not important in the early phases of training. Knight *et al.* (1991) trained horses on the treadmill for 6 weeks at 40 to 80% VO_{2max} and found only a 10% increase after 2 weeks but no further increase. Hinchcliff *et al.* (2002) found that 10 weeks of training at 92% VO_{2max} resulted in a 17% increase in VO_{2max}.

These finding were reinforced by the work of Tyler *et al.* (1996a, b). They studied horses in training over a 34 week period in which the first 7 weeks training at 60% VO_{2max} resulted in a 15% increase in VO_{2max}. In the following 9 weeks in which they trained three days per week at 80% VO2 and two days per week at 100% VO_{2max} there was only an additional 5% increase in VO_{2max} above the first 7 weeks of training values. They proposed that endurance based moderate intensity training is more important in inducing adaptations in VO_{2max} than high intensity training supporting the earlier work of Evans *et al.* (1995).

Metabolic responses to training

The animal is in a continual state of demand for energy to perform its tasks. All forms of work require the transfer of chemical energy to mechanical work. The energy component of the cell (muscle) is adenosine triphosphate (ATP). It is the only energy source that can be used for muscular contraction. However, muscle cells can store only limited amounts of ATP, therefore, metabolic means must exist within the muscle cell with the capability to produce ATP rapidly. Muscle cells can produce ATP by a number of means:
- Creatine Phosphate (CP) can provide the energy directly for the formation of ATP; and/or
- The energy for the formation of ATP can be supplied from the chemical breakdown of feed sources (glucose and/or fats) and by either aerobic or anaerobic (glycolysis) means.

Within skeletal muscle the primary sites of energy production are the cytoplasm for anaerobic and the mitochondria for aerobic. In high intensity exercise energy is provided principally from the ATP-CP glycolysis network. During lower intensity aerobic work the energy is provided via the Krebs Cycle within the mitochondria. The improvements in metabolic efficiency with training are the result of increased concentrations of the key regulatory enzymes within the different metabolic pathways. Phosphofructokinase (PFK) is recognized as the rate limiting enzyme in glycolysis with succinate dehydrogenase (SDH) and citrate synthase (CS) being the key controllers within the aerobic pathway. The responses and adaptations of these enzymes to training stimuli are very specific with high intensity exercise stimulating changes in glycolytic regulators and endurance based work stimulating changes in the aerobic pathway.

Geor *et al.* (1999) exercised horses for 10 consecutive days of moderate-intensity training at 55% VO_{2max} for 60 min per day (13-14 km/day) which resulted in 8.9% increase in VO_{2max} and 24% increase in run time to exhaustion but there was no effect on plasma epinephrine or activity of SDH, CS and 3 hydroxyacyl CoA dehydrogenase (HAD) indicating mitochondria oxidative state did not change. Similarly, Green *et al.* (1991) looked at a short training program of 2 hours per day at 59% peak VO_{2max} repeated for 10-12 consecutive days and reported no change in SDH, CS, HAD, hexokinase, phosphorylase, PFK and lactate dehydrogenase (LDH).

These studies highlight that to promote enzymatic adaptations at the mitochondrial level, the horse needs to be working at an intensity at least 60% VO_{2max} and for a period of approximately two weeks. This reinforces the need for programs to be designed to allow the same stimuli to be applied over at least two weeks allowing for adaptations before a higher intensity stimulus is applied.

Mitochondria

The mitochondria are frequently referred to as the power house of energy production as it is within the mitochondria that all aerobic energy production takes place. Mitochondria exist in all eukaryotic cells and contain the metabolic pathways for aerobic energy production. Approximately 80% of the inspired oxygen is consumed by mitochondria to meet the metabolic demands. The genotype of mitochondria therefore must be among the key factors that determine muscle utilization of oxygen and therefore are a powerful influencing factor of aerobic performance.

The development of the mitochondria is a key component of training. The mitochondria however, do not increase in specific activity, *i.e.* enzyme activity per unit of mitochondria, but they increase in number (Brooks *et al.*, 2005) with this adaptation resulting predominately from endurance based (Preload) training. The available research suggests that the increased oxidative capacity resulting from short-term training is regulated at the pre-translational step but the increase following long term training is the result of mitochondrial replication. Coyle *et al.* (1984) proposed that the magnitude of the increase in mitochondria is influenced by the duration of the exercise or training session. However, this is not a direct linear relationship for with additional training this factor becomes less important. He further proposed the best adaptations occur with/when intensity of training interacts with duration. Murakami *et al.* (1994) trained rats for 3, 6 and 12 weeks on a treadmill for 90 minutes a day 5 days per week. Training for 3, 6 and 12 weeks significantly increased activities of CS (31, 28 and 47%) ubiquinol-cytochrome-c oxidoreductase (61, 63 and 77%) and cytochrome oxidase (25, 26 and 32%) indicating changes in the aerobic metabolic energy pathway. The concentration of mitochondrial cytochrome b mRNA was elevated proportionally with enzymes activity while mitochondrial DNA remained unaltered at 3 and 6 weeks but did increase significantly after 12 weeks of training (35%). Tyler *et al.* (1996b) reported that the mitochondrial volume/density continued to increase over the 34 weeks of training and paralleled the increase in VO_{2max}. Further they reported that the greatest rate of increases in HAD and CS occurred in the first 10 weeks of training at an intensity of 60% VO_{2max}, these levels continued to increase when training at higher intensity although at a reduced rate. They proposed that endurance based moderate intensity training is more important in inducing peripheral adaptations than high intensity training.

Bone

The adaptation of bone is dependent on the nutritional status, in relation to the calcium/ phosphorus relationship, which affects mineralisation and the level of stress impacted on the bone *i.e.* the speed of the gallop. Bones will increase their density and mass thus becoming stronger if the stress applied is controlled (Jeffcott, 2000). However if the tissue is adversely stressed the bone may become weaker. In the initial stages of training the bone becomes weaker as there is resorption of bone minerals which is then followed by a period in which the previously resorbed bone is again laid down (Nielsen *et al.*, 1997). In the early stages of training the collagen tissue is being absorbed faster than it is formed therefore decreasing the bone's strength, however this process is reversed as the training progresses. It has been shown that this strength decrease of bone may persist for up to 50-60 days during the initial stages of training (Nielsen *et al.*, 1997), with this being dependent on the time phase that the horse was not in training prior to entering training. It is during this phase of training that the stress applied to the bone has to be controlled to prevent injury.

Lanyon (1990) in discussing the capacity of bone to adapt to stress outlined that bone has the capacity to withstand repetitive loading with the characteristics of the bone changing in response to the functional load bearing. The training regimen therefore needs to be designed so that the loads applied during training are appropriate to the level of bone development. In addition, Stone (1988) outlines that the volume intensity and load-bearing nature of the exercise training are also important in stimulating connective tissue adaptations.

Keller and Spengler (1989) suggested there was a loading threshold for positive bone change and they indicated that this needs to be greater than the 25% of the maximum effort. Biewener *et al.* (1986) performed a similar study with chicks training at 35% maximum speed, and reported similar findings to Keller and Spengler. Matsuda *et al.* (1986) exercised chicks at 70-80% of maximum aerobic capacity and found that runners had a greater cortical cross-sectional area. The results of these studies suggest that exercise below certain threshold intensity does not alter a predetermined strain state that bone attempts to maintain during remodeling.

Preliminary work by Hutchinson (unpublished) on yearling and early two year old Thoroughbreds has supported this threshold intensity concept. He has galloped horses on a treadmill at speeds between 32 to 42 km/hr at different grades, and examined the

Management of lameness causes in sport horses

changes in bone cortical thickness. His finding supported the earlier research in that there was no change below a certain galloping speed and that a small grade of only 2 degrees created more bone stimuli than a high grade of 6 degrees.

Some training tools

Treadmill

The treadmill provides an ideal tool for interval training, in that both distance and speed can be accurately controlled and time greatly reduced in comparison to track interval work. The treadmill traditionally has been used as a research tool or in clinical diagnostic testing. However with the development of the high-speed treadmill it has become more popular as a training tool. The uniqueness of the treadmill is that the intensity, volume and duration of the work interval can be controlled. This is a major advantage when doing high quality galloping work.

Research has shown that the inclined treadmill forces the hind limbs to carry more weight and to provide greater propulsion. This aspect provides an ideal approach to assist in the muscular development of the hind limbs during training.

Treadmill work can be introduced early in the training program as part of the slow work, however its major benefit comes with high speed interval work-outs. The intensity and duration of each gallop will vary depending on the level of fitness of the horse and its ability. The level of stress applied, speed and duration of gallops, with each work out can be monitored by the use of heart rate monitor or by measurements of blood lactate concentrations.

Several studies have investigated the effectiveness of the treadmill in stimulating physiological responses similar to those experienced on the training track. Courouce *et al.* (2000) in examining the physiological responses of track versus treadmill, found that at 2% incline on the treadmill horses produced similar responses to those reported following training on the track. Courouce *et al.* (2000) also reported that training on an un-inclined treadmill produced significant differences for the variables V200, V4 and VHRmax compared to that recorded on a track. Harkins *et al.* (1993) found a negative correlation between track running speed over distances of 1,200, 1,600 and 2000 m and treadmill gallop variables with the stronger correlation being between 1,600 m and 2,000 m with VLa4, VO_{2max} and V200 measured on the treadmill. Further Lucia and Greppi (1996) also found a correlation between racing performance and fitness parameters after exercise tests both on the treadmill and track in Standardbred racehorses. However, the fitness parameters calculated on the treadmill occurred at a significantly lower speed than for the same variable on the track. The speed at which VLa4 occurred was significantly higher (9.11 m/s *vs.* 8.17 m/s) on the track than for the treadmill. They concluded that despite the lower speeds the treadmill tests appear more strenuous compared with the track tests. The work of Davie (unpublished) however, has shown that for a typical Australian training gallop, the lactates are much higher than those for the treadmill. Following a single 1,200 m gallop lactate concentrations ranged from 14-18 mmol/L in comparison with 3 x 1,200 treadmill gallops with 5 min recovery periods lactates concentrations ranged from 5 to 16 mmol/L. Werkmann *et al.* (1996) looked at the conditioning effects in Thoroughbred horses exercising for 5, 15 or 25 minutes duration, on a treadmill at 6% incline at blood lactate concentrations at V2.5 or V4 for 11 exercise sessions with one day of rest between two consecutive exercise sessions. There was no effect of conditioning on V200 and V4 leading them to suggest that to exercise horses for up to 25 minutes at intensities that elicit blood lactates of 4 mmol/L may not be sufficient to stimulate adaptations in blood lactate responses. The research to date suggests that the intensity of exercise needed to stimulate adaptations on the treadmill may be different than that on the track and to equate work on the track with the treadmill needs to be treated with caution.

The difficulty with utilising some field tests such as the VL4 is that the speeds required are well below those that are routinely used by trainers, they are however able to be used effectively on the treadmill.

Swimming

In the human area the benefits of swimming training have long been known (Fry, 1986). In humans the mean arterial blood pressure during swimming tends to be higher than at the same heart rate during running, however, swimming training induces a reduction in resting blood pressure in hypertensive patients (Tanaka *et al.*, 1997) and has shown positive adaptations in stoke volume. The actual benefits or improvements in fitness in the human area are well known, however for the horse the actual benefits they obtain is rather an unknown entity. Misumi *et al.* (1995) reported that improvements do occur in aerobic capacity at the muscular level with a combination of running and swimming.

Swimming a horse is quite different from humans in relation to physiological responses to the exercise. Human studies have shown that the highest VO_2 attained during swimming averages approximately 90% of that attained during cycling. Blood lactates during maximum swimming have been shown to be in the same order as that during maximum cycling (10 mM). Asheim *et al.* (1970) examined horses swimming for three periods of four minutes with three minutes rest between swims. Lactates ranged from 3.0 to 9.3 mmol/L after the third swim with heart rates ranging from 158-210 bpm.

In contrast unpublished work by the author (Davie, unpublished) has shown heart rates and blood lactates in horses following 6 x one and half minutes swims with one minute rest periods between to be only in the order of 3 mM and 130 bpm respectively. It is believed that swimming training could elicit central adaptations as changes in ventricular mass and volume as a result of the after load training stimuli.

Designing training programs

One of the most underrated aspects of training (conditioning) is the design of the program itself. There will always be variations in what trainers do with a horse, depending on the age, nature and injury status of the horse, its response to work and the past experiences of the trainer. However, regardless of these variables it is important to have a sound basis on which to work. The transition from the paddock to the stage of moderate work is a high risk period. All trainers are aware of this and take a horse through the foundations of training, with initial long slow work, medium pace work and then finally the sprint work. What varies is the time period spent at each phase and the intensity and or duration of the work within each phase. This variation is based on sound judgment by the trainer in relation to both the past history of the horse and how well the horse copes with the existing work and the time period available to them before racing. It is the time period till racing that creates the most stress for the trainer. In terms of muscular, skeletal and mental adaptations, the time frame in which they are expected to have the horse prepared to race is generally unrealistic. For example bone density decreases with training and is not on an increase for some 50+ days after the commencement of training, this indicates that undue stress within this time period may increase the likelihood of injury. The design or structure of a training program needs to consider the following aspects:

- goals you have in mind in relation to the nature of the event the horse is being trained for;
- the time period that the horse has been turned out of training or the initial fitness status and age of the horse;
- training facilities;
- climate in which you live.

A training program needs to be soundly based and individualised with consideration to the above variables in an attempt to match the ability of the horse and the type of race it is being trained for.

The basis of any training program is to continually provide increased levels of stress to the muscle, heart and lungs to stimulate adaptations to improve fitness. The *Overload Principle* states that for continual adaptation, the level of stress needs to be continually increased. However, it is important to appreciate that there is a limit to the gains in fitness that can be achieved and that individual horses will differ in relation to how well they can cope with the stress (Smith *et al.*, 1999).

In applying the overload principle, it is important to understand that adaptations take time to occur (Seiler, 1996), as indicted by the work of Pilegaard *et al.* (2000) which showed that the transient increases in transcription from consecutive bouts results in accumulation of mRNA, which they suggest may represent the basis for adaptation. In the human area Moritani (1992) showed that strength gains were fast in the early stages of training due to neural adaptations, with later improvements in strength being more a result of muscle hypertrophy. The large adaptations in strength occur in the first six to eight weeks of training.

When the horse trains, damage to some cells will occur due to the stresses encountered therefore the recovery period needs to be adequate to allow for repair of this damage. This is because during hard gallops the muscle metabolism is up to 100 times that at rest, with the increased oxygen consumption resulting in free radical formation which causes muscle damage. Free radical formation is a normal response to the increased oxygen consumption that occurs with training. The rate of increase is controlled by anti-oxidant buffers, however when too much stress is applied the buffering system is exceeded and concentration increases. It has been shown that this damage can last for 48 to 96 hours (Duarte *et al.* 1993). The application of a further hard gallop in this time period is therefore likely to induce further damage and delay recovery.

After a training session the horse's body overreacts to fatigue and muscle damage and experiences a period of overcompensation to the original stress. The muscle then re-establishes itself but at a level slightly higher than the pre-training state (Bomba, 1994). This small increase is called the *adaptation*. The adaptation may take one or several formats including:
- an increased storage of muscle glycogen;
- an increased capacity to utilise feeds (glycogen and fats) as an energy source;
- an increased capacity of muscles to sustain a certain speed; or
- an increased capacity of muscle to take up and use oxygen.

Training then needs to be designed to incorporate the application of a stress to the horse and of equal importance to allow sufficient recovery time for overcompensation and adaptation to occur. The time period before exposure to the next training stimuli should be of sufficient duration to allow time for the training effect (adaptation) from the first session to occur (Rushall and Pike, 1990). If the next training session is applied without sufficient time for recovery, overcompensation and adaptation, then performance decrements occur in the form of earlier onset of fatigue. With repeated training sessions without sufficient recovery then the horse will become fatigued earlier in each training session and performance will decrease.

In bringing about these adaptations the intensity of training (aerobic *vs.* anaerobic), duration, number of training sessions and recovery period are all of paramount importance. When designing a training program it is important to firstly consider the distance of the race that the horse is primarily being trained for as the higher the intensity/speed of the event (1,000 m) the more the horse will be reliant upon anaerobic energy production. However, it has been shown that even for sprint races, the aerobic energy system contributes as much as 70-80 percent of the total energy (Eaton *et al.*, 1995; Tyler *et al.*, 1996a, b). Therefore even in training programs for sprinting races, training for aerobic as well as the anaerobic energy pathways is important.

Exposure of the muscle to a stress helps to develop adaptations to the horse's body systems, which serves to minimise the future impact of the stress. However, it needs to be understood that if the stress is too small in either intensity or duration, little or no adaptation is stimulated. But, if the stress is too severe, adaptation is delayed or even prevented.

The variations to the training program used to apply different levels of stress are:
- length of the training program;
- intensity;
- duration; and
- frequency.

Length of the program

Based on the time period for muscle hypertrophy, six to eight weeks and for bone adaptation (50+ days) it is apparent that the program needs to be structured to incorporate different levels of stress within a time frame of twelve to fifteen weeks.

Intensity

Intensity refers to the level of stress that is applied *i.e.* how fast the horse gallops. The greater the intensity the more stress applied to the muscles, heart and energy system. The level of stress needs to be closely monitored, as it is much more destructive to the horse's muscle cells as the intensity increases. As a result of the damage from high intensity gallops, longer recovery periods are needed. A major contributor to this damage is the formation of free radicals which increases oxidative stress. In the human field the effects of applying too much stress when the muscle is not conditioned for it, results in formation of free radicals which increases oxidative stress resulting in delayed onset of muscle soreness (DOMS).

In the initial four to seven weeks of training, during which the key factor is developing the cardio-respiratory system while at the same time keeping the stress on the bone and ligament structures to a minimum, the intensity of training is low. However, by week four the intensity every second day in increased to around 50% to 60% VO_{2max}. This intensity has shown improvements in VO_{2max} of up to 20% over this time period. In contrast Werkmann *et al.*. (1996) exercised horses for 25 minutes at an intensity of V_4 and found no changes in lactate responses to exercise re-enforcing the need to exercise above specific thresholds. In humans the training intensity needed to stimulate adaptations is varied with reported ranges from 70% HR_{max} or 58% VO_{2max} for the general healthy people to 90% HR_{max} or 85% VO_{2max} representing an upper limit for most adaptations to occur (McArdle *et al.*, 1996). Training can also be based on the top speed over set distances. Depending on the distance the speed can be set at between 75 to 90% of the best time over the relevant distance (Bosch and Klomp, 2005). For the horse, racing speeds vary from 16 to 17.5 m/s for distances between 1,200 to 2,000 m meters. The training intensity based on 75-90% max speed is 14 to 16 sec/200 m and 13 to 15 sec/200 m splits for distances of 2,000 m to 1,200 m respectively.

Duration

Duration refers to the total amount of work performed during the training session - the amount of time the stress (intensity) is applied. Changing the duration of the gallop is designed to improve the capacity of the horse to increase the amount of exercise it can do at a specific intensity or speed. In general the volume of work is increased by 10% per week over the first ten weeks during which period all workouts are at a controlled speed. Studies have shown that ten consecutive days of training has not been sufficient to stimulate adaptations in the key regulatory enzymes in the metabolic pathway. Therefore the increases in the volume of work need to be small over long periods of time to allow the suggested transient increases seen in mRNA to allow for new protein growth.

Frequency

Frequency of the application of the stress is the number of training sessions or repetitions of a gallop. In deciding how many times per week that a working gallop is performed the following needs to be considered. Because during hard gallops the muscle metabolism is up to 100 times that at rest, the increased oxygen consumption results in free radical formation which causes muscle damage. It has been shown that this damage can last for 48 to 96 hours (Duarte *et al.*, 1993). The application of a further hard gallop in this time period is most likely to induce further damage and delay recovery.

Summary

The ideal training program is one that maximises adaptation, while minimising cellular and systemic stress. Very hard training may result in damage, pain, fatigue and lower resistance to infection. In practical terms the ideal is to do the least training possible that achieves the maximum benefits. The key factors in this are the intensity, duration, frequency of gallops and recovery period.

The recovery time should be:
- long enough to allow repair and remodelling of muscle cells to occur; but
- not so long that reverting to the previous muscle cellular state could begin.

In planning the training program you also have to recognise that different adaptations respond at different rates. Plasma volume increases quickly while structural changes, such as blood vessel growth into muscles, occurs slowly. These factors will affect the relative amount of training you apply to achieve specific adaptations.

References

Asheim, A., O. Knudsen, A. Lindholm, C. Rülcker and B. Saltin, 1970. Heart rate and blood lactate concentrations of Standardbred horses during training and racing. J American Veterinary Medical Association 157: 304-312.

Baar, K., E. Blough, B. Dineen and K. Esser, 1999. Transcriptional Regulation in Response to Exercise. Exercise and Sport Sciences Reviews, Volume 27. J.O. Holloszy (Ed.). Pub Lippincott Williams & Wilkins.

Bakos, Z., K. Voros, T. Jarvinen and J. Reiczigel, 2002. Two-dimensional and M-mode echocardiographic measurements of cardiac dimensions in healthy standardbred trotters. Acta Veterinaria Hungarica 50: 273-282.

Biewener, A.A., S.M. Swartz and J.E. Bertram, 1986. Bone modeling during growth: dynamic strain equilibrium in the chick tibiotarsus. Calcified Tissue International 39, pp. 390-395.

Bomba, T.D., 1994. Theory and Methodology of Training: The key to athletic performance. 3rd Ed. Iowa: Kendall & Hunt Publication Company.

Bosch, F. and R. Klomp, 2005. Running. Biomechanics and Exercise Physiology Applied in Practice. Elsevier Churchill Livingstone Publications, London, pp 228-230.

Brooks, G.A., T.D. Fahey and K.M. Baldwin, 2005. Exercise Physiology: Human Bioenergetics and its Applications Fourth Edition. McGraw Hill Publications

Courouce, A., R. Corde, J.P. Volette, G. Cassiat, D. Hodgson and R. Rose, 2000. Comparison of some responses to exercise on the track and the treadmill. Veterinary Journal 159: 57-63.

Coyle, E., W.H. Martin, D.R. Sinacore, M.J. Joyner, J.M. Hagberg and J.O. Holloszy, 1984. Time course of loss of adaptations after stopping intense endurance training. Journal Applied Physiology 57: 1857-1864.

Duarte, J.A., H.J. Appell, F. Carvalho, M.L. Bastos and J.M. Soares, 1993. Endothelium-derived oxidative stress may contribute to exercise-induced muscle damage. International Journal Sports Medicine 14: 440-443.

Eaton, M.D., D.L. Evans, D.R. Hodgson and R.J. Rose, 1995. Maximal accumulated oxygen deficit in Thoroughbred horses. Journal Applied Physiology 78: 1564-1568.

Evans, D.L., 1994. Fitness tests in the racehorse. In: Proceedings 16th Bain-Fallon Memorial Lecture, pp. 127-141.

Evans, D.L. and R.J. Rose, 1987. Maximum oxygen uptake in racehorses: Changes with training state and prediction from submaximal cardiorespiratory measurements. Equine Exercise Physiology 2. J.R. Gillespie and N.E. Robinson, N.E. (Eds), Davis, California: ICEEP Publications, pp. 52-67.

Evans, D.L., J.E. Rainger, D.R. Hodgson, M.D. Eaton and R.J. Rose, 1995. The effects of intensity and duration of training on blood lactate concentrations during and after exercise. Equine Veterinary Journal Suppl. 18: 422-425.

Fry, A., 1986. The effect of weight training on the heart. NSCA Journal 8: 38-41.

Gauvreau, G.M., H. Staempfli, L.J. McCutcheon, S.S. Young and W.N. McDonell, 1995. Comparison of aerobic capacity between racing Standardbred horses. Journal of Applied Physiology 78: 1447-1451.

Geor, R.J., L.J. McCutcheon and H. Shen, 1999. Muscular and metabolic responses to moderate-intensity short-term training. Equine Veterinary Journal Supplement 30: 311-317.

Green, H.J., S. Jones, M.E. Ball-Burnett, D. Smith, J. Livesey and B.W. Farrance, 1991. Early muscular and metabolic adaptations to prolonged exercise training in humans. Journal of Applied Physiology 70: 2032-2038.

Harkins, J.D., R.E. Beadle and S.G. Kamerling, 1993. The correlation of running ability and physiological variables in Thoroughbred racehorses. Equine Veterinary Journal 25: 53-60.

Hinchcliff, K.W., M.A. Lauderdale, J. Dutson, R.J. Geor, V.A. Lacombe and L.E. Taylor, 2002. High intensity exercise conditioning increases accumulated oxygen deficit in horses. Equine Veterinary Journal 34: 9-16.

Jeffcott, L., 2000. Skeletal maturity in horses-why we should be racing 2 year olds. Equine Fitness The Olympic Way. Proceedings 329 Feb. 21-25, pp 107-117.

Keller, T.S. and D.M. Spengler, 1989. Regulation of bone stress and strain in the immature and mature rat femur. Journal of Biomechanics 22: 1115-1127.

Kriz, N.G., D.R. Hodgson and R.J. Rose, 2000. Changes in cardiac dimensions and indices of cardiac function during deconditioning in horses. American Journal of Veterinary Research 61: 1553-60.

Knight, P.K., A.K. Sinha and R.J. Rose, 1991. Effects of training intensity on maximum oxygen uptake. In: Equine Exercise Physiology 3, edited by S.G.B. Persson, A. Lindholm, and L.B. Jeffcott. ICEEP Publication, Davis CA. pp. 77-82.

Lanyon, L.E., 1990. The physiological basis of training the skeleton. The Sir Frederick Smith Memorial Lecture. Equine Veterinary Journal Supplement 9: 8-13.

Long, K.L., J.D. Bonagura and P.G.G. Darke, 1992. Standardised imaging technique for guided M-mode and Doppler echocardiography in the horse. Equine Veterinary Journal 24: 226-235.

Lord, P.F. and M.A. Croft, 1990. Accuracy of formulae for calculating left ventricular volume of the equine heart. Equine Veterinary Journal Supplement 9: 53-56.

Lucia, C. and G.F. Greppi, 1996. Correlation of racing performance with fitness parameters after exercise tests on treadmill and on track in Standardbred racehorses. Pferdeheilkunde 12: 466-469.

Lund, R.J. and A.J. Guthrie, 1995. Measurement of maximal oxygen consumption of thoroughbred horses at an altitude of 1250m using open-circuit flow-through calorimetry. Journal South African Veterinary Association 66: 239-243.

McArdle, W.D., F.I. Katch and V.L. Katch, 2001. Exercise Physiology Fifth Edition. Energy, Nutrition, and Human performance. Published by Lippincott Williams and Wilkins. Pp. 478-479.

MacDougall, J.D., H. Wenger and H. Green, 1991. Physiological testing of the high-performance athlete. 2nd ed. Illinois: Human Kinetics. 431 pp.

Matsuda, J.J., R.F. Zernicke, A.C. Vailas, V.A. Pedrini, A. Pedrini-Mille and J.A. Maynard, 1986. Structural and mechanical adaptations of immature bone to strenuous exercise. Journal of Applied Physiology 60: 2028-2034.

Menapace, F.J., W.J. Hammer, T.F. Ritzer, K.M. Kessler, H.F. Warner, J.F. Spann and A.A. Bove, 1982. Left ventricular size in competitive weight lifters: An echocardiographic study. Med. Sci. Sports Exerc. 14: 72-75.

Misumi, K., H. Sakamoto and R. Shimizu, R. 1995. Changes in skeletal muscle composition in response to swimming training for young horses. Journal of Veterinary Medical Science 57: 959-961.

Morganroth, J., B.J. Maron, W.L. Henry and S.E. Epstein, 1975. Comparative left ventricular dimensions in trained athletes. Annals of Internal Medicine 82: 521-524.

Moritani, T., 1992. Time course of adaptations during strength and power training. In: P.V. Komi (ed.). Chapter 9B, Blackwell Scientific Publications London, pp. 266-278.

Murakami, T., Y. Shimomura, N. Fujitsuka, N. Nakai, S. Sugiyama, T. Ozawa, M. Sokabe, S. Horai, K. Tokuyama and M. Suzuki, 1994. Enzymatic and genetic adaptations of soleus muscle mitochondria to physical training in rats. American Journal of Physiology 267(3 Pt 1): E388-395.

Nielsen, B., G. Potter, E. Morris, T. Odom, D. Senor, J. Reynolds, W. Smith and M. Martin, 1997. Modifications of the third metacarpal bone in young racing quarter horses as a result of training. Journal Equine Veterinary Science 17: 541-549.

Pilegaard, H., G.A. Ordway, B. Saltin and D. Neufer, 2000. Transcriptional regulation of gene expression in human skeletal muscle during recovery from exercise. Am J Physiol Endocrinal Metab 279: E806-E814.

Reef, V.B., 1995. Heart mumurs in horse: determining their significance with echocardiography. Review. Equine Veterinary Journal Suppl. 19: 71-80.

Rushall, B. and F. Pike, 1990. Training for sport and fitness. Melbourne: The Macmillan Company of Australia.

Seiler, S., 1996. The time course of training adaptations. www.krs.hia.no.

Smith, R.K., H. Birch, J. Patterson-Kane, E.C. Firth, L. Williams, W.W.R. van Cherdchutham and A.E. Goodship, 1999. Should equine athletes commence training during skeletal development? Changes in tendon matrix associated with development, ageing, function and exercise. Equine Veterinary Journal Supplement 30: 201-9.

Stone, M.H., 1988. Implications of connective tissue and bone alterations resulting from resistance exercise training. (Review). Medicine & Science in Sports & Exercise 20 (5 Suppl): S162-168.

Tanaka, H., D.R. Bassett Jr., E.T. Howley, D.L. Thompson, M. Ashraf and F.L. Rawson, 1997. Swimming training lowers the resting blood pressure in individuals with hypertension. Journal of Hypertension 15: 651-657.

Tyler, C.M., L.C. Golland, D.R. Evans, D.R. Hodgson and R.J. Rose, R.J. 1996a. Changes in maximum oxygen uptake during prolonged training, overtraining and detraining in horses. Journal Applied Physiology 81: 2244-2249.

Tyler, C.M., L.C. Golland, D.R. Evans, D.R. Hodgson and R.J. Rose, R.J. 1996b. Changes in fitness during prolonged training in Standardbred horses. Pferdeheilkunde 12: 480-481.

Von Wittke, P., A. Linder, E. Deegen and H. Sommer, 1994. Effects of training on blood lactate-running speed relationship in Thoroughbred racehorses. Journal Applied Physiology 77: 298-302.

Voros, K., 1997. Quantitative two dimensional echocardiography in the horse: review. Acta Veterinaria Hungarica 45: 127-36.

Young, L.E., D.J. Marlin, C. Deaton, H. Brown-Feltner, C.A. Roberts and J.L.N. Wood, 2002. Heart size estimated by echocardiography correlates with maximal oxygen uptake. Equine Exercise Physiology 6. Equine Veterinary Journal Suppl. 34: 467-471.

Werkmann, J., A. Lindner and H.L. Sasse, 1996. Conditioning effects in horses of exercise of 5, 15 or 25 minutes duration at two blood lactate concentrations. Pferdeheilkunde 12: 474-479.

Diagnosis of osteoarthritis and traumatic joint disease

Michael W. Ross
University of Pennsylvania, New Bolton Center, 382 West Street Road, Kennett Square, PA 19348-1692, USA

Clinical characteristics of horses with osteoarthritis and traumatic joint disease

Anamnesis

There are few characteristics that accurately separate anamnesis in horses with osteoarthritis (OA) and traumatic joint disease (TJD) from other lameness conditions such as stress related bone injury of long bones and soft tissue injuries. Horses with chronic OA may warm out of lameness (lameness becomes less apparent with exercise) although in most horses lameness eventually becomes progressive (horses warm into lameness) during the exercise period. Horses with chronic OA may perform better if "raced from a field" (chronic turn out situation in which horses can freely move about in between races) but most horses managed in this manner do not undergo high speed training between races (usually older racehorses) and it is likely better performance is related to this aspect of management rather than constant movement associated with turn out.

Acute, severe lameness is often seen in horses with TJD caused by fractures involving the actual articular surface or subchondral bone. Unless fractures are displaced and there are obvious clinical signs associated with joint involvement (peri-articular swelling in horses with displaced fractures, effusion, lameness noticed at the walk, pointing the limb, and pain on flexion) horses with TJD caused by incomplete fractures may have a history of warming out of lameness within a few days from the time acute, severe lameness is seen. In some horses with dorsal frontal (hindlimbs) or mid-sagittal (usually hindlimb) fracture of the proximal phalanx training and racing may continue for days to weeks, but horses are intermittently prominently lame and eventual diagnosis includes radiographic changes showing marked proliferation of new bone and radiolucenct changes adjacent to the original fracture line, indicating the presence of chronic fracture involving the articular surface and subchondral bone (Figure 1).

A common history in racehorses with early OA and TJD is poor performance and high speed lameness. Often clinical signs referable to the involved joint are subtle or lacking when horses are examined after work particularly in young racehorses with non or mal-adaptive bone remodeling affecting the metatarsophalangeal (MTPJ) and metacarpophalangeal (MCPJ) joints (see below). Lameness after training or racing that resolves quickly is common in horses with stress related bone injury of cancellous (subchondral) and cortical bone.

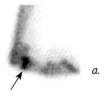 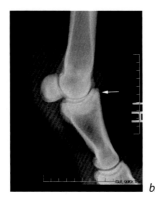 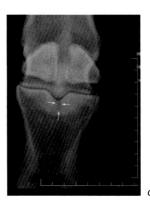

Figure 1. Flexed lateral delayed phase scintigraphic image (a) and lateromedial (b) and dorsoplantar digital radiographic projections of a 3-year-old Standardbred pacer with chronic LH lameness abolished using low plantar analgesia. In this horse intraarticular analgesia did not abolish lameness. Notice a focal area of moderate increased radiopharmaceutical uptake of the proximal phalanx (black arrow, a) and corresponding proliferative changes associated with the dorsal proximal aspect of the proximal phalanx (white arrow, b) indicating fracture was present for several weeks. In the DP projection (c) note radiolucent changes associated with the original short incomplete mid-sagittal fracture (small white arrows).

Lameness examination

Palpation

Clinical signs of OA and TJD can range from obvious to subtle or lacking. It is important to understand that there can be considerable damage to subchondral bone but no or minimal accompanying clinical signs. In older racehorses and in non-racehorse sport horses such as jumpers and dressage horses with chronic OA clinical signs of effusion, reduction in flexion range, joint capsule and surround soft tissue fibrosis and a positive response to joint flexion tests are commonly present. In fact, in these horses false positive palpation findings are possible since many horses perform quite well with chronic OA particularly if OA is bilateral and symmetrical. On the other hand if horses are examined immediately after articular fracture clinical signs lag behind signs of acute lameness, leading to false negative clinical examination findings. After initial first aid is given re-evaluation may reveal effusion and swelling not previously noted just minutes to a few hours before.

There is a distinct difference in clinical signs between horses with chronic OA and those with early OA or TJD in which the disease process involves subchondral (cancellous) bone. Subchondral bone plays a huge role in the development of joint disease, and hence I prefer to use the term OA rather than degenerative joint disease. The term OA implies there is inflammation (deterioration) of bone (osteo) and the joint (arthro). Osteoarthritis describes the overall degenerative process occurring in subchondral bone, overlying articular cartilage and the synovial membrane, and allows for the importance of the subchondral bone to be recognized. This is particularly important in young racehorses in which subchondral bone changes can be substantial. Understanding the role of subchondral bone is crucial in the diagnosis of injury, particularly early diagnosis in young racehorses and helps to explain to clients, trainers, and colleagues, lameness without classic clinical or radiographic changes. For instance, common clinical findings of synovitis (effusion) or radiographic changes such as marginal osteophytes occur late in horses with OA, yet in many of these patients obvious scintigraphic findings and subtle radiographic changes such as sclerosis of subchondral bone or mild radiolucency will be present. It is now well accepted that many of the common articular fractures such as carpal chip fractures and third metacarpal bone (McIII) and third metatarsal bone (MtIII) condylar fractures occur in pathologic bone. Fractures are not single event injuries originating from a "bad step" or "hole in the racetrack" but rather are a terminal event in a pathologic process of bone remodeling. Horses can have TJD from incomplete fractures of the distal condyles of McIII/MtIII, proximal sesamoid bones (PSBs), proximal and distal phalanges (Figure 2), third carpal bone (C3) and third and central tarsal bones without effusion although the skin surface over the involved joint may feel warm (a reliable but non-specific clinical sign). In racehorses the common practice of applying paints and blisters makes interpretation of warmth over joints difficult because in these skin temperature is usually elevated and horses are painful to direct palpation.

Movement

Determination in which limb(s) the horse is lame is critical to accurate detection of OA and TJD particularly in horses with early disease (Ross, 2002). In horses with bilateral forelimb or hindlimb lameness obvious head nod or pelvic hike may be lacking but a short, choppy gait (often unexpected for a good sized well-conformed horse) is

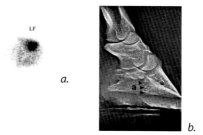

a.

b.

Figure 2. Solar delayed phase scintigraphic image (a) and dorsolateral palmaromedial oblique xeroradiographic view (b) of the LF distal phalanx in a 3-year-old Standardbred filly. Increased radiopharmaceutical uptake (IRU) in the subchondral bone of the distal phalanx was seen 6 months before these images were taken but radiographs were negative. The filly was rested and returned to work only to develop acute pronounced lameness localized by palmar digital analgesia. Intense IRU in subchondral bone of the distal phalanx (a) corresponds to the incomplete fracture (a, arrowheads) seen in the horizontal oblique xeroradiographic projection (2b). (Source: Ross, 2003).

commonly observed. Short, choppy gait is often present in racehorses with early OA from non or mal-adaptive bone remodeling particularly those with involvement of all four fetlock joints. Upper level performance or racehorses often have compensatory lameness making interpretation of findings during movement confusing, since lameness in more than one limb is commonly found. There are no consistent findings during movement useful to differentiate horses with OA and TJD from those with other lameness conditions but careful evaluation of limb flight might be useful in defining from where pain is originating.

Gait deficits in the lame horse: Can you tell from where the pain is originating?

Lameness diagnosticians have passed down much information about equine lameness from generation to generation, most of which has stood the test of time (Ross, 2001). In fact, little about the basic lameness examination has changed in the last century. Once the source of pain has been localized, however, our ability to define and characterize lesions has greatly expanded, mainly because of the recent advances in ancillary imaging modalities. Arthroscopic evaluation of articular injuries and the addition of ultrasonography, scintigraphy, xeroradiography, computed and digital radiology, computed tomography, magnetic resonance imaging, and thermography have enabled us to define a myriad of diagnoses previously unknown. Still, the most important aspect of lameness examination in the horse is the clinical relevance of abnormal findings.

Supporting and swinging limb lameness: Is there a difference?

Supporting limb lameness is a term that has been used to describe a weight-bearing lameness, one that is painful during the actual weight-bearing portion of the stride. Most lameness conditions are of this type. Supporting limb lameness has also been referred to as stance phase lameness. However, the term stance phase is used frequently in descriptions of gait analysis and describes only the phase of the stride during which the limb is actually on the ground. As you will see, most horses with supporting limb lameness alter the stride in such a way as to affect not only the actual stance phase of the stride but also the swing phase.

Swinging limb lameness is a term that is used to describe lameness that primarily affects the way the horses carries or swings the lame limb. If this term were only used to describe mechanical gait deficits it would be appropriate. The problem with this term is that most horses that have painful lameness conditions alter the swing phase of the stride in a typical and repeatable fashion and a clear separation between supporting and swinging limb lameness is difficult to make. Swinging limb lameness should be a term reserved for mechanical defects of gait such as fibrotic myopathy, upward fixation of the patella, stringhalt, or other lameness conditions causing a mechanical restriction of gait. In these horses there is lameness manifested in the swing phase of the stride, but no apparent pain. Unfortunately, the term swinging limb lameness is often used inappropriately to describe the gait deficit in horses that have painful, supporting limb lameness. The most

Management of lameness causes in sport horses

vivid example is a horse with bicipital bursitis or OCD of the scapulohumeral joint. I often hear practitioners describe a horse's gait as swinging limb lameness simply because of a marked shortened cranial phase of the stride.

However, dramatic improvement in the cranial phase of the stride can be achieved by performing diagnostic analgesia, eliminating pain associated with lameness. Thus, the gait deficit is the direct result of pain (and not from gait restriction due to mechanical causes) and no clear differentiation between a supporting and swinging limb lameness can be made. Horses with painful forelimb lameness almost always shorten the cranial phase of the stride, although perhaps not to the extreme as does a horse with authentic scapulohumeral joint lameness or bicipital bursitis. Since the terminology is confusing and often erroneous, I prefer to avoid use of these terms and simply describe lameness as accurately as possible. For instance, saying a horse has 2 out of 5 LF lameness with a marked shortening of the cranial phase of the stride reminiscent of other horses I have seen with shoulder region lameness gives the most accurate and useful information.

Is there a relationship between upper limb lameness and exacerbation of clinical signs when the lame limb is on the outside of the circle?

In conversations I have had with fellow practitioners I have learned there is a tendency for many to equate swinging limb lameness with one that is more evident when the lame limb is on the outside of a circle. Most of the time upper limb lameness is presumed yet not confirmed using diagnostic analgesia. It does make sense that if a horse is reluctant to swing the limb forward, that the lameness may be most prominent when the horse is asked to go in the circle and the lame limb is on the outside. Once again, however, many horses with painful weight-bearing lameness will show more pronounced lameness with the limb on the outside of the circle, a finding that neither suggests the lameness originates from the upper limb nor indicates a swinging limb lameness is present at all. It has been my experience that most lameness conditions can be considered mixed lameness. In other words, there are characteristics that are manifested during actual weight bearing or the stance phase and those seen during the swing phase of the stride. While in some horses it may be clinically useful to differentiate what portion of the stride is being affected by the current lameness problem, without the use of high-speed gait analysis techniques, it may be impossible to know for sure what is indeed abnormal. With the exception of mechanical defects in gait I have not been able to categorise clinical characteristics of most equine lameness conditions into the swinging or supporting limb types. Finally, a shortened cranial phase of the stride is such a common characteristic in horses with both forelimb and hindlimb lameness that it should not be misinterpreted as pathognomonic neither for the location nor type of lameness.

Are there characteristics of gait that can be reliably used to determine the source of pain?

Can you tell the location of pain (where is the horse lame?) by simply watching the horse move? I have often been in awe of legendary lameness diagnosticians who were said to be able to simply look at how a horse moves and tell where it was lame. In general, however,

I have been disappointed in attempts to categorise lameness based on how a horse moves, at least on a clinical basis. In the future, it may be possible to use gait analysis to more carefully define lameness location. In the forelimbs, lame horses typically have a shortened cranial phase of the stride, but usually travel (track) straight during limb advancement. While it is true those horses with severe shoulder region lameness will have a marked shortening of the cranial phase of the stride and may appear to "drag" the limb, those with more mild pain will show no definite characteristics allowing the observer to pinpoint the source of lameness.

Carpal lameness – as good as it gets
Some (but not all) horses with carpal region (most consistently middle carpal) pain (not carpal sheath) have a characteristic way of moving. These horses travel wide, appearing to abduct the limb during limb advancement. On closer examination the limb is actually placed more laterally than expected during the late protraction phase of the stride (the limb does not actually swing unless advanced OA severely restricts carpal flexion). Lameness is often most pronounced with the limb on the outside of a circle and may be less evident with the limb on the inside. Some horses with pain originating more proximally in the limb (humeral stress fractures, elbow joint pain) may also travel similarly. It has been my experience that horses with shoulder region pain tend to guard the limb and actually travel straight or slightly narrow, but not wide.

Hindlimb lameness
In the hindlimb, I believe it is equally difficult to determine the precise source of pain based on gait characteristics. All horses with hindlimb lameness have a shortened cranial phase of the stride at the trot. Some horses with injury of the tuber ischii will have dramatic shortening of the cranial phase, and of course those with fibrotic myopathy have a classic gait deficit associated with the termination of the cranial phase of the stride. However, there is clinical value in observing horses with hindlimb lameness at the walk and comparing the cranial and caudal phases of the stride. For instance, at the walk, horses with pelvic fractures or OA involving the coxofemoral joint or those with severe hoof pain (usually, but not always at the toe) will have a shortened caudal phase of the stride, only to reverse stride characteristics at the trot. Horses with a "stabby" hindlimb gait (leg moves medially and then stabs laterally during advancement) are usually thought to have distal hock joint pain, but in my experience, this gait is typically seen in horses with pain originating anywhere from the distal tibia to the hoof. In racehorses, the most common location of pain with this type of hindlimb gait is the MTPJ. Some, but not all, horses with stifle pain, will swing the limb laterally (abduct) during advancement or place the limb more laterally than expected or simply place the limb straight ahead (rather than "stab"). Other subtle characteristics of horses with stifle lameness include subtle external rotation of the limb during advancement that results in the stifle appearing "prominent" on the affected side. Unfortunately, diagnostic analgesia used in some horses suspected of having stifle lameness localizes the source of pain as the MTPJ. It is not unusual to have concomitant ipsilateral pain in both the stifle and MTPJ regions (intralimb compensatory lameness). Plaiting is an unusual gait abnormality usually seen in horses with bilateral hindlimb lameness. Plaiting is most common in horses with upper limb lameness such

as bilateral pelvic fractures or OA of the coxofemoral joint, but is also seen in those with bilateral severe suspensory desmitis.

More on the effects of circling on the clinical manifestation of pain

Where is the source of pain if lameness is worse with the limb on the inside outside of the circle? It is important to realize that the observation that lameness is worse with the limb on the outside of the circle means neither the horse has "swinging limb lameness" nor that the source of pain is in the upper limb. In the forelimb, the most common sources of pain in horses with lameness worse with the limb on the outside are the foot and the carpus. Horses with proximal suspensory desmitis can also be worse with the limb on the outside of the circle. Horses with forelimb lameness conditions, including those involving the shoulder joint, are worse with the limb on the inside of the circle. Horses with medially located carpal pain may be better with the limb on the inside of the circle. Most horses with hindlimb lameness are worse with the limb on the inside of the circle. Possible exceptions are proximal suspensory desmitis and stifle pain (unusual in my experience, but anecdotal evidence from others).

Stride differences between the walk and trot

Careful observation of differences in stride characteristic between the walk and the trot can help determine the source of pain in horses with hindlimb lameness. Fetlock drop is a characteristic of gait used to determine the lame limb in horses at a trot. In general, horses have greater fetlock excursion, or drop, when weight bearing in the sound limb and less fetlock drop in the lame limb. For example, at a trot a horse lame in the LH will have more pronounced fetlock drop in the RH. Differences in fetlock drop are more difficult to perceive at a walk. In general horses with soft tissue injuries such as suspensory desmitis, gastrocnemius injury, or severe tendonitis may exhibit excessive fetlock drop in the affected limb at the walk; however, when trotted, the same horse will revert to excessive fetlock drop in the unaffected limb (unless the injury is bilateral). This reversal or differential gait manifestation between the walk and trot can be useful to diagnose hindlimb soft tissue injury.

Most horses with hindlimb lameness will shorten the cranial phase of the stride at the trot, a gait characteristic that can be marked in those with severe lameness. At the walk the shortened cranial phase of the stride is less obvious. Horses with severe lameness as the result of pelvic fractures involving the coxofemoral joint (such as acetabular fractures) and those with lameness in the foot (dorsally located pain such as laminitis or hoof abscessation) walk with an exaggerated cranial phase of the stride, only to trot with a marked shortened cranial phase. This disparity in cranial phase of the stride can be a useful observation to locate lameness in one of these 2 areas.

How and when can hindlimb lameness be confused with forelimb lameness?

It is important to understand how a horse with unilateral hindlimb lameness modifies its gait so that hindlimb lameness can mimic forelimb lameness at the trot. When the lame limb hits the ground the horse shifts its weight cranially to transfer load away from the lame limb. This causes the head and neck to shift forward and nod down at the same time. The contralateral forelimb bears weight simultaneously with the lame hindlimb and the head nod coincides, thus mimicing lameness in the forelimb ipsilateral to the lame hindlimb. Head and neck movement in horses with hindlimb lameness is not always observed. In order to see compensatory head and neck movement horses must generally have prominent (≥3 out of 5, see below) hindlimb lameness. At the pace, a lateral gait, LH lameness mimics RF lameness and RH lameness mimics LF lameness.

Horses can have a head and neck nod from singular forelimb lameness, from singular ipsilateral hindlimb lameness, or concurrent forelimb and ipsilateral hindlimb lameness. A prominent head nod is seen in horses with simultaneous LF and LH lameness. The examiner must first determine whether both limbs are affected. Problems arise since a horse with only LF lameness may shorten the LH stride at the trot, leading the examiner to question whether or not LH lameness also exists. Horses with only LH lameness can have a rather pronounced head nod, so the examiner may question the existence of LF lameness. Although a horse with LF lameness may have a compensatory shortened stride of the LH, in the absence of lameness there should not be a marked pelvic hike. A head nod seen consistent with a LF lameness may be inappropriately severe to be caused by mild LH lameness. If a horse has simultaneous LF and LH lameness it is essential to nerve block the hindlimb first, because moderate to severe hindlimb lameness produces head and neck nod that will not be abolished unless the hindlimb lameness is resolved. With resolution of the hindlimb lameness you expect to see resolution of the pelvic hike and reduction in the head nod.

Simultaneous lameness of a diagonal pair of limbs is less common than simultaneous ipsilateral lameness, except in trotters, since many horses perform at gaits that induce compensatory lameness either in the contralateral or ipsilateral limb. With simultaneous LH and RF lameness the head nod reflects the forelimb component, a mandatory clinical sign for perception of RF lameness. The horse may drift away from the LH and have a shortening of the cranial phase of the stride. The horse may have a short, choppy stride, both in the forelimbs and hindlimbs. The horse may have a rocking gait. It cannot shift weight or compensate from stride-to-stride in the usual fashion, so it tends to rock back and forth from the hindlimbs to the forelimbs.

Diagnostic analgesia

Identification of the authentic source of pain requires careful, basic lameness detective work that cannot be replaced by advanced imaging modalities. Remaining now, and in the future, is the most important basic principle in lameness diagnosis – to identify the primary or baseline lameness using diagnostic analgesia. There is no substitute for elimination of a head nod or pelvic hike, or improving the horse's gait or performance, using diagnostic analgesic techniques, and thus, proving in a clinical sense, the actual cause of lameness.

There remain a number of clinical assumptions about lame horses that should be challenged, or at least deserve discussion and thought, since they have been the source of confusion.

The days of thinking that palmar digital analgesia ONLY abolishes pain in the palmar/plantar aspect of the foot are over!

Palmar Digital Analgesia (Ross, 2005)

The most common cause of lameness in all types of racehorse and non-racehorse sport horses involves the foot or digit and can be abolished by palmar digital analgesia (PDA) (Ross and Dyson, 2003). I have long disagreed with the common perception that PDA only abolishes pain associated with the palmar 1/3 of the foot. In my clinical impressions, PDA abolishes pain from a majority of the foot and pastern region and can abolish pain associated with conditions of the fetlock joint such as mid-sagittal fractures of the proximal phalanx, fractures of the PSBs and Mt/McIII condylar fractures (Ross *et al.*, 1992; Ross, 1998). Of 164 racehorses and non-racehorse sport horses in which lameness was abolished using PDA, findings included non-adaptive remodeling/fracture of the distal phalanx (41 racehorses), subchondral trauma/remodeling (20 non-racehorses), combination of navicular disease/subchondral trauma (19 non-racehorses), soft-tissue injuries of the foot (7 horses), OA of the distal interphalangeal joint (7 horses), OA of the proximal interphalangeal joint (6 horses), undiagnosed foot soreness (6 horses), laminitis (4 horses), old wing fractures of the distal phalanx (4 horses), dorsal laminar trauma of the distal phalanx (3 horses), mid-sagittal fractures of the proximal phalanx (2 horses), IRU of the cartilages of the foot and proximal aspect of the distal phalanx (2 horses) and 1 horse each with trauma of the proximal palmar aspect of the middle phalanx, navicular bone fracture and distal phalangeal extensor process fracture (Ross, 1998). Pain was not limited to the palmar aspect of the foot and in fact, conditions involving the dorsal aspect of the foot and pastern were numerous, confirming my clinical suspicion that PDA is a comprehensive block capable of abolishing pain from a majority of the foot, pastern and in some horses fetlock region (Figure 3). Recent studies have confirmed PDA abolishes pain from a majority of the foot including the toe region and that differential blocking of horses with lameness in this region is problematic because of communications between synovial cavities, the close proximity of nerves to synovial structures and potential diffusion of local anesthetic solution (Keegan *et al.*, 1996; Schumacher *et al.*, 2000, 2001; Dyson, 1995; Bowker *et al.*, 1993).

Bone scintigraphy has been invaluable to me in diagnosis of horses with lameness abolished with PDA. In my referral practice horses with abnormalities of bone far outnumber those with soft tissue injuries but in many horses the sources of pain may be multifocal. The early results with MRI suggest there is often more than one lesion

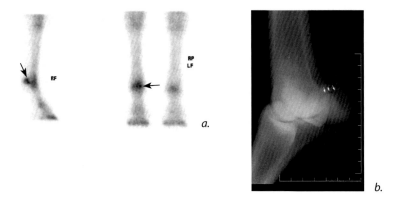

Figure 3. Lateral (left image) and dorsal (right images) delayed phase scintigraphic images (a) and a dorsomedial palmarolateral oblique digital radiographic projection of the fetlock joint (b) of a 4-year-old Standardbred pacer with RF lameness localized to the digit by palmar digital analgesia. Focal mild-to-moderate increased radiopharmaceutical uptake (IRU) can be seen in the RF fetlock region (a, arrows), involving the medial proximal sesamoid bone. A non-displaced apical fracture of the medial PSB (arrows) can be seen (b).

and this modality will undoubtedly be useful in correlating the clinical and other imaging information. I urge practitioners who are pioneering MRI to keep in mind the importance of bone, in particular the subchondral bone of the distal phalanx and navicular bone when developing image sequences to evaluate this complex area and to opine a final diagnosis.

Further information regarding the distal phalanx

Our recent retrospective study of racehorses with fractures of the distal phalanx confirmed the most common distribution of distal phalangeal fractures is the lateral aspect of the LF and the medial aspect of the RF (Rabuffo and Ross, 2002). Medial fractures are most common in the hindlimb (Rabuffo and Ross, 2002). In some racehorses with "sore front feet" I have found mild-to-intense IRU in the central and palmar aspects of the distal phalanx in lateral aspect of the LF and the medial aspect of the RF, the same distribution as found in horses with distal phalangeal fractures (Figure 2; Ross, 1998; Rabuffo and Ross, 2002). Increased radiopharmaceutical uptake of the distal phalanx was seen in horses examined for poor performance or lameness that later developed fractures in the distal phalanx in the same location, a finding that has led us to believe forelimb distal phalangeal fractures are the result of a continuum of stress related bone injury (stress fractures) rather than single-event traumatic injuries (Ross, 1998; Rabuffo and Ross, 2002). The distal phalanx appears prone to the effects of mal or non-adaptive remodeling and in the forelimbs distribution may be determined by the effects of counterclockwise racing. Focal areas of IRU in subchondral bone of the distal phalanx are likely similar to those in the distal aspect of Mt/McIII and may lead to fracture of the distal phalanx or OA of the distal interphalangeal joint (Figure 2).

Horses with OA and TJD may NOT "block out" with intra-articular analgesia

The concept that horses can have articular pain, incomplete fracture, subchondral bone pain or other manifestations of OA and TJD and not "block out" with intra-articular (IA) analgesia is difficult for many practitioners to accept. While this concept is deep-rooted in the equine world it should change. These are my clinical impressions:
- Horses with early OA as a result of non or mal-adaptive bone remodeling of subchondral bone, a common finding in young racehorses, may not block out with IA analgesia, or will have an incomplete response leading practitioners to look elsewhere for a source of pain.
- Horses with advanced OA, those with radiographic evidence of "bone-on-bone", will not block out with IA analgesia. Practitioners may be incredulous with this clinical finding since radiographic changes are advanced but often resort to perineural analgesic techniques or look elsewhere for a source of pain.
- Horses with incomplete fractures that may appear to extend into a joint may have incomplete or no response to IA analgesia only to block out with perineural techniques above the affected joint. Often practitioners look elsewhere for a source of pain unless perineural techniques are used (Figure 1). False negative results can delay accurate diagnosis.
- Incomplete fractures or other forms of TJD may not be visible radiographically on initial examination but obvious radiographic changes develop 2-3 weeks later. This finding in combination with lameness abolished using perineural but not IA analgesic techniques and lack of common clinical signs of articular involvement is common in racehorses.
- IA analgesia is easier to perform (involves a single injection) than are many of the perineural techniques and practitioners are likely to be more familiar and comfortable with landmarks associated with IA injection sites.
- IA analgesia is more specific than is perineural analgesia but likely lacks clinical sensitivity since false negatives occur frequently. IA analgesia rules in articular involvement if lameness is abolished, but does NOT rule out articular involvement if it fails to abolish lameness.

Why does this occur? There are several possible explanations. Subchondral bone pain plays a critical role in horses with OA and TJD. There is poor or incomplete analgesia of subchondral bone when using the IA approach. Additional time is needed to allow diffusion of local anesthetic solution to sensory neural elements involved in innervation of subchondral bone; but, most often a quick response is expected. Worry about diffusion of local anesthetic solution to affect periarticular or nearby structures (IA analgesia of the distal interphalangeal joint and potential confusion with navicular disease or other painful conditions of the foot; IA analgesia of the middle carpal joint and the potential confusion with proximal suspensory desmitis or other conditions of the proximal palmar aspect of McIII) often prompt practitioners to wait only 5-10 minutes to assess response to IA analgesia, leading to false negative results. IA analgesia is effective at abolishing pain associated with synovits/capsulitis but may be ineffective at abolishing pain associated with subchondral bone. Fractures, non or mal-adaptive bone remodeling or other forms of TJD may not initially cause overlying cartilage defects or damage; IA analgesia is ineffective at abolishing pain associated with subchondral defects. From the clinical perspective confusion most often occurs with the MTP and MCP joints.

Subchondral bone pain in the fetlock joint

I have been quite interested in a clinical syndrome involving the MTP and MCP joints. The MTPJ has historically been under-recognized as a source of hindlimb lameness but in my practice was equal in importance to the tarsus and in fact, one of the most important sources of pain in the Standardbred (STB) racehorse (Ross *et al.*, 1992a, b). In the mid-to-late 1980's I recognized a perplexing problem in STBs in which clinical signs consistently including decreased performance and a short-choppy gait or stride in horses with bilateral lameness, mild to moderate lameness in horses with unilateral hindlimb lameness, but effusion of the MTPJ and a positive response to lower limb flexion tests were absent or inconsistent. Historically, horses could be "blocked sound" but not "injected sound" according to trainers and referring veterinarians. Low plantar perineural diagnostic analgesia was most consistent in abolishing pain but in some horses intra-articular analgesia was effective, or partially so. Conventional radiographs and xeroradiographs were negative or equivocal in most horses, but occasionally mild sclerosis of the subchondral bone of the third metatarsal bone (MtIII) was seen. Scintigraphy provided the answer; Focal areas of IRU in the subchondral bone of MtIII were the hallmark of this clinical syndrome (Ross, 1995, 1998, 2003). The most common area of IRU involved the distal, plantarolateral aspect of MtIII and often IRU was bilateral (Figure 4). But, what is it?

Stress remodeling and non or mal-adaptive remodeling

The name "non or mal-adaptive bone remodeling" has been used but remodeling is a difficult concept to explain. The concept that bone changes shape and strength, modeled and remodeled, in response to the magnitude and direction of strain (Wolff's Law) explains many of the changes in bone morphology seen in the sport horse, particularly

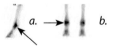

Figure 4. Lateral (a) and plantar (b) delayed phase scintigraphic images of a 4-year-old trotter with mal or non-adaptive bone remodeling of the distal, plantarolateral aspect of the left third metatarsal bone (MtIII). Focal increased radiopharmaceutical uptake (arrows) in the subchondral bone of MtIII is the most common scintigraphic finding in the metatarsophalangeal joint (With permission, Ross MW. The Standardbred. In: Dyson SJ, Pilsworth RC, Twardock AR, Martinelli MJ. Equine Scintigraphy. Newmarket UK: Equine Veterinary Journal 2003;153-189.).

in young racehorses. Repetitive cyclic loading of bone in racehorses causes predictable change in both cortical and cancellous bone, although those of cortical bone are better understood. Stress fractures of cortical (long) bones can lead to catastrophic bone failure and breakdowns. Adaptive changes in bone in response to repetitive cyclic loading include modeling, micro-modeling, and remodeling (Pool, 1994). Modeling is the change in shape of a bone and the most familiar is dramatic change in the dorsal cortex of McIII in Thoroughbreds due to the addition of normal lamellar or abnormal fiber bone in response changes in strain (Pool, 1994; Numamaker, 1994). Micro-modeling occurs in cancellous bone, and is the normal process by which trabecular bone strengthens and changes shape resulting from compressive and tensile forces. This process results in subchondral sclerosis and if accelerated results in deposition of biomechanically inferior woven rather than lamellar bone (Figure 5; Pool, 1994). Bone remodeling is the process by which formed bone in both regions undergoes resorption and replacement by mature lamellar bone. During resorption, bone porosity increases and stiffness decreases. When microdamage or microfracture formation outpaces bone deposition in the remodeling process, both cortical and cancellous bone are subject to fracture. In cortical bone of McIII, high strain cyclic fatigue has been proposed to cause decreased stiffness, which in turn, causes the bone to strengthen (Nunamaker, 1994). Dorsal cortical fracture or stress fracture may develop if high strain cyclic fatigue occurs when the remodeling process of bone resorption is dominant (Nunamaker, 1994).

In the clinical situation, the concept of a continuum of stress related bone change in both cortical and cancellous bone is useful in understanding the pathogenesis of predictable stress related bony injury that ultimately leads to the development of lameness, fractures and OA. This process is sometimes referred to as adaptive bone change in the normal

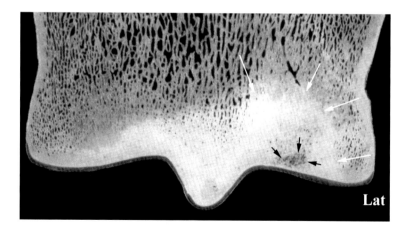

Figure 5. Microradiograph (100 µm) of distal third metatarsal bone in a Standardbred racehorse with non or mal-adaptive remodeling (lateral [Lat] is to the right). Extensive subchondral sclerosis (white arrows), more extensive in the lateral condyle, surrounds an area of resorption (black arrows) or necrotic subchondral bone. Cartilage overlying the lateral condyle appears intact.

portion of the spectrum and non-adaptive when the process becomes pathologic. It is proposed that normal bone undergoes modeling and remodeling as a response to training in order to strengthen and endure cyclic fatigue. Cortical thickening and subchondral sclerosis are normal events, but when the process becomes pathologic, sequential bone changes of stress reaction, stress fracture, and catastrophic fracture sometimes occur. Stress reaction is a term used to indicate abnormal bone remodeling which is scintigraphically, but not radiographically apparent, and is thought to precede stress fracture. Recent studies of the dorsal cortex of McIII, and in other long bones such as the tibia, humerus, and ilium, show stress related bone changes exist before fracture. Microfractures and periosteal callous indicative of stress fracture preceded complete fracture in both the humerus and pelvis (Stover *et al.*, 1992; Johnson *et al.*, 1994). Stress related changes of cortical bone are familiar radiographically, as thickened areas of cortex, linear areas of radiolucency corresponding to new periosteal bone formation, proliferative changes, and oblique fracture lines, representing stress fracture.

Stress related changes of cancellous bone, however, are more difficult to see radiographically, and diagnosis can be challenging. A remodeling scheme of distal McIII and MtIII similar to that seen in cortical bone has been proposed to account for subchondral bone changes, and later overlying cartilage damage and fracture (Ross, 1995, 1998; Stover *et al.*, 1994). The term traumatic osteochondrosis was suggested to account for the remodeling process of distal McIII/MtIII in Thoroughbreds (Pool *et al.*, 1990). This disease has also been termed osteochondritis dissecans (OCD) of McIII, implying the problem is developmental in nature, but this term is misleading since it appears the injury is an acquired stress related lesion (Pool *et al.*, 1990; Hornof *et al.*, 1981). While the distal aspect of McIII/MtIII remains a common region subject to stress related bone changes, the carpal bone, in particular the third carpal bone (C-3), and the distal tarsal bones are also commonly affected (Pool *et al.*, 1990).

In summary, stress related subchondral bone changes are thought to be a normal adaptive response of cancellous bone to training. However, the process often becomes mal or non-adaptive. Ischemia (controversial) of dense subchondral bone, microtrauma or microfractures, mechanical trauma to overlying cartilage caused by dense subchondral bone, and weakened subchondral bone caused by intense resorption predispose to the development of articular fracture (such as chip or condylar fractures) or OA.

Bone scintigraphy is of tremendous value in identifying early stress related changes in bone and in monitoring healing. Focal, mild-to-intense areas of IRU in cortical or subchondral bone indicate active bone remodeling and possible fracture. Predictable sites of stress reaction or stress fracture occur in young racehorses undergoing intense race training. In cortical bone these sites such as McIII, the humerus, tibia and pelvis are well known and accepted. In cancellous bone the common sites include C3, the distal aspect of McIII (medial > lateral) and the distal aspect of MtIII (lateral > medial). In the continuum of events that lead from the normal adaptive response of cortical or cancellous bone to a non or mal-adaptive process (pathologic bone) and subsequent fracture or OA abnormal scintigraphic findings often precede lameness, which in turn precedes radiographic evidence of remodeling changes or fracture. In subchondral bone, scintigraphic evidence of focal areas of IRU can help the clinician identify regions of sclerosis or radiolucency, particularly if special radiographic views are used to evaluate subchondral bone. I find it interesting that lameness is more likely to be abolished using perineural rather than intra-articular analgesia. This finding supports the idea that overlying cartilage damage occurs relatively late in this process and pain is emanating from subchondral bone. This could also explain the lack of clinical signs such as effusion and a positive response to flexion tests and the lack of response to intra-articular medication. Client communication can be difficult in young horses with stress related subchondral bone injury, simply because the classic signs of OA or fracture do not exist either clinically or radiographically. This process may be best understood by clients by referring to quotes such as "…he was making progress faster than his bones were keeping up (Bramlage)" or simply "…he outran his bones (Searcy)[1]."

The fetlock joint: Differences between racehorses and non-racehorses

The above discussion highlighted the common changes of subchondral bone in racehorses, the earliest lesion in the development of OA. Chronic stress related subchondral bone injury is the most common cause of fractures but single event injury may occur. Stress remodeling of distal Mc/MtIII and the PSBs likely predispose to fracture of these bones. Lateral condylar fractures of Mc/MtIII occur most commonly in areas of subchondral sclerosis where modeling/remodeling and microfractures exist before complete fracture. Information regarding the role of existing damage to subchondral bone and subsequent fracture of the PSBs is lacking but likely a similar process to that found in Mc/MtIII exists. We have found the existence of a spectrum of subchondral bone injury in MtIII that likely precedes fracture but similar stress related injury of the proximal phalanx is not recognized (Ross *et al.*, 1992a, b; Ross, 1995, 1998, 2003). Mid-sagittal fracture of the proximal phalanx is likely a single event injury and not the result of stress related subchondral bone injury (Ross, personal observations 1981-2006). Dorsal frontal fracture of the proximal phalanx, however, may occur as the result of a process of stress related bone injury since in both Standardbred and Thoroughbred racehorses scintigraphic evidence of bone modeling is often seen bilaterally even if radiographic evidence of fracture exists unilaterally (Ross, personal observations 1981-2006). Furthermore, at the time of initial diagnosis of dorsal frontal fracture of the proximal phalanx (more common in the right hindlimb) there is often proliferative changes seen radiographically that predate acute onset of lameness (Ross, personal observations 1981-2006).

In racehorses subchondral bone injury far outpaces other classical clinical and radiographic evidence of OA. Horses can have substantial lameness without obvious clinical signs. The development of radiographically apparent marginal osteophytes and enthesophyte formation at capsular attachments appears to develop late in OA at least in the MCP and MTP joints. Subchondral sclerosis and radiolucent defects and overlying cartilage damage can be extensive with minimal radiographic evidence of osteophyte formation.

---

[1] From the Philadelphia Inquirer, March 15, 1997.

In non-racehorses the opposite is found. Classic clinical signs of OA are commonly present and in fact pre-date the onset of lameness in many horses. Chronic joint capsule enlargement, osteophyte formation, synovitis and effusion is often found without evidence of lameness or poor performance. Scintigraphic evidence of subchondral bone involvement is minimal and has a different appearance to that seen in racehorses (see below) but radiographically apparent marginal osteophyte formation and ethesous new bone are commonly seen.

Fracture and other forms of TJD occur uncommonly in non-racehorses. Mid-sagittal fracture of the proximal phalanx and acute, subchondral bone injury (focal areas of IRU seen scintigraphically, similar to that found in racehorses) of distal Mc/MtIII occur.

Imaging

Radiography

Well-positioned and well-exposed radiographic projections are extremely important in the diagnosis of OA and TJD but have the aforementioned limitations. Digital radiographs are useful in the critical evaluation of subchondral bone and in seeing incomplete fractures.

Bone scintigraphy and radiography/radiology

Bone scintigraphy has taught me the importance of detailed radiographic examination, has prompted me to take additional, sometimes designer radiographic views and has sharpened my radiological interpretation. There is nothing like a "hot spot" on a bone scan to allow liberal imagination on interpretation of a radiograph (put on your imaginoscope).

Seeing focal areas of IRU in the distal Mc/MtIII (Figure 4) prompted the acquisition of "down angled" oblique radiographic views in order to adequately evaluate the condyles of Mc/MtIII for sclerotic and radiolucent changes (Figure 6). These views are now routinely taken and have improved our ability to evaluate the palmar/plantar aspect of the MCPJ/MTPJ; but, beware that small osteochondral fragments in the dorsal aspect of these joints can be missed on the down-angle oblique projections. On conventional horizontal oblique views the PSBs obscure the ability to evaluate the distal aspect of Mc/MtIII and in fact, in the hindlimb, there is often overlap of the distal aspect of the PSBs and the proximal aspect of the proximal phalanx. Flexed dorsopalmar/plantar views are useful in the radiographic evaluation of non or mal-adaptive bone injury.

Recognition of focal areas of IRU in subchondral bone of the distal phalanx representing areas of non or mal-adaptive bone remodeling and stress fractures in racehorses and areas of subchondral bone injury associated with OA of the distal interphalangeal joint in non-racehorses prompted us to re-think radiographic evaluation of the foot. Rather than rely only on elevated, down-angled views of the wings of the distal phalanx, in

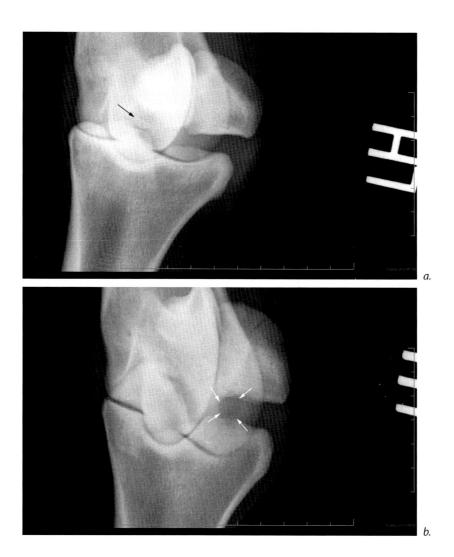

Figure 6. Dorsolateral plantaromedial digital radiographic view of the metatarsophalangeal joint (a) taken with the conventional horizontal radiographic beam and a dorsolateral 25-30° proximal plantaromedial (down-angle) oblique digital radiographic view (b). With a horizontal radiographic beam the lateral proximal sesamoid bone overlaps a lesion involving the distal third metatarsal bone (MtIII) whereas with the down-angled radiographic beam the space between the PSBs and the proximal phalanx is opened-up to allow evaluation of radiolucent and sclerotic changes (b, white arrows) associated with mal or non-adaptive bone remodeling of the distal medial aspect of MtIII. A small osteochondral (OCD) fragment involving the medial plantar process of the proximal phalanx can be seen (a, black arrow).

horses in which lameness is abolished using PDA we now acquire standard oblique views using a horizontally directed radiographic beam with the foot elevated on a block (Figure 2; Dyson, 1995; Rabuffo and Ross, 2002). Horizontal oblique views are advantageous to evaluate subchondral bone of the distal phalanx for the presence of radiolucent defects, to evaluate the distal phalanx for the presence of incomplete fractures, to evaluate the margins of the distal interphalangeal joint for osteophyte formation and to evaluate the dorsal aspect of the distal phalanx for proliferative changes associated with chronic inflammation (dorsal laminar tearing; Ross, 1998).

Modeling of the navicular bone was a common scintigraphic finding in the study of horses with lameness abolished using PDA and confirmed the importance of the palmar proximal palmar distal (skyline, tangential) radiographic view (Ross, 1998). Often, conventional views of the navicular bone will be negative or equivocal but sclerotic and radiolucent changes in the medullary cavity of the navicular bone, blending of the medullary cavity and palmar cortex and palmar cortical changes can only be seen on this radiographic view. This view is now routinely taken in horses in which lameness is abolished using PDA.

The dorsoproximal dorsodistal (skyline, tangential) radiographic view of the distal row of carpal bones is now considered routine in the radiographic evaluation of the carpus. Dorsal, lateral, flexed lateral and flexed dorsal scintigraphic views of the carpus can be used to pinpoint lesions to the radial fossa of C3 and critical review of skyline projections can be done with this information in mind. Careful positioning and exposure of the radial fossa are key in the diagnosis of non or mal-adaptive bone remodeling of C3 in young racehorses and the differentiation of this problem from the more advanced changes associated with incomplete fracture or subchondral lucency of C3.

In horses with early OA of the tarsometatarsal and distal intertarsal joints and in those with frontal slab fractures of the third tarsal bone (T3) scintigraphic examination routinely reveals IRU in the dorsolateral aspect of the distal tarsus (Else et al., 2001). The dorsomedial palmarolateral oblique (DMPLO) view is the most important radiographic view for evaluation of subtle changes associated with early OA and incomplete T3 slab fractures.

Chronic, severe OA

Racehorses can develop severe lameness and end-stage OA without the development of classic radiographic signs of OA (marginal osteophyte and enthesophyte formation). This occurs most commonly in the MCP joint but can also occur in the middle carpal and medial femorotibial joints. In the fetlock joints global narrowing of the joint space between Mc/MtIII and the proximal phalanx seen on the dorsopalmar/plantar projection is a subtle radiographic sign of widespread cartilage damage (Figure 7). More commonly narrowing of the medial joint space causes tilting normal arrangement of the median sagittal ridge of McIII and the sagittal groove of the proximal phalanx and can proceed to ominous findings of "bone-on-bone." Narrowing of the joint space between the PSBs and

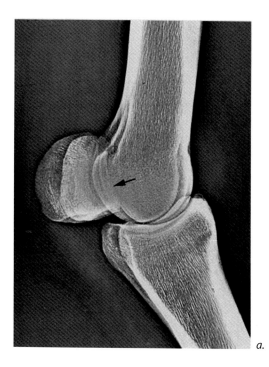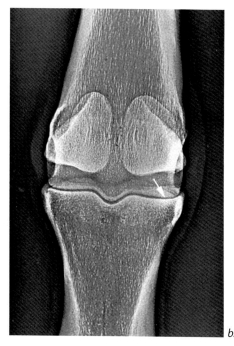

a.

b.

Figure 7. Lateromedial (a) and dorsopalmar (b) xeroradiographic projections of a 6-year-old TB stallion with severe RF. The horse was referred for scintigraphic evaluation because intraarticular analgesia failed to alleviate lameness and obvious radiographic changes associated with osteoarthritis (OA) were not seen. In these views subtle changes of OA can be seen including a reduction in joint space between the palmar condyles of the third metacarpal bone (McIII) and proximal sesamoid bones (a, black arrow) and narrowing of the joint space between McIII and the proximal phalanx (b, white arrow) on the medial aspect of the joint. Obvious signs of OA such as the presence of enthesophytes and marginal osteophytes cannot be seen.

the palmar/plantar aspects of Mc/MtIII occurs but can be difficult to evaluate without a well-positioned lateromedial view (Figure 6).

Ultrasonograpic examination

Ultrasonographic examination of joints can be useful to image soft tissue structures of joints and cartilaginous surfaces (Denoix, 2002). Collateral desmitis (numerous joints), patellar desmitis and meniscal injury in the stifle joint, proliferative synovitis (MCPJ), intersesamoidean ligament injury, articular cartilage defects (sagittal ridge and condyles – MCPJ/MTPJ; medial femoral condyle – subchondral cysts) can be seen. Ultrasonographic evaluation can be useful in establishing diagnosis and prognosis associated with OA and TJD.

More on scintigraphic examination

Bone scintigraphy is invaluable in the diagnosis of OA and TJD. Using scintigraphy diagnosis of subchondral bone injury can be made in racehorses with non or mal-adaptive bone remodeling causing poor performance, in those with lameness localized to a joint but in which radiographic findings are negative or equivocal, in those with fractures not yet visible radiographically, or in those with severe OA but with confusing clinical signs (Figures 1-7). An ominous scintigraphic finding is focal IRU of the palmar/plantar aspect of distal McIII/MtIII indicating the presence of severe cartilage and subchondral bone damage regardless of radiographic findings (Figure 8). Scintigraphy easily provides an answer in horses with negative or equivocal radiographic signs but with clinical signs consistent with incomplete articular fracture. The scintigraphic appearance of chronic OA in non-racehorses is completely different than in racehorses (Figure 9). In the fetlock joint focal areas of mild to moderate IRU in the central and dorsal aspect of the joint are most commonly seen and often correspond to advanced radiographic signs of OA (marginal osteophyte formation) and arthroscopic evidence of extensive cartilage damage most prominent in the distal, dorsal, medial aspect of McIII/MtIII.

While I used the fetlock joint to illustrate the value of scintigraphy in the diagnosis of OA and TJD the modality is equally useful in most other joints. Sensitivity is high but specificity is low, meaning it is difficult to differentiate the conditions of fracture and sclerosis. For example, in C3 a focal area of IRU involving the dorsal medial aspect of the bone could indicate the presence of non or mal-adaptive bone remodeling and sclerosis, an incomplete small (chip) osteochondral fragment, a complete displaced small osteochondral fragment, frontal slab fracture or sagittal slab fracture. Focal IRU on one side of a joint is seen in horses with non or mal-adaptive remodeling or fracture, whereas IRU involving both sides

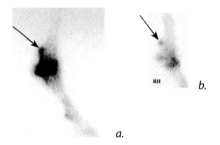

Figure 8. Lateral delayed phase scintigraphic image of the RF fetlock region in the horse depicted in Figure 7 showing intense increased radiopharmaceutical uptake (IRU) of the subchondral bone consistent with severe osteoarthritis (OA). An ominous scintigraphic finding is IRU of the palmar aspect of the distal third metacarpal bone (a, arrow). Increased radiopharmaceutical uptake in this region is only seen in horses with severe OA, such as that seen in the 5-year-old STB trotter with severe RH lameness depicted in Figure 8b. Focal IRU in the plantar pouch is seen as was severe collapse of the medial joint space in the dorsoplantar radiographic view, and yet lameness did not improve after intraarticular analgesia.

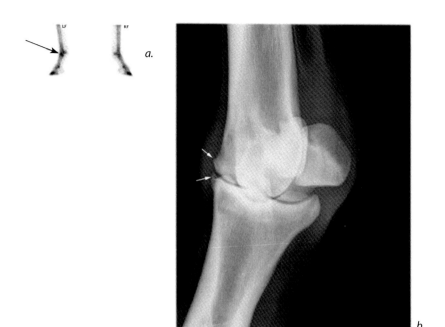

Figure 9. Lateral delayed phase scintigraphic images of the left front (LF) and right front (RF) fetlock region (a) and a dorsolateral palmaromedial oblique digital radiographic view (b) in a 9-year-old TB jumper with mild LF lameness as the result of chronic osteoarthritis (OA) of the metacarpophalangeal joint. Notice mild, focal increased radiopharmaceutical uptake involving the central and dorsal aspects of the fetlock joint (a, arrow), a much different scintigraphic appearance than is seen in racehorses (see Figure 4). Advanced radiographic signs of OA (b, marginal osteophyte formation, arrows) can be seen. In non-racehorses scintigraphic evidence of OA is usually mild and most often involves the central and dorsal aspects of the joint and is usually less impressive than are radiographic findings.

is consistent with advanced OA. Scintigraphy must be used in combination with anamnesis, clinical examination findings and results of other imaging modalities such as radiology and MR imaging to determine the difference between bone bruising (bone contusion, an acute injury) and chronic mal or non-adaptive bone remodeling (chronic injury, a common abnormality). Magnetic resonance imaging will likely become the modality of choice in differentiating these conditions (see below).

Accuracy is improved by using numerous views. For example, in the carpus accurate determination of location of IRU can be made by using a flexed lateral and a flexed dorsal view in combination with routine standing lateral and dorsal views. Numerous views are mandatory to prevent false negative scans. In lateral views medially located lesions are difficult to "see" scintigraphically and additional views are necessary (caudal view to see the medial femorotibial joint, a common location of chronic OA; solar and dorsal/plantar views to see the medial aspect of the distal phalanx, a common location for the development of fractures of this bone).

In general intensity of IRU is inversely proportional to the duration of injury and the presence of radiographic changes. Horses with acute injury are more likely to have intense IRU and equivocal radiographic changes, whereas those with chronic disease are more likely to have less than impressive scintigraphic but impressive radiographic abnormalities. Focal uptake even if it involves 1 or 2 "pixels" may indicate the presence of short, incomplete fractures or well-localized subchondral bone injury as the result of non or mal-adaptive bone remodeling.

Magnetic resonance imaging

In the diagnosis of OA and other TJD in horses MR imaging is in its infancy. Magnetic resonance imaging could be useful to differentiate subchondral bone injury from other forms of TJD caused by soft tissue injuries. Chronic, repetitive subchondral bone injury associated with non or mal-adaptive bone remodeling is the most common form of subchondral bone injury and in a limited number of horses MR images show reduced signal intensity on T1, T2 and STIR sequences in the area of IRU and sclerotic changes seen radiographically. In horses with bone bruising or bone contusion increased signal intensity on STIR images in combination with low signal intensity on T1 images has been seen. Marginal osteophyte formation, synovitis, joint capsule thickening, collateral ligament changes, and periarticular ligamentatous and tendinous changes (such as the suspensory branches and the fetlock joint) have been seen in horses with chronic OA. Cartilage damage (thickness) is difficult to determine because of anatomic details of equine joints (particularly the fetlock joint) and problems associated with positioning of joints with horses under general anesthesia.

Arthroscopic examination

The best way to examine articular surfaces, grade cartilage damage, diagnose hidden osteochondral fragments not seen radiographically or when there are equivocal radiographic findings and to intervene surgically, currently, is using arthroscopic evaluation. While it would be ideal to have a way to evaluate articular cartilage damage using non-invasive techniques this technology is currently unavailable (see MRI above). In young racehorses arthroscopic evaluation is unrewarding in the diagnosis of subchondral bone injury but useful in those horses with occult cartilage damage or osteochondral fragmentation. The palmar/plantar condyles of Mc/MtIII can be difficult to evaluate but cartilage damage is generally worse in the palmar/plantar aspect of the fetlock joint. In non-racehorses cartilage damage is generally most pronounced in the dorsal aspect of the fetlock joint, particularly on the distal, dorsal medial aspect of Mc/MtIII. Arthroscopic evaluation of the medial femorotibial joint in non-racehorses is often quite useful to corroborate clinical, radiographic and ultrasonographic findings and the most common lesion is cartilage damage of the distal medial femoral condyle and fraying of the axial aspect of the medial meniscus. Extensive cartilage damage of the talus is often seen in horses with chronic lameness localized to the tarsocrural joint but in which radiographic findings are not pronounced.

References

Bowker, R.M., S.J. Rockershouser, K.B. Vex, I.M. Sonea, J.P. Caron and R. Kotyk, 1993. Immunocytochemical and dye distribution studies of nerves potentially desensitized by injections into the distal interphalangeal joint or the navicular bursa of horses. J. Am. Vet. Med. Assoc. 203: 1707-1714.

Denoix, J-M., 2002. Ultrasonographic examination of joints. In: M.W. Ross and S.D. Dyson (eds.), Diagnosis and Management of Lameness in the Horse. Philadelphia, Saunders, pp. 189-194.

Dyson, S.J., 1995. Comparison of responses to analgesia of the navicular bursa and intra-articular analgesia of the distal interphalangeal joint in 102 horses. Proceedings. Am. Assoc. Equine Practnr. 41: 234-239.

Elce, Y.A., M.W. Ross, A.M. Woodford and C.M.M. Arensberg, 2001. A review of central and third tarsal bone slab fractures in 57 horses. Proceedings. Am. Assoc. Equine Practnr. 47: 488-490.

Hornof, W.J., T.R. O'Brien, R.R. Pool, 1981. Osteochondritis dissecans of the distal metacarpus of the adult racing thoroughbred horse. Vet. Radiol. 22: 98-105.

Johnson, B., A. Ardans, S.M. Stover, et al., 1994. California racehorse postmortem program: A 4-year overview. In: Proceedings. 40th Ann. Conv. Am. Assoc. Equine Practnr: 167-169.

Keegan, K.G., D.A. Wilson, J.M. Kreeger, M.R. Ellersieck, K.C. Kuo and Z. Li, 1996. Local distribution of mepivacaine after distal interphalangeal joint injection in horses. Am. J. Vet. Res. 57: 422-426.

Nunamaker, D.M., 1994. Bucked shin complex. In: Proceedings 22nd Ann. Surg. Forum, Am. Coll. Vet. Surg. 1994, pp. 157-159.

Pool, R.R., 1994. Cyclic loading: Stress remodeling of cancellous bone in young race horses. In: Proceedings. 22nd Ann. Surg. Forum, Am. Coll. Vet. Surg. 1994, pp. 185-189.

Pool, R.R. and D.M. Meagher, 1990. Pathologic findings and pathogenesis of racetrack injuries. Vet. Clin. N. Amer. [Equine Pract.] 6: 1-30.

Rabuffo, T.S. and M.W. Ross, 2002. Fractures of the distal phalanx in 72 racehorses: 1990-2001. Proceedings Am. Assoc. Equine Practnr. 45: 375-377.

Ross, M.W., 1995. Classification of scintigraphic findings in the metatarsophalangeal joint in Standardbreds - correlation with clinical and radiographic characteristics: 114 horses (1993- 1995). In: Proceedings 41st Ann. Conv. Am. Assoc. Equine Practnr., pp. 88-89.

Ross, M.W., 1998. Observations in horses with lameness abolished by palmar digital analgesia. Proceedings Am. Assoc. Equine Practnr. 41: 230-232.

Ross, M.W., 1998. Scintigraphic and clinical findings in the Standardbred metatarsophalangeal joint: 114 cases (1993-1995). Equine Vet. J. 30: 131-138.

Ross, M.W., 2001. Lameness: Fact or Fiction? In: Proceedings 29th Annual Surgical Forum, 2001, pp. 54-56.

Ross, M.W., 2002. Movement. In: M.W. Ross and S.D. Dyson (eds), Diagnosis and Management of Lameness in the Horse. Philadelphia, Saunders, 2002, pp. 60-73.

Ross, M.W., 2003. The Standardbred. In: S.J. Dyson, R.C. Pilsworth, A.R. Twardock and M.J. Martinelli, Equine Scintigraphy. Newmarket UK: Equine Veterinary Journal, pp. 153-189.

Ross, M.W., 2005. Bone Scintigraphy: Lessons Learned from 5000 Horses. In: Proceedings 51st Ann. Conv. Am. Assoc. Equine Practnr. 2005, pp. 6-20.

Ross, M.W. and S.J. Dyson, 2003. Diagnosis and management of lameness in the horse. Philadelphia, Saunders.

Ross, M.W., Nolan P.M. and J.A. Palmer, 1992. The importance of the metatarsophalangeal joint in Standardbred lameness. In: Proceedings 37th Annu Conv Am Assoc Equine Practnr. pp. 741-756.

Ross, M.W., P.M. Nolan, J.A. Palmer, et al., 1992. The importance of the metatarsophalangeal joint in Standardbred lameness. Vet. Surg. 21: 404.

Schumacher, J., J. Schumacher, F. De Graves, R. Steiger, M. Schramme, R. Smith and M. Coker, 2001. A comparison of the effects of two volumes of local analgesic solution in the distal interphalangeal joint of horses with lameness caused by solar toe or solar heel pain. Equine Vet. J. 33: 265-268.

Schumacher, J., R. Steiger, J. Schumacher, F. Degraves, M. Schramme, R. Smith and M. Coker, 2000. Effects of analgesia of the distal interphalangeal joint or palmar digital nerves on lameness cause by solar pain in horses. Vet. Surg. 29: 54-58.

Stover, S.M., B.J. Johnson, B.M. Daft, D.H. Read, M. Anderson, B.C. Barr, H. Kinde, J. Moore, J. Stoltz and A. Ardans, 1992. An association between complete and incomplete stress fractures of the humerus in racehorses. Equine Vet. J. 24: 260-263.

Stover, S.M., D.H. Read, B.J. Johnson, et al., 1994. Lateral condylar fracture histomorphology in racehorses. In: Proceedings 40th Ann Conv. Am. Assoc Equine Practnr., pp. 173.

Management of osteoarthritis and traumatic joint disease

C. Wayne McIlwraith

Barbara Cox Anthony University Chair, Colorado State University, Ft. Collins, CO, USA

A recent survey suggested that 60% of lameness problems are related to osteoarthritis (OA) (Caron and Genovese, 2003), stressing the importance of advancements of both medical and surgical treatment options. This section reviews medical options currently used for treating joint disease, emphasizing recent and/or future perspectives. The section after this will address the surgical options.

The aim of treatments for acute synovitis, with or without accompanying capsulitis, is to return the joint to normal as quickly as possible. In addition to bringing relief to the patient and allowing it to return to normal work, suppression of synovitis and capsulitis is important in order to prevent the products of inflammation from compromising the articular cartilage and leading to osteoarthritis. In addition to the potential deleterious effects of synovitis on articular cartilage, it is important to provide pain relief and minimize the potential microinstability associated with excessive synovial effusion. It has also been shown experimentally in the rabbit that joint inflammation weakens intra-articular ligaments in addition to affecting the cartilage.

In all traumatic entities in the joint, the goal in addition to returning the joint to normal as quickly as possible is to prevent the occurrence or reduce the severity of osteoarthritis. In other words, there are two goals: 1) reduce pain (lameness), and 2) minimize progression of joint deterioration. While this section addresses medical treatments, it is important to note that timely removal of osteochondral chip fragments, timely and appropriate reduction of fixation of large intra-articular fractures, accurate diagnosis of ligamentous and meniscal injuries with arthroscopy and the appropriate treatment of osteochondritis dissecans entities are all critical treatments to prevent OA. The remainder of this sections deals with treatments where progress, knowledge, or new treatments have been developed in the past 10 years.

Physical therapy and shock wave therapy

Swimming and underwater treadmills are popular rehabilitation tools following arthroscopic surgery for joint injury and also, to a lesser degree, rehabilitation of non-surgical injuries. Underwater treadmills have become increasing available and decrease the weight-bearing while potentially providing a massaging effect on the limbs and preventing fibrosis of the joint capsule. Controlled work with some evidence basis for the relative usefulness of these modalities would be an excellent contribution to our knowledge.

The only non-medical or non-surgical physical therapy tool that has been looked at in a controlled fashion in the horse is that of extracorporeal shock wave therapy (ESWT). An equine specific controlled OA study has been done comparing ESWT to Adequan® and a sham treatment group (Frisbie *et al.*, 2004). The study used our established short-term (70 day) OA model, where an osteochondral fragment is created at time 0 and treatments are initiated 14 days later. ESWT was administered on days 14 and 28 using the VersaTron machine (High Medical Technologies) and a 12 mm probe, and a sham shock wave procedure was performed on the control horses on days 14 and 28 (Frisbie *et al.*, 2004). A positive control group involved IM Adequan® treatment every 4 days for 28 days. The shock wave energy was delivered mainly to the middle carpal joint capsular attachments, but some energy was delivered to the area of fragmentation. Significant improvement in clinical lameness, decreased synovial fluid TP (as a marker of synovitis), and less glycosaminoglycan (GAG) levels in the serum (a biomarker of early osteoarthritic change) was observed with ESWT compared to both control and Adequan® treated horses (Frisbie *et al.*, 2004). These results imply promise for this type of therapy in localized joint disease in horses, but clinical studies with sufficient numbers still need to be reported.

Non-steroidal anti-inflammatory drugs (NSAID's)

The term NSAID's is used to describe anti-inflammatory agents that inhibit some components of the enzyme system that converts arachidonic acid into prostaglandins and thromboxain's. Their use in the horse was well reviewed in 1996 (May and Lees, 1996). All NSAID's inhibit cyclooxygenase activity to some degree (May and Lees, 1996; Vane, 1971), but more recently two different isoenzymes for cyclooxygenase (COX) called COX-1 and COX-2 have been reported and this has potential importance in the horse. COX-1 has been associated with the "good" or "housekeeping" functions of the cyclooxygenase pathway (Frisbie, 2004). It has constitutively produced and has been shown to be important in the balance of normal physiologic function of the gastrointestinal and renal system, while having a lesser role in the inflammatory COX cascade. COX-2 has mainly been associated with inflammatory events, especially those driven by macrophages and synovial cells it is attributed with only minor roles in normal physiology, thus its "bad" or "inducible" role. There have been developments of drugs that preferentially inhibit COX-2 enzyme. While it appears logical that inhibition should minimize side effects, there has been some suggestion that complete inhibition of COX-2 may not be optimal for the joint or the patient (Frisbie, 2004). It is felt at this stage that while COX-1 is mainly responsible for the protective functioning of prostaglandins, COX-2 also plays some accessory role, or is, at least, more important than previously thought. The mainstream still feels that the beneficial effects of selective COX-2 inhibition in joint disease are ideal. Anecdotally we have used carprofen (Rimadyl™) at the Orthopaedic Research Center at CSU in horses that have developed high creatinine levels and diarrhea in association with phenylbutazone use. The disappearance of these side effects when the horse is placed on carprofen implies a protective effect with a drug that has more preferential COX-2 inhibiting activity than phenylbutazone.

A new development has been the licensing of a topical NSAID preparation (1% diclofenac sodium cream). Research in humans had previously indicated that the topical NSAID's application could be clinically beneficial, while reducing systemic side effects. Anti-inflammatory effects were shown in experimentally induced subcutaneous inflammation (Caldwell et al., 2004). A clinical field trial of the topically applied diclofenac liposomal cream for the relief of joint inflammation showed promising results (Bertone et al., 2002). The product is now licensed.

A relatively recent paper also raised the issue of whether NSAID's are deleterious to articular cartilage. The topic is not a new one and in 1993 there was a suggestion that inhibition of the E group of prostaglandins could have long-term unfavorable effects on cartilage metabolism (Dingle, 1993). In vitro work in the horse had initially shown no evidence of deleterious effects on cartilage metabolism (Jolly et al., 1995), but in a more recent paper based on administering phenylbutazone for 14 days to horses and then testing the serum on articular cartilage explants in vitro concluded there was decreased proteoglycan synthesis to a degree similar to that with rhIL-1β (Beluche et al., 2001). Until in vivo deleterious effects have been demonstrated the author feels that in the absence of any clinical associations between the use of phenylbutazone and articular cartilage degeneration, continued appropriate use of NSAID's is justified.

Intra-articular corticosteroids

The use of intra-articular corticosteroids for equine joint disease was extensively reviewed in 1996 (Trotter, 1996a). More recent clarification of the benefits and deleterious side effects of intra-articular corticosteroids in the horse represent a good example of clinical observation leading to scientific inquiry. Based on the authors observation of an apparent lack of correlation between the prior use of betamethasone esters (Betavet Soluspan®) and articular cartilage degradation during arthroscopic surgery for osteochondral chip removal, experimental studies were initiated of the three most commonly used intra-articular corticosteroids, namely methylprednisolone acetate (Depo-Medrol®; Pharmacia and Upjohn Co., Kalamazoo, MI 49001), triamcinolone acetonide (Vetalog®; Bristol Myers Squibb for Fort Dodge, Fort Dodge, IA 50501), and betamethasone esters (Betavet Soluspan®; Schering-Plough Animal Health Corp., Union, NJ 07083). They were evaluated using the osteochondral fragment model (Frisbie et al., 1998; Foland et al., 1994; Frisbie et al., 1997). The first product studied was Betavet Soluspan® (later discontinued but then available as Celestone Soluspan®, and this has since been discontinued). Osteochondral fragments were created arthroscopically on the distal aspect of both middle carpal joint in 12 horses and one joint was treated with 2.5 mls of Betavet Soluspan® at 14 days after surgery and repeated in 35 days. The opposite joint was injected with saline as a control. No deleterious side effects to the articular cartilage were demonstrated and exercise also did not have any harmful effects in the presence of corticosteroid administration (Foland et al., 1994).

The other studies with intra-articular corticosteroids (all studies with this model except betamethasone esters) were modified so that the opposite joint was not used as a control and also the chip fragment model was modified to more effectively produce early osteoarthritic change.

Depo-Medrol® and Vetalog® were tested using three groups (Trotter, 1996a; Frisbie et al, 1997). Eighteen horses were randomly assigned to each of 3 groups (6 horses/group). Both middle carpal joints in the placebo control group (CNT) horses were injected intra-articularly (IA) with polyionic fluid. The corticosteroid control group horses (i.e. MPA CNT or TA CNT) were injected with corticosteroid in the middle carpal joint without an osteochondral fragment and the opposite middle carpal joint was injected with a similar volume of polyionic fluid. The corticosteroid treated group horses (MPA TX or TA TX) were treated with corticosteroid in the joint that contained the osteochondral fragment and the opposite middle carpal joint was injected with a single volume of polyionic fluid. All horses were treated intra-articularly on days 14 and 28 after surgery and exercised on a high-speed treadmill for 6 weeks, starting on day 15.

In joints containing an osteochondral fragment and treated with MPA there was lower, although not significant reduction in the degree of lameness; however there was a significantly lower PGE_2 concentration in the synovial fluid and lower scores for intimal hyperplasia and vascularity (no effect on cellular infiltration in the synovial membrane compared to placebo treated joints). Of more importance, modified Mankin scores (a score of histopathological change in the articular cartilage) were significantly increased in association with MPA, suggesting deleterious effects of intra-articular administration of MPA. This is in contrast to the results with triamcinolone acetonide (TA or Vetalog®). Using the same experimental design, 12 mg of TA was used with each injection. Horses that were treated intra-articularly with TA in a joint containing a fragment (TA TX) were less lame than horses in the CNT and TA CNT groups. Horses treated with TA in either joint had lower protein and higher HA and GAG concentrations in synovial fluid. Synovial membrane from CNT and TA CNT had less inflammatory cell infiltration, intimal hyperplasia and subintimal fibrosis. Analysis of articular cartilage morphologic parameters evaluated using a standardized scoring system were significantly better from TA CNT and TA TX groups irrespective of which joint received TA. The results overall supported favorable effects of TA on degree of clinically detectable lameness and on synovial fluid, synovial membrane, and articular cartilage morphological parameters, both with direct intra-articular administration and remote site administration as compared to placebo injections (Foland et al., 1994). Repetitive intra-articular administration of MPA to exercising horses has been shown to alter the mechanical integrity of articular cartilage (Murray et al., 1998), but had no effect on subchondral or cancellous bone (Murray et al., 2002).

These in vivo studies, coupled with some in vitro work, have fueled the recommendation that the use of triamcinolone acetonide especially in high motion joints is ideal. There have been some options on "low" dose corticosteroid administration alleviating negative effects of MPA. However, based on in vitro titrations studies, it appears that the lower doses that are commonly used are unlikely to have the same effects and a greater concentration of corticosteroid is needed to inhibit the catabolic compared to the anabolic effects in articular cartilage (Dechant *et al.*, 2003). On the other hand, clinical improvement is more important to the clinician than *in vivo* data.

An area of concern is that no form of intra-articular betamethasone esters is available as licensed medication in the US. While compounded product is available, there are concerns on using compounded drugs intra-articularly because of the recent FDA stance on bulk compounding but, more importantly, risk of liability in case of a reaction and a malpractice suit. An unfortunate sequel to this has been a return of some practitioners to more use of Depo-Medrol®. The availability of a generic betamethasone esters preparation would help the situation immensely and human rheumatologists are attempting to do this.

Fear of laminitis has also caused less use of triamcinolone acetonide by some equine practitioners, despite scientific studies demonstrating its effectiveness, as well as its chondroprotective properties. There has been anecdotal associations made and maximum doses established based on a report of no cases of laminitis in 1,200 horses treated when a dose did not exceed 18 mg (Genovese, 1983). A recent publication provides the first follow-up study with data on the potential for triamcinolone acetonide to produce laminitis and the conclusion was that there was no association between the occurrence of laminitis and the intra-articular use of triamcinolone acetonide (McCluskey and Kavenagh, 2004). Another traditional cliché has been that while it is better not to use Depo-Medrol® in high-motion joints, its use in low-motion joints (such as the distal tarsal joints) is appropriate. The implication has been made that we don't care about the state of the articular cartilage in these joints and may be able to promote ankylosis. There is no evidence yet that we can promote ankylosis in this fashion and the other side of this argument is that we should preserve articular cartilage whenever we can.

Intra-articular corticosteroids have commonly been combined with hyaluronan and there has been a perception that it might be protective against the effects of corticosteroid. This perception has been based on tradition rather than scientific proof, but has become common thinking amongst equine practitioners.

Another study suggested that the effect of intra-articular MPA on joint metabolism was different between inflamed and normal joints and also highlighted the potential for introducing *in vitro* culture artifacts (in addition to the effect of inflammation) when investigating the effective intra-articular corticosteroids on chondrocyte function.

Using a model of synovitis based on injection of lipopolysaccharide into carpal joints it was demonstrated that acute synovitis prevented changes produced by intra-articular MPA alone (Todhunter *et al.*, 1998). It also needs to be pointed out, however, that in other studies with synovitis based on chip fragmentation, MPA was shown to be deleterious.

Hyaluronan (sodium hyaluronate)

Hyaluronan is non-sulfated glycosaminoglycan and the biological characteristics and therapeutic use of hyaluronan in an equine osteoarthritis have been reviewed previously

(McIlwraith *et al.*, 2001; Howard and McIlwraith, 1996). Hyaluronan has modest analgesic effects (Gotoh *et al.*, 1993), but more emphasis has been placed on its anti-inflammatory effects that may be physical (steric hindrance) or pharmacological (inhibition of inflammatory cells and mediators) (Howard and McIlwraith, 1996). Various *in vivo* and *in vitro* studies have shown protection against IL-1, driven prostaglandin synthesis, as well as inhibition of free radicals, but the ability of hyaluronan to inhibit the activity of MMPs is questionable (Lynch *et al.*, 1998; Clegg *et al.*, 1998). It has also been pointed out that, because several inflammatory mediators can augment the production of HA by synovial fibroblasts *in vitro*, elevated synthesis of HA in early osteoarthritis may constitute a protective response by the synovium to joint inflammation (Howard and McIlwraith, 1996). While providing a rationale for exogenous administration, it may explain the elevated levels of HA in response to intra-articular injection of a number of medications (Frisbie *et al.*, 1998; Foland *et al.*, 1994).

It has been the authors clinical impression that HA alone is useful for mild to moderate synovitis, but for the treatment of most clinical cases, adjunctive use of a corticosteroid is necessary. It has also been claimed that HA preparations of molecular weight exceeding 1×10^6 daltons may provide superior clinical and chondroprotective events, but this is a controversial claim (Aviad and Houpt, 1994; Smith and Gosh, 1987).

A randomized, double-blind, and placebo controlled clinical study in 77 Standardbred trotters with moderate to severe lameness has been reported. Horses were randomized for treatment with HA, polysulfated glycosaminoglycan (PSGAG) or placebo for 3 weeks. The mean and initial lameness score was significantly reduced during treatment and at the last examination in all three groups ($p<0.01$) (Gaustad and Larsen, 1995). Additionally, the prevalence of sound horses increased significantly from 1-3 weeks of treatment into the last examination in all three groups. Comparison of the two treatment groups with regard to the development of the lameness curve and time until soundness indicated a small, non-significant difference in favor of HA. No significant difference was detected between the two treatment groups in the prevalence or accumulative incidences of soundness. The study detected a superior effect on the two drugs (250 mg of PSGAG intra-articularly 4 times of 20 mg of HA intra-articularly twice) compared to placebo for reduction of lameness score during the treatment period and the total study period, time until soundness, and the prevalence of sound horses at the last examination. All three treatments were effective in the treatment of clinical traumatic arthritis in horses, but HA and PSGAG gave better results than placebo. In a second paper, the same group compared intra-articular saline with rest alone in 38 Standardbreds with traumatic arthritis. The mean lameness was significantly lower when 2.0 mls of 0.9% NaCl solution was injected. This raises the question: is this effect due to withdrawing fluid and/or placing a needle in the joint (Gaustad *et al.*, 1999)?

The use of intravenous (IV) HA in the treatment of joint disease is now common. An experimental study documented a significant improvement in clinical lameness, decreased PGE_2 and total protein levels in the synovial fluid, and decreased synovial membrane hyperemia and cellular infiltration (Kawcak *et al.*, 1997).

In a recent survey of questionnaires sent to 20 members of AAEP (14 responses) it was uncommon for the respondents to administer IA HA initially or alone, particularly in horses with established osteoarthritis. Twelve of 14 supplemented HA injections with other forms of treatment (usually IA corticosteroids). Most clinicians reported being unimpressed by the efficacy of IV HA, particularly when used alone. They considered effects on osteoarthritic signs to be not dramatic and duration to be short (Caron and Genovese, 2003).

The prophylactic use of IV HA has been studied in both Quarter Horse and Thoroughbred racehorses. One hundred forty horses were entered in the Quarter Horse study and received either IV saline or HA every 2 weeks for the duration of the 9 month study (McIlwraith *et al.*, 1998). Trends for HA treated horses to race longer, require an intra-articular injection of corticosteroid earlier, have a better speed index, higher average number of starts, and more money earned were observed when compared to placebo treated horses. A similar study has been conducted in Thoroughbred racehorses using synovial fluid markers and starting with horses without musculoskeletal problems. No significant differences were found, but anecdotal reports from trainers and various equine disciplines have been positive regarding the prophylactic use of IV HA.

Polysulfated glycosaminoglycan

Polysulfated glycosaminoglycan (PSGAG) belongs to a group of polysulfated polysaccharides and includes, in addition to PSGAG (Adequan®, Luitpold Pharmaceuticals Inc, Animal Health Division, Shirley, NY 11967), pentosan polysulfate, as well as glycosaminoglycan peptide complex (Rumalon®). These drugs have been referred to as chondroprotective, or a more recent definition, slow-acting disease modifying osteoarthritic drugs (SAMOD). Because of this PSGAG has been traditionally used where cartilage damage is considered to be present rather than in the treatment of acute synovitis (Trotter, 1996b). Therapy with such drugs is either meant to prevent, retard, or reverse the morphologic cartilaginous lesions of osteoarthritis with the major criteria for inclusion being prevention of cartilage degeneration. The principal GAG present in PSGAG is chondroitin sulfate and the product is made from an extract of bovine lung and trachea modified by sulfate esterification.

Adequan® was reviewed extensively in 1996 (Trotter, 1996b). At that time there had been a number of *in vitro* studies, including one demonstrating that PSGAG was the only drug tested (others included phenylbutazone, flunixon, betamethasone, and hyaluronan) that inhibited stromelysin (Sokoloff, 1979). There had been three other *in vitro* studies on the effect of PSGAG on equine cartilage that were somewhat contradictory. Initially it was reported that PSGAG caused increased collagen and glycosaminoglycan synthesis in both articular cartilage explants and cell cultures from normal and osteoarthritic equine articular cartilage (Glade, 1990). However, other work had found a dose dependent inhibition to proteoglycan synthesis, little effect on proteoglycan degradation, and no effect on proteoglycan monomer size (Caron *et al.*, 1991). Various *in vivo* studies have supported the value of intra-articular (250 mg) PSGAG in equine joint disease;

including a clinical study (Tew, 1982), a study using a Freund's adjuvant-induced model (a study in dogs) (Altman *et al.*, 1989) and another equine carpal model using sodium monoiodoacetate ((Yovich *et al.*, 1993). In the latter study, there was significant reduction of articular cartilage fibrillation erosion, less chondrocyte death, and markedly improved Safranin O staining. At the same time, PSGAG had no benefit in healing articular cartilage lesions that were already present.

A second study using intramuscular PSGAG (500 mg every 4 days for 7 treatments) showed relatively insignificant effects with treatment (limited to slightly improved Safranin O staining in sodium monoiodoacetate joints when PSGAG was used) (Trotter *et al.*, 1989). In a more recent unpublished experimental study where IM PSGAG was used as a positive control (administered every 4th day for 28 days starting 14 days post OA induction), there was some improvement in clinical lameness 56 days after initiation of treatment and decreased GAG levels in the serum 14 days post-treatment (GAG is a marker of disease in this OA model) (Frisbie *et al.*, 2004). However, there was more impressive improvement in the third test group (shock wave group therapy; discussed previously) (Frisbie *et al.*, 2004).

Although a survey to assess the perceived efficacy of PSGAG in 1996 reported that PSGAG was considered more effective than HA for the treatment of sub-acute degenerative joint disease and less effective for idiopathic joint effusion and acute synovitis (Caron, 1996) and the author has used IM PSGAG routinely post-surgically it now appears that there is very weak evidence for clear cut efficacy with IM administration. It has been reported that articular cartilage concentrations of PSGAG after IM administration are capable of inhibiting some cartilage degrading enzymes (Burba *et al.*, 1993), but the duration of effective concentration is unclear. A number of degradative enzymes known to be present in articular tissue has been shown to be reduced with *in vitro* and *in vivo* studies in other animal models (Howell *et al.*, 1986), but direct evidence of effectiveness in the horse is lacking.

A principal driving force of the persistent use of IM PSGAG in preference for intra-articular PSGAG has been the work demonstrating a slightly increased risk of infection (compared to corticosteroids and HA) (Gustafson *et al.*, 1989a). Apparently receiving less notice is a companion paper reporting all risks could be obviated with concurrent IA administration of 125 mg (0.5 ml) of amikacin sulfate (Gustafson *et al.*, 1989b). The author still feels that post-operative IA PSGAG when there is significant exposure of subchondral bone (loss of articular cartilage) is a successful treatment. The main clinical observation is reduction of hemarthrosis, synovial effusion, and improvement in viscosity. There is some insinuation from experimental work that the endogenous repair of cartilaginous lesions can be reduced with PSGAG (Todhunter *et al.*, 1993). This is a potential (but yet to be demonstrated clinically significant) caveat.

Pentosan polysulfate

The use of this drug in the treatment of joint disease was reviewed in 1996 (Little and Gosh, 1996). PPS could also be considered as a disease modifying osteoarthritic drug (DMOAD) and it was pointed out in the review article that PPS unlike NSAID's do not possess analgesic activity (Little and Gosh, 1996). The conclusion was that in order to provide symptomatic relief and efficacy, a drug such as PPS must be capable of correcting the pathobiological imbalances that are present within the OA joint and the authors at that time felt that PPS fulfilled these requirements. However, at this stage the only reports of its use in the horse were anecdotal.

PPS is a heparinoid compound but is unique in that it is derived from beechwood hemicellulose instead of animal sources. Commercial products available include Cartrophen Vet® (licensed in small animals in Australasia, but not in horses) and more recently Pentosan Equine Injection® (pentosan polysulfate sodium 250 mg/ml) which is licensed in Australasia. In studies in sheep, weekly intra-articular injections of PPS for 4 weeks improved joint function and reduced mean radiographic scores and Mankin histologic scores of articular cartilage damage in the femoral condyle (Gosh *et al.*, 1993).

Recent work from our laboratory has demonstrated favorable results. Using the osteochondral fragment-treadmill model of equine OA in the carpus, there was significant decrease in articular cartilage fibrillation and a strong trend for overall cartilage histologic appearance (modified Mankin Score). Furthermore, most other parameters showed numerical improvements (including lameness, joint flexion, synovial fluid TP, synovial fluid collagen degradation products, and aggrecan synthesis) although statistical significance less than 0.05 were not obtained. In this study PPS was given at a dose of 3 mg/kg body weight once weekly for 4 weeks (Platinum Performance®, Platinum Performance Inc., PO Box 990, Buellton, CA 93427). This is the current recommendation for treating horses with mild or early stage OA, particularly with multiple joint involvements (being a systemic drug). On the other hand, based on the previously cited study, there has been some discussion of potentially increasing the dose frequency to 3 mg/kg once every 5 days, for a total of 7 injections.

Oral joint supplements

It is important to recognize that none of the oral supplements or oral nutraceuticals is licensed and proof of efficacy is generally lacking. Most products include glucosamine and/or chondroitin sulfate along with other added ingredients. Historically the oral glycosaminoglycan products initially available for the horse included a chondroitin sulfate product from bovine trachea (Flex-Free®) and a complex of glycosaminoglycans and other nutrients from the sea mussel, *Perna canaliculus* (Syno-Flex®). More recently a combination of glucosamine hydrochloride, chondroitin sulfate, manganese, and Vitamin C has been marketed as a nutraceutical (Cosequin®) and a number of other products have simulated Cosequin®. Since that time, other products have attempted to compete on the basis of decreased cost (with no demonstration of comparable efficacy) or other added ingredients. With regard to the commonly used practice of combinations of using glucosamine and/or chondroitin sulfate, glucosamine sulfate is a precursor of the disaccharide subunits of cartilage proteoglycans. While glucosamine salts have been reported as well absorbed after oral absorption in man (Setnikar *et al.*, 1993), one study has reported an oral bioavailability of glucosamine hydrochloride in horses to be 2.5%, with a large volume of distribution, which the authors interpreted as poor absorption from the intestinal tract but extensive tissue uptake (Adebowale *et al.*, 2003). A second study in dogs concluded that glucosamine is absorbed orally, albeit low (12%), and it is most likely due to extensive first pass metabolism in the gastrointestinal tract and/or liver prior to systemic availability (Adebowale *et al.*, 2002).

More recent work on the quantification of glucosamine in serum and synovial fluid after nasogastric or intravenous administration of glucosamine hydrochloride to horses questions effective absorption of glucosamine hydrochloride in the horse (Laverty *et al.*, 2005). Eight adult female horses with no evidence of joint disease were randomly assigned to two different groups (n=4) for a cross over study. Glucosamine hydrochloride (20 mg/kg) was administered by nasogastric intubation or IV injection and blood samples were collected. Glucosamine was assayed by fluorescence assisted carbohydrate electrophoresis (FACE) with glucosamine achieving a maximum concentration of 288 ± 53 μM following IV dose and 5.8 ± 1.7 μM following nasogastric dose. Synovial fluid reached a peak concentration at 250 μM post-IV dosing and 0.3-0.7 μM post-nasogastric dosing. It was concluded that the levels of glucosamine obtained in synovial fluid following nasogastric administration with clinically recommended doses are lower than those that have been studied *in vitro* to elucidate glucosamine action on joint cells.

Chondroitin sulfate consists of alternating disaccharide subunits of glucuronic acid and sulfated N-acetylgalactosamine molecules and is a principal glycosaminoglycan of aggregating proteoglycan (aggrecan). Chondroitin sulfate is less sulfated, but resembles PSGAG in structure and mechanism of action. Oral absorption of a chondroitin sulfate has been tested in horses. A low molecular weight chondroitin sulfate (0.80 kDa) has been evaluated by quantifying the disaccharide content using a validated method that combined enzymatic digestion of plasma followed by fluorescence HPLC (Du *et al.*, 2004). Low molecular weight chondroitin sulfate was absorbed to a higher extent compared with glucosamine and it was also demonstrated that its absorption may be influenced by the molecular weight of the polymer (Du *et al.*, 2004).

In vitro studies can potentially help determine at what concentrations glucosamine or chondroitin sulfate may inhibit the catabolic response in equine cartilage explants. One study done with cartilage discs incubated with lipopolysaccharide in the varying concentrations of glucosamine, chondroitin sulfate, or both revealed that glucosamine concentrations as low as 1 mg/ml decreased NO production relative to LPS stimulated cartilage, but that chondroitin sulfate at either 0.25 or 0.50 mg/ml did not inhibit NO production. Glucosamine concentrations as low as 0.5 mg/ml decreased PGE_2 production, where as CS did not affect PGE_2. The combination decreased MMP-9 activity, but has no effect on MMP-2 and there was a trend for decreasing MMP-13 protein concentrations (Fenton *et al.*, 2000).

In vitro dose titration studies of glucosamine hydrochloride (GU) and chondroitin sulfate (CS) alone and in combination have recently been reported based from work in our laboratory. There were no detrimental effects of GU, GS, or GU plus GS on normal cartilage metabolism. Higher doses of GU, CS and GU plus CS appeared to limit total GAG release into the media, where as intermediate doses enhanced GU, CS, and GU plus CS enhanced GAG synthesis and total cartilage content (Dechant *et al.*, 2005).

The same dosages tested on IL-1 conditioned articular cartilage explants revealed no treatment effects for GU or CS alone, but a protective effect of high dosages of GU plus CS for total GAG release into the media. The study suggested that GU plus CS might be beneficial to cartilage metabolism by preventing GAG degradation. However the question of effective concentration of GU after oral administration is still an issue (Laverty *et al.*, 2005) and clear *in vivo* demonstration of reduction and degradation would be ideal information.

Other oral joint supplements used include Platinum Performance® (Platinum Performance Inc., PO Box 990, Buellton, CA 93427), which is a combination of rare earth minerals and omega-3 fatty acids (making it somewhat unique). Omega 3 fatty acids have been shown to inhibit aggrecanase (Curtis *et al.*, 2000). This has been used post-operatively but all information is anecdotal. Similarly, oral HA products are new to the market and a recent controlled study in our laboratory did not demonstrate effectiveness in our equine OA model (Frisbie DD, McIlwraith CW, Kawcak CE, *et al.* Unpublished data 2004). Recently another experimental study using the CSU equine OA model has demonstrated value for an oral supplement containing soy and avocado. This is the first well controlled scientific study demonstrating a positive effect with an oral nutraceutical.

Summary

Conventional medications still form a large part of the equine veterinarians' armamentarium. Increased attention is being paid to physical therapy regimens and positive results demonstrated with shock wave therapy can perhaps decrease the use of medication for equine joint disease. COX-2 inhibitors are going to be useful to the veterinarian when the patient is not tolerating phenylbutazone well. Intraarticular corticosteroids continue to be the principal intra-articular therapy. The use of methylprednisolone acetate has decreased appropriately and the value of betamethasone esters and triamcinolone acetonide recognized. Continued availability of licensed medication is a challenge. Intra-articular HA continues to be used in conjunction with corticosteroids. Recent research challenges the degree of value gained from intramuscular Adequan, but all scientific research has been very positive with intra-articular use of the drug. It is predicted that pentosan polysulfate will become a licensed medication and its value has been documented scientifically. Oral nutraceuticals continue to be somewhat of a "black box" as far as efficacy is concerned, but positive results in a controlled study with the product of Vétoquinol is exciting.

New biologic therapies

The knowledge gained from improved understanding of critical mediators in equine traumatic arthritis and OA has lead to the identification of new targets for therapy. Two obvious targets identified include metalloproteinases (MMPs) and IL-1.

Inhibition of metalloproteinases as a therapeutic approach

Metalloproteinase inhibitors include peptide-based inhibitors (including hydroxamic acids), non-peptidal inhibitors (this includes chemically modified tetracycline's such as doxycycline), and naturally occurring inhibitors (such as N-3 fatty acids, *i.e.* fish oils). Recent work has demonstrated that N-3 fatty acids, as found in fish oils, will inhibit MMPs and aggrecanase (which as discussed before, is a key enzyme in the degradation of aggrecan) (Curtis *et al.*, 2000).

In vitro in our laboratory with the MMP inhibitor Bay-12-9566 using equine and canine articular cartilage explants in an IL-1 degradation model and using the COL2-3/4C$_{short}$ immunoassay showed that there were significant dose dependent reductions in the catabolic effect of IL-1α on the release of proteoglycans and type II collagen from articular cartilage explants exposed to 10 fold increases in concentrations (1nM:10 μM) (Billinghurst *et al.*, 1999). No *in vivo* work has been done in the horse; however, an *in vivo* study in experimental OA in the dog, failed to demonstrate efficacy with an MMP inhibitor (Trumble, 2003) and the prospect for these being a valuable biological therapy for horses seems low.

Novel methods of administering therapeutic proteins (including Gene Therapy)

The functional unit of DNA is the gene which can be defined as the set of DNA sequences that are required to produce a single polypeptide (protein). The gene sequence codes for a specific messenger RNA (mRNA) molecule that, in turn, carries the genetic information from the nucleus to the cytoplasm for translation into amino acid sequence (*i.e.* a protein). While many recognized diseases relate to a lack of or a defect in or an imbalance of a particular protein (S) and since the gene is the basal unit ultimately responsible for protein production, it is also a logical therapeutic target (Frisbie and McIlwraith, 2001). At the moment most gene therapy protocols (at least the ones we have evaluated) are directed towards increasing levels of selected therapeutic proteins in an attempt to alter specific disease dysfunction. Depending on the natural function of the protein we might be able to enhance or repress certain direct effects on specific cellular processes.

The key component is the efficient transfer and expression of therapeutic genes (and the example used in our laboratory is IL-1ra) by inserting the manipulated gene sequence into a vector. One such example is interleukin-1 receptor antagonist (IL-1ra), which we have used in our laboratory. Previous work when the protein was isolated and administered to laboratory animals with induced OA showed that it inhibited the progression of OA.

After the gene sequence of the equine IL-1ra molecule was deduced in our laboratory (Howard *et al.*, 1998), the value of gene therapy with IL-lra using an adenoviral vector in the treatment of equine OA was investigated (Frisbie and McIlwraith, 2001; Frisbie *et al.*, 2002).

Proof of principal experiments demonstrating *in vitro* expression of an active equine IL-1ra protein following gene transfer of the equine IL-1ra gene sequence to cultured equine synoviocytes using an adenoviral vector were first performed (Frisbie and McIlwraith, 2001, 2000). Following confirmation that the adenoviral vector could infect equine synoviocytes and produce a biologically active IL-1ra protein, an *in vivo* dose titration study was done. Using the same adenoviral vector carrying the equine IL-1ra gene (AdeqIL-1ra) the optimal vector concentration to provide peak concentrations and duration of IL-1ra protein expression without significant side effects was determined. Next, using our established experimental model of equine OA this gene therapy treatment was tested and shown to significantly reduce lameness and synovial effusion in the arthritic/fragmented joints. The horses receiving gene therapy also had significantly less pathologic change noted on gross examination of the joints compared to placebo treated arthritic/fragmented joints and microscopically there was also significant improvement in the articular cartilage compared to the controls.

Since that time gene therapy, again with IL-1ra but combined with IGF-1, has been tested for its capability of improving cartilage healing and a gene therapy protocol using BMP-2 shown to aid healing in the presence of osteomyelitis in rabbits (Southwood *et al.*, 2004).

Diagnostic and surgical arthroscopy – Progress in the last 15 years

The arthroscope began by 1975 to achieve real clinical use in human orthopedics and diagnostic arthroscopy of equine carpal joints in three horses was reported in 1975 (Hall and Keeran, 1975). The acquisition of an arthroscope and development of expertise in it started with the author seeing it as a possible way to monitor the development of synovitis in an experimental study. It is another example of the inter-relationship between science and clinical applications, as while initial work in experimental equine arthritis led to an initial exploration of arthroscopy, experience with the limitations of what could be achieved with arthroscopy surgery (McIlwraith, 1990a; McIlwraith and Brmlage, 1996) has fed back into attempts to developing novel treatment techniques, as well as recognizing the need for early diagnosis and prevention of injury.

The application of arthroscopic techniques to the horse has revolutionized the treatment of traumatic joint injuries. The first detailed paper on diagnostic arthroscopy in the horse was published in 1978 (McIlwraith and Fessler, 1978), and it is important to recognize that arthroscopic surgery is the diagnostic method of choice to evaluate articular cartilage and remains the gold standard to assessing pathologic joints. As in human orthopedics, use of the arthroscope in horses extended into surgical practice as technology and techniques of triangulation developed. These techniques were first detailed in textbook form in 1984 (McIlwraith, 1984). Diagnostic arthroscopy is especially valuable when response to medical treatment of a joint is suboptimal. In many instances articular cartilage lesions are most extensive than what is insinuated on radiographs, but these lesions can sometimes be better related to physical examination and the extent of clinical signs.

By 1990, arthroscopy in the horse had gone from being a diagnostic technique used by a few veterinarians to the accepted way of performing joint surgery (McIlwraith, 1990a). Prospective and retrospective data substantiated the value of the technique in the treatment of carpal chip fractures (McIlwraith et al., 1987), fragmentation of the dorsal margin of the proximal phalanx (Yovich and McIlwraith, 1986), carpal slab fractures (Richardson, 1986), osteochondritis dissecans (OCD) of the femoropatellar joint (Martin and McIlwraith, 1985; McIlwraith and Martin, 1985), OCD of the shoulder (Bertone et al., 1987), and subchondral cystic lesions of the femur (Lewis, 1987) (The results with tarsocrural OCD were published by McIlwraith et al., 1991). During this period, the use of diagnostic arthroscopy led to the recognition of previously undescribed articular lesions, many of which are treated using arthroscopic techniques.

Since 1990 there has been further sophistication of techniques: new ones have been developed and treatment principals have been changed based on new pathobiologic knowledge and further prospective and retrospective studies defining the success of various procedures. Many of these advances have been recorded in a recent publication (McIlwraith, 2002a). For example, there has been further documentation of success rates following arthroscopic removal of fragments from the dorsoproximal margin of the proximal phalanx (Norrdin et al., 1998; Kawcak et al., 2001). Advances and understanding of the pathogenesis of osteochondral disease and fragmentation in the carpus and fetlock have been reported (Kawcak and McIlwraith, 1994; Colon et al, 2000), which naturally led to progression and diagnosis and treatment. Parameters for the surgical treatment of joint injury have been carefully defined (McIlwraith and Bramlage, 1996). Arthroscopic treatment of fractures in the previously considered inaccessible palmar aspect of the carpus have been described (Wilke et al., 2001), together with arthroscopy of the palmar aspect of the distal interphalangeal joint (Brommer et al., 2001; Vacek et al., 1992). Arthroscopy has also led to understanding of the contribution of soft tissue lesions to joint disease. In the carpus, tearing of the medial palmar intercarpal ligament (MPICL) was first reported in 1992 (McIlwraith, 1992) and its implications discussed by Phillips and Wright (1994) and Whitton et al. (1997a, b, c).

In the fetlock joints success rates following arthroscopic removal of osteochondral fragments of the palmar/plantar aspect of the proximal phalanx have now been documented (Foerner et al., 1987; Fortier et al., 1995). Results for arthroscopic treatment of osteochondritis dissecans for the distal/dorsal aspect of the third metacarpal/metatarsal bones (McIlwraith and Vorhees, 1990) and results of arthroscopic surgery to treat apical, abaxial, and basilar fragments of the sesamoid bones have also been reported (Southwood and McIlwraith, 2000; Southwood et al., 1998).

The results of arthroscopic surgery for the treatment of OCD in the tarsocrural joint have been documented (McIlwraith et al., 1991), and the arthroscopic approach and intra-articular anatomy of the plantar pouch of this joint have also been described (Zamos *et al.*, 1994).

Considerable advances have been made in arthroscopic surgery of the stifle joint. Results of arthroscopic surgery for the treatment of OCD of the femoropatellar joint were reported in 1992 (Foland *et al.*, 1992), and the syndrome of fragmentation of the distal apex of the patellar recognized and its treatment reported in the same year (McIlwraith, 1990b). The use of arthroscopic surgery for treating certain patellar fractures was discussed in 1990 and reported in the refereed literature in 2000 (Marble and Sullins, 2000).

In the femorotibial joints the use of arthroscopic surgery to treat subchondral cystic lesions of the medial condyle of the femur (Howard *et al.*, 1995) and proximal tibia (Textor *et al.*, 2001) have been reported. Research has led to alternative methods of treating subchondral cystic lesions. After an initial demonstration that subchondral cystic lesions could develop on the medial condyle after 3 mm deep, 5 mm wide penetration of the subchondral bone plate (Ray *et al.*, 1996), examination of the fibrous tissue of subchondral cystic lesions in horses demonstrated that it produced local mediators and neutral metalloproteinases and causes bone resorption *in vitro* (Von Rechenberg *et al.*, 2000a). Production of nitric oxide (NO), PGE2 and MMPs in media of explant cultures of equine synovial membrane and articular cartilage has also been demonstrated in normal and osteoarthritic joints (Von Rechenberg *et al.*, 2000b). Injection of corticosteroids into the lining membrane of subchondral cysts has therefore been carried into the clinical arena.

Cartilage lesions of the medial femoral condyle have been described (Schneider *et al.*, 1997). Arthroscopy has allowed great advances in the recognition and treatment of meniscal tears and cruciate injuries (Walmsley, 1995, 2002; Walmsley *et al.*, 2003). Successful treatment of grade I and grade II meniscal tears has been achieved and documented as well as lack of success recognized with lesions that are not completely accessible. Arthroscopy has also been used to remove fragments from the intercondylar eminence of the tibia (Mueller *et al.*, 1994), and internal fixation of one case has been reported (Walmsley, 1997). Techniques have also been developed for diagnostic and surgical arthroscopy of the caudal pouches of the femorotibial joints (Stick *et al.*, 1992; Hance *et al.*, 1993; Trumble *et al.*, 1994).

Diagnostic and surgical arthroscopy of the coxofemoral joint has been described, lesions identified and some surgical treatments performed (Honnas *et al.*, 1993; Nixon, 1994). The use of the arthroscope is no longer confined to the limbs and the arthroscopic anatomy of the temporomandibular joint has been described recently (Weller *et al.*, 2002).

The use of arthroscopy in assisting repair with internal fixation of articular fractures has become routine. This includes fractures of the metacarpal/metatarsal condyles and carpal slab fractures (Richardson, 2002; Bassage and Richardson, 1998; Zekas *et al.*, 1999). These techniques can be used in both non-displaced and displaced fractures. Techniques have been described for evaluation and treatment of problems in smaller joints such as the distal and proximal interphalangeal joints (Boening, 2002; Boening *et al.*, 1990; Vail and McIlwraith, 1992; Schneider *et al.*, 1994). In addition joints in which lameness is less commonly encountered, such as the elbow, have been examined and treated arthroscopically.

The use of the arthroscope for the evaluation and treatment of tendon sheath problems have been another area of major advance. The arthroscope has been used to assess and treat tenosynovitis of the digital flexor sheath, and techniques for endoscopically assisted annular ligament release have been described (Nixon, 1990, 2002a; Nixon *et al.* 1993; Fortier *et al.*, 1999). Intrathecal longitudinal tears of the digital flexor tendon have also been described and treated arthroscopically (Wright and McMahon, 1999; Wilderjans *et al.*, 2003). The arthroscope has been used increasingly for carpal sheath conditions (McIlwraith, 2002b; Nixon *et al.*, 2003). Removal of radial osteochondroma's and physeal remnants using arthroscopic visualization has produced excellent results (McIlwraith, 2002b; Nixon *et al.*, 2003), and superior check ligament desmotomy (Southwood *et al.*, 1999; Nixon, 2002; Kretz, 2001) is now done arthroscopically, as well as release of the carpal canal (Textor *et al.*, 2003). Techniques for tenoscopy of the tarsal sheath have been described. Arthroscopy of the synovial bursae has also been reported with the principal conditions being the treatment of contamination and infection.

The general advantages of arthroscopic surgery include:
1. An individual joint can be examined accurately through a small (stab) incision and with greater accuracy then was previously possible. The availability of such an atraumatic technique allows numerous lesions and "new' conditions that are not detected radiographically to be recognized.
2. All types of surgical manipulations can be performed through stab incisions under arthroscopic visualization. The use of this form of surgery is less traumatic, less painful, and provides immense cosmetic and functional advantages.
3. Surgical intervention is now possible in situations where it would not have been attempted previously. The decreased convalescence time, with earlier return to work and improved performance is a significant advantage in the management of equine joint problems. The need for palliative therapies has decreased, as has the number of permanently compromised joints.

It is to be recognized that, although the technique appears uncomplicated and attractive to the inexperienced surgeon, some natural dexterity, good 3-dimensional anatomical knowledge, and considerable practice are required for the technique to be performed optimally. Experience and good case selection are of paramount importance. The statement made in 1987 by a prominent human orthopedic surgeon is worth remembering: "*of those 9,000 North American surgeons and the other surgeons of the world performing arthroscopy, many are ill-prepared and are therefore, not treating their patient fairly. Overuse and abuse by a few is hurting the many surgeons that are contributing to orthopedic surgery by lowering patient's morbidity, decreasing the cost of healthcare, shortening the necessary time of patient's returning to gainful employment, and adding to the development of a skill that has made profound change in the surgical care of the musculoskeletal system*" (Nixon, 2002).

Back to positive connotations, arthroscopy remains the most sensitive and diagnostic modality for intra-synovial evaluation in the horse. This is somewhat different to human orthopedics where arthroscopy predominately is used for surgical interference and much of its diagnostic function has or is being replaced by magnetic resonance imaging (MRI). Arthroscopy has continued to be of great benefit in the horse, with increased recognition of soft tissue lesions in joints, tendons, sheaths, and bursa. However, as stated above, while there are many benefits gained from arthroscopy it is technically demanding and the need for training remains.

Last, but not least, with the development and successful treatment of many conditions with arthroscopy, the limitations that are left by articular cartilage degradation and erosion has been recognized. In fact, the recognition of the limitations of arthroscopy because of residual osteoarthritis and lack of articular cartilage is another example of clinical observation leading us back to scientific research.

References

Adebowale, A.O., D.S. Cox, I. Linang *et al.*, 2003. Analysis of glucosamine and chondroitin sulfate content in marketed products and CACO-2 permeability of chondroitin sulfate raw materials. J Am Nutraceuticals Assoc 3: 37-44.

Adebowale, A.O., J. Du, I. Liang *et al.*, 2002. The bioavailability and pharmacokinetics of glucosamine hydrochloride and low molecular weight chondroitin sulfate after single and multiple doses to beagle dogs. Bio Pharm Drug Dispos 23: 217-225

Altman, R.D., D.D. Dean, O. Muniz *et al.*, 1989. Prophylactic treatment of canine osteoarthritis with glycosaminoglycan polysulfuric acid ester (abstr). Arth Rheum 32: 759-766.

Aviad, A.D. and J.B. Houpt, 1994. The molecular weight of therapeutic hyaluronan (sodium hyaluronate): How significant is it? J. Rheumatol 21: 297-239.

Bassage, L.H. II and D.W. Richardson, 1998. Longitudinal fractures of the condyles of the third metacarpal and metatarsal bones in racehorses: 224 cases (1986-1995). J Am Vet Med Assoc 212: 1757-1764.

Beluche, L.A., A.L. Bertone, D.E. Anderson and C. Rohde, 2001. Effects of oral administration of phenylbutazone to horses on *in vitro* articular cartilage metabolism. Am. J. Vet. Res. 62: 1916-1921.

Bertone, A.L., C.W. McIlwraith, B.E. Powers, G.W. Trotter and T.S. Stashak, 1987. Arthroscopic surgery for the treatment of osteochondrosis in the equine shoulder joint. Vet Surg 16: 303-311.

Bertone, J.J., R.C. Lynn, N.J. Vatistas *et al.*, 2002. Clinical field trial to evaluate the efficacy of topically applied diclopenac liposomal cream for the relief of joint lameness in horses. In: Proceedings, 48th Annual Convention of AAEP, pp. 190-193.

Billinghurst, R.C., K. O'Brien, A.R. Poole and C.W. McIlwraith, 1999. Inhibition of articular cartilage degradation in culture by a nonpeptidic matrix metalloproteinase inhibitor. Ann NY Acad Sci 878: 594-597.

Boening, K.J., 2002. Arthroscopic surgery of the distal and proximal interphalangeal joints. Clin Equine Pract 1: 218-225.

Boening, K.J., F.C. Saldern, I. Leendertse and F. Rahlenbeck, 1990. Diagnostic and surgical arthroscopy of equine coffin joints. Proc Am Assoc Equine Pract 36: 331-317.

Brommer, H., A.M. Rijkenhuizen, H.A.M. van den Belt *et al.*, 2001. Arthroscopic removal of an osteochondral fragment at the palmaroproximal aspect of the distal interphalangeal joint. Equine Vet Educ 13: 294--297.

Burba, D.J., M.A. Collier, L.E. Default *et al.*, 1993. *In vivo* kinetic study on uptake and distribution of intramuscular titanium-labeled polysulfated glycosaminoglycan in equine body fluid compartments and articular cartilage in an osteochondral defect model. J Equine Vet Sci 13: 696.

Caldwell, F.J., P.O. Mueller, R.C. Lynn *et al.*, 2004. Effect of topical application of diclopenac liposomal suspension on experimental induced subcutaneous inflammation in horses. Am. J. Vet. Res. 65: 271-276.

Caron, J.P. and R.L. Genovese, 2003. Principal and practices of joint disease treatment. In: M.W. Ross and S.J. Dyson (eds.), Diagnostics and Management of Lameness in the Horse. 1st edition, Philadelphia, Elsevier Science, pp. 746-763.

Caron, J.P., J.B. Kaneene and R. Miller, 1996. Results of a survey of equine practitioners on the use and efficacy of polysulfated glycosaminoglycan. Am J Vet Res 209: 1564-1568.

Caron, J.P., S.W. Eberhart and R. Nachreiner, 1991. Influence of polysulfated glycosaminoglycan on equine articular cartilage in explant culture. Am J Vet Res 52: 1622-1625.

Clegg, P.D., M.D. Jones and S.D. Carter, 1998. The effect of drugs commonly used in the treatment of equine articular disorders on the activity of equine matrix metalloproteinases-2 and 9. J Vet Pharmacol Ther. 21: 406-413.

Colon, J.L., L.R. Bramlage, S.R. Hance and R.M. Embertson, 2000. Qualitative and quantitative documentation of the racing performance of Thoroughbred racehorses after arthroscopic removal of dorsoproximal first phalanx osteochondral fractures (1986-1995). Equine Vet J 32: 475-481.

Curtis, C.L., C.E. Hughes, C.R. Flannery *et al.*, 2000. n-3 fatty acids specifically modulate catabolic factors involved in articular cartilage degradation. J Biol Chem 275: 721-724.

Dechant, J.E., G.M. Baxter, D.D. Frisbie *et al.*, 2003. Effects of dosage titration of methylprednisolone acetate and triamcinilone acetonide on interleukin-1-conditioned equine articular cartilage explants *in vitro*. Equine Vet J. 35: 444-450.

Dechant, J.E., G.M. Baxter, D.D. Frisbie *et al.*, 2005. Effects of glucosamine hydrochloride and chondroitin sulfate, alone an in combination, on normal and interleukin-1 conditioned equine articular cartilage explant metabolism. Equine Vet J 37:227-231.

Dingle, J.T., 1993. Prostaglandins in human cartilage metabolism. J Lipid Mediat. 6: 303-312.

Du, J., I. Liang, A.O. Adebowale *et al.*, 2004. The bioavailability and pharmockinetics of glucosamine hydrochloride and chondroitin sulfate after oral, intravenous single dose administration in the horse. Bio Pharm Drug Dispos 25: 109-116.

Fenton, J.I., K.A. Chlebek-Brown, T.L. Peters *et al.*, 2000. Glucosamine HCl reduces equine articular degeneration in explant cultures. Osteo Cart 6: 258-265.

Foerner, J.J., W.P. Barclay, T.N. Phillips *et al.*, 1987. Osteochondral fragments of the palmar/plantar aspect of the fetlock joint. Proc Am Assoc Equine Pract 33: 739-744.

Foland, J.W., C.W. McIlwraith and G.W. Trotter, 1992. Arthroscopic surgery for osteochondritis dissecans of the femoropatellar joint of the horse. Equine Vet J 24: 419-423.

Foland, J.W., C.W. McIlwraith, G.W. Trotter *et al.*, 1994. Effect of betamethasone and exercise on equine carpal joints with osteochondral fragments. Vet. Surg. 23: 369-376.

Fortier, L.A., J.J. Foerner and A.J. Nixon, 1995. Arthroscopic removal of axial osteochondral fragments of the plantar/palmar proximal aspect of the proximal phalanx in horses: 119 cases(1988-1992)..J Am Vet Med Assoc 206: 71-74.

Fortier, L.A., A.J. Nixon, N.G. Ducharme *et al.*, 1999. Tenoscopic examination and proximal annular ligament desmotomy for treatment of equine 'complex' digital sheath tenosynovitis. Vet Surg 28: 429-435.

Frisbie, D.D., 2004. Current and future treatments of equine joint disease. In: Proceedings AAEP 2004, Focus on joints.

Frisbie, D.D. and C.W. McIlwraith, 2000. Evaluation of gene therapy as a treatment for equine traumatic arthritis and osteoarthritis. Clin Orthop 3795: S273-87.

Frisbie, D.D. and C.W. McIlwraith, 2001. Gene therapy: Future therapies in osteoarthritis. In, AAEP Proceedings 47: 211-216.

Frisbie, D.D., S.C. Ghivizzani, P.D Robbins et al., 2002 Treatment of experimental equine osteoarthritis by an in vivo delivery of the equine-1 receptor antagonist gene. Gene Therapy 9: 12-20.

Frisbie, D.D., C.E. Kawcak, G.M. Baxter et al., 1998. Effects of 6α-methylprednisolone acetate on an in vivo equine osteochondral fragment exercise model. Am. J. Vet. Res. 59: 1619-1628.

Frisbie, D.D., C.E. Kawcak and C.W. McIlwraith, 2004. Evaluation of extracorporeal Shock Wave Therapy for osteoarthritis. In: Proceedings 50th Annual Meeting of the Am Assoc. Equine Practitioners, pp. 261-263.

Frisbie, D.D., C.E. Kawcak, G.W. Trotter et al., 1997. Effects of triamcinolone acetonide on an in vivo osteochondral fragment exercise model. Equine Vet. J. 29: 349-359.

Gaustad, G. and S. Larsen, 1995. Comparison of polysulfated glycosaminoglycan in sodium hyaluronate with placebo in treatment of traumatic arthritis in horses. Equine Vet. J. 27: 356-362.

Gaustad, G., N.I. Dolvik and S. Larsen, 1999. Comparison of intra-articular injection of 2 mls of 0.9% NaCl solution with rest alone for treatment of horses with traumatic arthritis. Am. J. Vet. Res. 60: 1117-1121.

Genovese. R.L., 1983. The use of corticosteroids in racetrack practice. In: Proceedings Symposium Effective Use of Corticosteroids in Veterinary Practice, pp. 56-65.

Ghosh, P.M., S. Armstrong, R. Read et al., 1993. Animal models of early osteoarthritis: Their use for the evaluation of potential chondroprotective agents. In: W.B. VandenBerg, P.M. van der Kraan and P.L.E.M. van Lent (eds.), Joint destruction in arthritis and osteoarthritis. Austin, TX: Birkhauser, pp. 195-206.

Glade, M.J., 1990. Polysulfated glycosaminoglycan accelerates net synthesis of collagen and glycosaminoglycans by arthritic equine cartilage tissues and chondrocytes. Am J Vet Res 51: 779-785.

Gotoh, S, J. Onya, M. Abe, K. Miyazaki, A. Hamai, K. Horic and K. Tokuyasu, 1993. Effects of the molecular weight of hyaluronic acid and its action mechanisms on experimental joint pain in rats. Ann. Rheum. Dis. 52: 817-822.

Gustafson, D.B., C.W. McIlwraith and R.L. Jones, 1989b. Further investigations into the potentiation of infection by intra-articular injection of polysulfated glycosaminoglycan and the effect of filtration and intra-articular injection of Amikacin. Am J Vet Res 50: 2018-2022.

Gustafson, S.B., C.W. McIlwraith and R.L. Jones, 1989a. Comparison of the effect of polysulfated glycosaminoglycan, corticosteroids, and sodium hyaluronate in the potentiation of a subinfective dose of Staphylococcus aureus in the middle carpal joint of horses. Am J Vet Res 50: 2014-2017.

Hall, M.E. and R.J. Keeran, 1975. Use of the Arthroscope in the Horse. Vet Med Small Animal Clin 70: 705-706.

Hance, R., R.K. Schneider, R.M. Embertson et al., 1993. Lesions of the caudal aspect of the femoral condyles in foals: 20 cases (1980-1990). J Am Vet Med Assoc 202: 637-646.

Honnas, C.M., D.T. Zamos and T.S. Ford, 1993. Arthroscopy of the coxofemoral joint of foals. Vet Surg 22: 115-121.

Howard, R.D. and C.W. McIlwraith, 1996. Hyaluronan and its use in the treatment of equine joint disease. In: C.W. McIlwraith and G.W. Trotter (eds.), Joint Disease in the Horse, Philadelphia WB Saunders.

Howard, R.D., C.W. McIlwraith and G.W. Trotter, 1995. Arthroscopic surgery for subchondral cystic lesions of the medial femoral condyle in horses: 41 cases (1988-1991) J Am Vet Med Assoc 206: 846-850.

Howard, R.D., C.W. McIlwraith, G.W. Trotter and J.F. Nyborg, 1998. Cloning of equine interleukin-1 alpha and equine interleukin-1 receptor antagonist and determination of their full length cDNA sequence. Am J Vet Res 57: 704-711.

Howell, D.S., M.R. Carreno, J.P. Palletta et al., 1986. Articular cartilage breakdown in a lapine model of osteoarthritis: Action of glycosaminoglycan polysulfate ester (GAGPS) on proteoglycan enzyme activity, hexuronate, and cell count. Clin Orthop 213: 69-76.

Jolly, W.T., T. Whittem, A.C. Jolly and E.C. Firth, 1995. The dose-related effects of phenylbutazone and methylprednisolone acetate formulation (Depo-Medrol®) on cultured explants of equine carpal articular cartilage. J. Vet. Pharmaco.l Therap. 18: 429-437.

Kawcak, C.E. and C.W. McIlwraith, 1994. Proximodorsal first phalanx osteochondral chip fragments in 320 horses. Equine Vet J 26: 392-396.

Kawcak, C.E., D.D. Frisbie, C.W. McIlwraith et al., 1997. Effects of intravenous administration of sodium hyaluronate on carpal jonts in exercising horses after arthroscopic surgery and osteochondral fragmentation. Am. J. Vet. Res. 58: 1132-1140.

Kawcak, C.E., C.W. McIlwraith, R.W. Norrdin, R.D. Park and S.D. James, 2001. The role of subchondral bone in joint disease: A review. Equine Vet J 33: 120-126.

Kretz, M.R., 2001. Clinical evaluation of 49 tenoscopically assisted superior check ligament desmotomies in 27 horses. Proc Am Assoc Equine Pract 47: 484-487.

Laverty, S., J.D. Sandy, T. Celeste, P. Vachon et al., 2005. Synovial fluid levels and serum pharmacokinetics in a large animal model following treatment withoral glucosaminoglycan at clinically relevant doses. Arthritis Rheum 52: 181-191.

Lewis, R.B., 1987. Treatment of subchondral bone cysts of the medial condyle of the femur using arthroscopic surgery. Proc Am Assoc Equine Pract 33: 887-893.

Little, C. and P. Ghosh, 1996. Potential use of pentosan polysulfate for the treatment of equine joint disease. I. In: C.W. McIlwraith and G.W. Trotter (eds.), Joint Disease in the Horse, Philadelphia WB Saunders, pp. 281-292.

Lynch, T.M., J.P. Caron, S.P. Annoczky et al., 1998 Influence of exogenous hyaluronan on synthesis of hyaluronan and collagenase by equine synoviocytes. Am J Vet Res 59: 888-892.

Marble, G.P. and K.E. Sullins, 2000. Arthroscopic removal of patellar fracture fragments in horses: 5 cases (1989-1998). J Am Vet Med Assoc 216: 1799-1801.

Martin, G.S. and C.W. McIlwraith, 1985. Arthroscopic anatomy of the equine femoropatellar joint and approaches for treatment of osteochondritis dissecans. Vet Surg 14: 99-104.

May, S.A. and P. Lees, 1996. Nonsteroidal anti-inflammatory drugs. In: C.W. McIlwraith and G.W. Trotter (eds.), Joint Disease in the Horse. Philadelphia, WB Saunders, pp. 223-237.

McCluskey, M.J. and P.D. Kavenagh, 2004. Clincial use of triamcinolone acetonide in the horses (205 cases) and the incidence of glucocorticoid-induced laminitis associated with its use. Equine Vet Educ 2004: 108-115.

McIlwraith, C.W., 1984. Diagnostic and surgical arthroscopy in the horse. Lenexa, Veterinary Medicine Publishing Co.

McIlwraith, C.W., 1990a. Diagnostic and surgical arthroscopy in the horse. 2nd edition. Philadelphia, Lea & Febiger.

McIlwraith, C.W., 1990b. Osteochondral fragmentation or the distal aspect or the patella in horses. Equine Vet J 22: 157-163.

McIlwraith, C.W., 1992. Tearing of the medial palmar intercarpal ligament in the equine mid-carpal joint. Equine Vet J 24: 367-371.

McIlwraith, C.W. (ed), 2002a. Arthroscopy - An Update. Clinical Techniques in Equine Practice, Vol. 1, No.4, W.B. Saunders December: pp. 199-281.

McIlwraith, C.W., 2002b. Osteochondromas and physeal remnant spikes in the carpal canal. Proc. 12th Ann Vet Symp (ACVS), pp. 168-169.

McIlwraith, C.W. and L.R. Bramlage, 1996. Surgical treatment of joint injuries. In, McIlwraith CW, Trotter GW, ed: Joint Disease in the Horse. Philadelphia, 1996, WB Saunders.

McIlwraith, C.W. and J.F. Fessler, 1978. Arthroscopy in the diagnosis of equine joint disease. J Am Vet Med Assoc 172: 263-268.

McIlwraith, C.W. and G.S. Martin, 1985. Arthroscopic surgery for the treatment of osteochondritis dissecans in the equine femoropatellar joint. Vet Surg 14: 105-116.

McIlwraith, C.W. and S.M. Vorhees, 1990. Management of osteochondritis dissecans of the dorsal aspect of the distal metacarpus and metatarsus. Proceedings 36th Annual Meeting Am Assoc Equine Pract 36: 547-550.

McIlwraith, C.W., J.F. Foerner and D.M. Davis, 1991. Osteochondritis dissecans of the tarsocrural joint; results of treatment with arthroscopic surgery. Equine Vet J 23: 155-162.

McIlwraith, C.W., D.D. Frisbie and C.E. Kawcak, 2001. Current treatments for traumatic synovitis, capsulitis, and osteoarthritis. In: Proceedings 47th Annual Meeting AAEP pp. 180-206.

McIlwraith, C.W., N.L. Goodman and D.D. Frisbie, 1998. Prospective study on the prophylactic value of intravenous hyaluronan in 2-year old racing Quarter horses. In: Proceedings 44th Annual Convention of the AAEP. pp. 269-271.

McIlwraith, C.W., J.V. Yovich and G.S. Martin, 1987. Arthroscopic surgery for the treatment of osteochondral chip fractures in the equine carpus. J Am Vet Med Assoc 191: 531.540.

Mueller, P.O.E., D. Allen, E. Watson et al., 1994. Arthroscopic removal of a fragment from an intercondylar eminence fracture of the tibia in 2-year-old horse..J Am Vet Med Assoc 204: 1793-1795.

Murray, R.C., N. Znaor, K.E. Tanner et al., 2002. The effect of intra-articular methylprednisolone acetate and energy on equine carpal subchondral and cancellous bone microhardness. Equine Vet J 34: 306-310.

Murray, R.C., R.M. DeBowes, E.M. Gaughn et al., 1998. The effects of intra-articular methylprednisolone and exercise on the mechanical properties of articular cartilage in the horse. Osteo Cart 6: 106-114.

Nixon, A.J., 1990. Endoscopy of the digital flexor tendon sheath in horses. Vet Surg 19: 266-271.

Nixon, A.J., 1994. Diagnostic and operative arthroscopy or the coxofemoral joint in horses. Vet Surg 1994:23:377-385.

Nixon, A.J., 2002. Arthroscopic surgery or the carpal and digital tendon sheaths. Clin Tech in Equine Pract 1: 245-256.

Nixon, A.J., A.E. Sams and N.G. Duchame, 1993. Endoscopically assisted annular ligament release in horses. Vet Surg 22: 501-507.

Nixon, A.J., B.L. Schachter and R.R. Poole, 2003. Caudal radial exostosis as a cause of carpal sheath tenosynovitis and lameness in horses. J Am Vet Med Assoc 224: 264-270.

Norrdin, R.W., C.E. Kawcak, B.A. Capwell and C.W. McIlwraith, 1998. Subchondral bone failure in an equine model of overload arthrosis. Bone 22: 133-139.

Phillips, T.J. and I.M. Wright, 1994. Observations on the anatomy and pathology of the palmar intercarpal ligaments in the middle carpal joints of Thoroughbred racehorses. Equine Vet J 26: 486-491.

Ray, C.S., G.M. Baxter, C.W. McIlwraith et al., 1996. Development of subchondral cystic lesions after articular cartilage and subchondral bone damage in young horses. Equine Vet J 28: 225-232.

Richardson, D.W., 1986. Technique for arthroscopic repair of third carpal bone slab fractures in horses. J Am Vet Med Assoc 188: 288-291.

Richardson, D.W., 2002. Arthroscopically assisted repair of articular fractures. Clin Equine Pract 1: 211-217.

Schneider, R.K., C.A. Ragle, B.G. Carter *et al.*, 1994. Arthroscopic removal of osteochondral fragments from the proximal interphalangeal joint of the pelvic limbs in three horses. J Am Vet Med Assoc 207: 79-82.

Schneider, R.K., P. Jenson and R.M. Moore, 1997. Evaluation of cartilage lesions on the medial femoral condyle as a cause of lameness in horses: 11 cases (1988-1994). J Am Vet Med Assoc 210: 1649-1652.

Setnikar, I., R. Palumbo, S. Canalis and G. Zanolo, 1993. Pharmacokinetics of glucosamine in man. Arzneimittelforschung 43:1109-1113.

Smith, M.M. and P. Ghosh, 1987. The synthesis of hyaluronic acid by human synovial fibroblasts is influenced by the extracellular environment. Rheumatol Int. 7: 113-122.

Sokoloff, L., 1979. Pathology and Pathogenesis of Osteoarthritis. In: D.J. McCarty (ed), Arthritis and Allied Conditions. 9th ed. Philadelphia,, Lea and Febiger, pp. 1135-1153.

Southwood, L.L. and C.W. McIlwraith, 2000. Arthroscopic removal of fracture fragments involving a portion of the base of the sesamoid bone in horses. J Am Vet Med Assoc 217: 236-240.

Southwood, L.L., C.W. McIlwraith, D.D. Frisbie, C.E. Kawcak *et al.*, 2004. Evaluation of Ad-BMP-2 enhancing fracture healing in an infected non-union fracture in a rabbit model. J Orthop Res 22: 66-72.

Southwood, L.L., T.S. Stashak, R.A. Kainer *et al.*, 1999. Desmotomy of the accessory ligament of the superficial digital flexor tendon in the horse with the use of a tenoscopic approach to the carpal sheath. Vet Surg 28: 99-105.

Southwood, L.L., G.W. Trotter and C.W. McIlwraith, 1998. Arthroscopic removal of abaxial fracture fragments of the proximal sesamoid bone in horses: 47 cases (1989-1997). J Am Vet Med Assoc 213: 1016-1021.

Stick, J.A., L.A. Borg, F.A. Nickels *et al.*, 1992. Arthroscopic removal of osteochondral fragment from the caudal pouch of the lateral femorotibial joint in a colt. J Am Vet Assoc 200: 1695-1697.

Tew, W.P., 1982. Demonstration by synovial fluid analysis of the efficacy in horses of an investigational drug (L-1016). J Equine Vet Sci: 42-50.

Textor, J.A., A.J. Nixon and L.A. Fortier, 2003. Tenoscopic release of the equine carpal canal. Vet Surg 32: 278-284.

Textor, J.A., a.j. Nixon, J. Lumsden *et al.*, 2001. Subchondral cystic lesions of the proximal extremity or the tibia in horses: 12 cases (1983-2000). J Am Vet Med Assoc 218: 408-413.

Todhunter, H.J., S.L. Fubini, V. Vernier-Singer *et al.*, 1998. Acute synovitis in intra-articular methylprednisolone acetate in ponies. Osteoarthritis Cartilage 6: 94-105.

Todhunter, R.J., R.R. Minor, J. Wootton *et al.*, 1993. Effects of exercise and polysulfated glycosaminoglycan on repair of articular cartilage defects in the equine carpus. J Orthop Res 11: 782-795.

Trotter, G.W., 1996a. Intra-articular corticosteroids. In: C.W. McIlwraith and G.W. Trotter (eds.), Joint Disease in the Horse. WB Saunders, Philadelphia, pp. 237-256.

Trotter, G.W.. 1996b. Polysulfated glycosaminoglycan (Adequan®). In: C.W. McIlwraith and G.W. Trotter (eds.), Joint Disease in the Horse, Philadelphia WB Saunders, pp. 270-280.

Trotter, G.W., J. Yovich, C.W. McIlwraith *et al.*, 1989. Effects of intramuscular polysulfated glycosaminoglycan on chemical and physical defect in equine articular cartilage. Can J Vet Res 43: 224-230.

Trumble, T.N., 2003. PhD dissertation; Colorado State University, Ft. Collins, CO.

Trumble, T.N., A.J. Stick, S.P. Arnoczky *et al.*, 1994. Consideration of anatomic and radiographic features of the caudal pouches of the femorotibial joints of horses for the purpose of arthroscopy. Am J Vet Res 55: 1682-1689.

Vacek, J.R., R.D. Welch and C.M. Honnas, 1992. Arthroscopic approach and intra-articular anatomy of the palmaroproximal and plantaroproximal aspect of distal interphalangeal joints. Vet Surg 4: 257-260.

Vail, T.B. and C.W. McIlwraith, 1992. Arthroscopic removal of an osteochondral fragment from the middle phalanx of a horse. Vet Surg 4: 269-272.

Management of lameness causes in sport horses

Vane, J.R., 1971. Inhibition of prostaglandin synthesis as a mechanism of action for aspirin-like drugs. Nature 231: 232-235.

Von Rechenberg, B., H. Guenther, C.W. McIlwraith *et al.*, 2000a. Fibrous tissue of subchondral cystic lesions in horses produce local mediators in neutral metalloproteinases and cause bone resorption *in vitro*. Vet Surg 29: 420.429.

Von Rechenberg, B., C.W. McIlwraith and M. Akens, 2000b. Spontaneous production of nitric oxide (NO) prostaglandins (PGE$_2$) in neutral metalloproteinases (MMPs) in media of explant cultures of equine synovial membrane and articular cartilage from normal and osteoarthritic joints. Equine Vet J 32: 140-150.

Walmsley, J.P., 1995. Vertical tears in the cranial horn of the meniscus and its cranial ligament in the equine femorotibial joint: 7 cases and their treatment by arthroscopic surgery. Equine Vet J 27: 20-25.

Walmsley, J.P., 1997. Fracture of the intercondylar eminence of the tibia treated by arthroscopic internal fixation. Equine Vet J 29: 148-150.

Walmsley, J.P., 2002. Arthroscopic surgery of the femorotibial joint. Clin Tech Equine Pract 1: 226-233.

Walmsley, J.P., T.J. Philips and H.G.G. Townsend, 2003. Meniscal tears in horses: an evaluation of clinical signs and arthroscopic treatment of 80 cases. Equine Vet J 35: 402-406.

Weller RR, Maieler LJ, Bowen IM. May SA, Liebich H-G. The arthroscopic approach and intra-articular anatomy of the equine temporomandibular joint. Equine Vet J 34: 421-424.

Whitton, R.C. and R.J. McCarthy Rose, 1997a. The intercarpal ligaments of equine mid-carpal joint. Part I: the anatomy of the palmar and dorsomedial intercarpal ligaments of the mid-carpal joint. Vet Surg 26: 359-366.

Whitton, R.C. and R.J. Rose, 1997b. The intercarpal ligaments of the equine mid-carpal joint. Part II: the role of the palmar intercarpal ligaments in the restraint of dorsal displacement of the proximal row of carpal bones. Vet Surg 26: 367-373.

Whitton, R.C., N.J. Kannegieter and R.J. Rose, 1997c. The intercarpal ligaments of the equine mid-carpal joint. Part III: clinical observations in 32 racing horses with mid-carpal joint disease. Vet Surg 26: 374-381.

Wilderjans, H., B. Boussaw, K. Madder and O. Simon, 2003. Tenosynovitis of the digital flexor tendon sheath and annular ligament constriction syndrome caused by longitudinal tears in the deep digital flexor tendon: a clinical and surgical report of 17 cases in Warmblood horses. Equine Vet J 35: 270-275.

Wilke, M., A.J. Nixon and J. Malark, 2001. Fractures of the palmar aspect of carpal 7 bones in horses: 10 cases (1984-2000). J Am Vet Med Assoc 219: 801-804.

Wright, I.M. and P.J. McMahon, 1999. Tenosynovitis associated with longitudinal tears of the digital flexor tendons in horses: a report of 20 cases. Equine Vet J 31: 12-18.

Yovich, J., G.W. Trotter, C.W. McIlwraith *et al.*, 1993. Effects of polysulfated glycosaminoglycan on repair of articular cartilage defects in the equine carpus. J Orthop Res 11: 782-795.

Yovich, J.V. and C.W. McIlwraith, 1986. Arthroscopic surgery for osteochondral fractures of the proximal phalanx of the metacarpophalangeal and metatarsophalangeal (fetlock) joints in horses. J Am Vet Med Assoc 188: 243-279.

Zamos, D.T., C.M. Honnas and A.G. Hoffman, 1994. Arthroscopic approach and intra-articular anatomy of the plantar pouch of the equine tarsocrural joint. Vet Surg 23:161-166.

Zekas, L.J., L.R. Bramlage, R.M. Embertson *et al.*, 1999. Characterization of the type and location of fractures of the third metacarpal/metatarsal condyles in 135 horses in Central Kentucky (1986-1994). Equine Vet J 31: 304-308.

How are osteoarthritis & traumatic joint disease managed in human athletes?

Harald Roos
Karl X Gustavs gata 67B, 254 40 Helsingborg, Sweden

Age is the most important risk factor for osteoarthritis (OA). Sex, race, obesity, biomechanical factors, inherited susceptibility, use and abuse of joints, as well as joint trauma also influence the development of OA. Soccer is a sport that combines high joint loading and a considerable risk for injuries, especially knee injuries. Since soccer is the most popular sports activity in the world with about 40 million participants it is a useful model for studying OA. An increased risk of hip and knee OA has been shown in former top level soccer players regardless of injuries (Lindberg *et al.*, 1992; Roos *et al.*, 1994). There has been much focus on major knee injuries and the risk of posttraumatic knee OA and joint trauma is considered the most important cause of early OA (Gelber *et al.*, 2000). A major knee trauma is often associated with an anterior cruciate ligament (ACL) injury, and this injury has been studied both concerning the short and long term effects.

Anterior cruciate ligament injury

The incidence of ACL injury in western countries ranges from 0.3-1 per 1000 inhabitants per year and is highest between 15 to 25 years of age (Fridén *et al.*, 1995; Myklebust *et al.*, 2003; Frobell *et al.*, 2006). The risk for an ACL injury in soccer is much higher than in the general population,1.8-2.7/1000 (Roos *et al.*, 1995), but the risk may be even higher in team handball (Myklebust *et al.*, 2003). It is clearly shown that female players in soccer, handball, basket ball have a 6-8 times higher risk to sustain an ACL injury than their male counterparts (Arendt *et al.*, 1999). The reason for this is not known, but anatomic, neuromuscular and hormonal differences between men and women have been discussed as possible reasons.

OA after ACL injury

Of the population aged 35-54 years, 5% have radiographic knee OA, and the large majority of these individuals has had a previous knee injury (Roos, 2005). Most studies report radiographic OA in approximately half of ACL injured patients regardless if they are surgically reconstructed or not (Segawa *et al.*, 2001; Myklebust *et al.*, 2003, Lohmander *et al.*, 2004; Von Porat *et al.*, 2004). In the studies from Sweden all ACL injured patients were soccer players who sustained their injuries when participating in organized soccer play 1986 (Roos *et al.* 1995, Lohmander *et al.* 2005, Von Porat *et al.* 2005). The players had radiographs taken 12-14 years after the injury and the prevalence of OA was 45%. The mean age for the female players at follow up was 31 years and for the males 36 years. The majority of the players had considerable knee symptoms.

It is estimated that the cost for ACL injuries in the USA will be rising to $3 billion annually, however the cost for subsequent knee OA, as a result of previous knee injury, is by far greater.

Isolated meniscal tear and the resulting surgery is also a well-recognized risk factor for OA of the knee (Englund *et al.*, 2003). An ACL injury is commonly associated with injuries to other ligaments, menisci, and or joint cartilage (Fridén *et al.*, 1995; Fithian *et al.*, 2002; Daniel *et al.*, 1994). About 50% of all acute ACL injuries are accompanied by a meniscal tears. In chronic ACL-injured patients with symptoms rendering an arthroscopy approximately 4 out of 5 had a meniscal lesion (Fithian *et al.*, 2002). Due to the risk of chronic instability and secondary meniscal injuries, ACL reconstruction is widely advocated for the young active individual with a fresh ACL injury, but so far no studies have showed a reduced risk of OA by reconstructive surgery (Daniel *et al.*, 1994; Lohmander *et al.*, 2004, Von Porat *et al.*, 2004). A recent study concluded a possible preventive effect of reconstructive knee ligament surgery, but this study used the old radiographic classification system of Ahlbäck and is thus not quite comparable to some of the other studies (Hart *et al.*, 2005). A personal interpretation of that study is that the importance of intact menisci is verified but if the films had been graded according to the Kellgren-Lawrence classification system, the prevalence might have been as high as in other studies (Lohmander *et al.*, 2004; Von Porat *et al.*, 2004). However, there are evidences for a decreased risk of secondary meniscus tears after ACL reconstruction compared to non-reconstructed knees, which indirectly will reduce the risk of OA (Andersson *et al.*, 1991).

Interestingly, in two recently reported studies on the long-term effects of an ACL injury (Engebretsen, personal communication 2006; Neuman *et al.*, 2005), the prevalence of OA after ACL injury is lower than previously reported. In the study by Engebretsen and co-workers a cohort of surgically treated ACL injuries, all involved in a previously reported randomized trial (Grontvedt *et al.*, 1996) have been examined after 16 years. The postoperative regime in these patients was, compared to modern treatment modalities, very conservative with fixation in knee braces and partial weight bearing. According to the Ahlbäck classification the prevalence of OA was 11% at follow up. It must be taken in mind that, as discussed above, this radiographic classification underestimates the signs of OA compared to the more commonly used classification by Kellgren-Lawrence. In the other cohort (Neuman *et al.*, 2005) all patients were primarily non-operatively treated and followed for 15 years. Initially all knees were arthroscopically examined and the ACL injury was verified and at that time associated injuries were treated. All the patients were thoroughly controlled by physiotherapists at certain time intervals during the rehabilitation period and they had a muscular training program (Zätterström *et al.*, 2000). Importantly, all patients were also advised to avoid contact sports. After 15 years 23 had been reconstructed due to either a longitudinal meniscus tear or severe problems with knee instability. The prevalence of OA in the entire group was 16%, but if ACL reconstructed patients and patients with associated meniscus injuries were excluded, none was found to have definite OA. The radiographic classification was comparable to the cohorts of ACL injured soccer players, who had a more conventional treatment of the injury. The prevalence of OA was as mentioned earlier 45% after the same time interval in these cohorts (Lohmander *et al.*, 2004; Von Porat *et al.*, 2004).

Prevention of ACL injuries

The best way of preventing OA after knee injuries is obviously to avoid the injuries. One randomized study on Italian soccer players reported a considerable preventive effect of a training program (Caraffa *et al.*, 1996) and a Norwegian study on handball players also described a significant lower incidence of ACL injuries in elite players after a neuromuscular training program (Holm *et al.*, 2004). When the preventive intervention was stopped, the injury rate went back to previous levels again.

Prevention of OA after knee injury

Different factors could be responsible for the development of OA after a knee injury. The bone marrow oedema visible on MR scans directly after the trauma indicates a blunt intra-articular trauma that may involve the articular cartilage. The high concentration of proteoglycanfragments seen in joint fluid, as long as 15 months after the trauma or a surgical procedure, may indicate an ongoing reparative process in the cartilage matrix (Dahlberg *et al.*, 1994; Beynnon *et al.*, 2005). It could be speculated that the cartilage thus is vulnerable to high loading as long as this process persists. This is supported by the finding of a low glucose-amino-glycan (GAG) content in the ACL injured knee 12 months after the trauma, according to the results of contrast enhanced MR study by Tiderius *et al.* (2005).

General physical activity and specific exercises may prevent or delay osteoarthritis. Results from animal studies and preliminary data from humans support the hypothesis that moderate exercise is beneficial for the cartilage in subjects at risk of osteoarthritis (Galois *et al.*, 2003; Otternes *et al.*, 1998; Roos and Dahlberg, 2006). Reduced muscular performance is a risk factor for osteoarthritis development in the middle-aged, and quadriceps dysfunction is present in subjects at risk before developing osteoarthritis (Becker *et al.* 2004). Also, epidemiologic data support moderate exercise being preventive of severe osteoarthritis requiring total knee replacement (Manninen *et al.*, 2001).

Since there obviously are differences in OA prevalence between different cohorts of ACL injured patients of about the same age 15 years after the injury, the development of OA seems to be dependent of the regime after the injury. Factors that may influence on the course are for example how associated injuries are treated, how and when different activities are introduced in the rehabilitation phase and if this is associated with pain and or swelling. When and if at all, high loading such as soccer and comparable activities should be introduced after an ACL injury is unknown.

With the knowledge today, it could really be questioned, due to ethical reasons, to recommend a young ACL injured 18 year old girl to return to soccer, independent on how successful the reconstruction of her ACL has been.

Treatment of early OA

First of all the definition of OA must be clear. The normal definition is the presences of radiographic features fulfilling the criteria for OA according to the Kellgren-Lawrence classification, associated with symptoms. In early OA with moderate symptoms a training program and patient information is the fist step. Several studies have shown positive effects of exercise (Ettinger *et al.*, 1997). The second step adds medical treatment, such as ordinary pain killers like paracetamol. NSAIDs could be questioned but are widely used. Steroids have some short term benefits and hyaloronic acid may have some symptomatic effect, comparable with NSAIDs (Bellamy *et al.*, 2005). A recent study questions the effect of glucosamin (Clegg *et al.*, 2006).

Unloading braces definitely have some place and lateral shoe support could also be tried.

Different kinds of arthroscopic procedures, such as lavage, shaving, *etc.* , have not been shown to have an effect that is better than placebo (Moseley *et al.*, 2002). Major surgical procedures are effective, and in unicompartemental OA in younger patients high tibial osteotomy is recommended (Magyar *et al.*, 1999). In the more advanced cases, total knee replacement is an intervention with a very high success rate.

Summary

After a major knee injury OA is seen in about 50% of all knees after 15 years. Since this injury often occurs when the players are around 20 years of age, there is a considerable risk of early symptomatic knee OA long before these players have reached 50 years of age. There are treatment options well worth trying before it is time for major surgical procedures. However, some new knowledge that may indicate a possibility to reduce the risk of OA after a major knee injury is discussed.

References

Andersson, C., M. Odensten and J. Gillquist, 1991. Knee function after surgical or nonsurgical treatment of acute rupture of the anterior cruciate ligament: a randomized study with a long-term follow-up period. Clin Orthop Relat Res. 264: 255-263.

Arendt, E.A., J. Agel and R. Dick, 1999. Anterior Cruciate Ligament Injury Patterns Among Collegiate Men and Women. J Athl Train. 34: 86-92

Becker, R., A. Berth, M. Nehring *et al.*, 2004. Neuromuscular quadriceps dysfunction prior to osteoarthritis of the knee. J Orthop Res 22: 768–773.

Bellamy, N., J. Campbell, V. Robinson, T. Gee, R. Bourne and G. Wells, 2005. Intraarticular corticosteroid for treatment of osteoarthritis of the knee. Cochrane Database Syst Rev. CD005328

Beynnon, B.D., B.S. Uh, R.J. Johnson, J.A. Abate, C.E. Nichols, B.C. Fleming, A.R. Poole and H. Roos, 2005. Rehabilitation after anterior cruciate ligament reconstruction: a prospective, randomized, double-blind comparison of programs administered over 2 different time intervals. Am J Sports Med. 33: 347-359.

Caraffa, A., G. Cerulli, M. Projetti, G. Aisa and A. Rizzo, 1996.Prevention of anterior cruciate ligament injuries in soccer. A prospective controlled study of proprioceptive training. Knee Surg Sports Traumatol Arthrosc. 4: 19-21.

Clegg, D.O., D.J. Reda, C.L. Harris *et al.*, 2006. Glucosamine, chondroitin sulfate, and the two in combination for painful knee osteoarthritis. N Engl J Med. 354: 795-808.

Dahlberg, L., H. Roos, T. Saxne, D. Heinegård, M. Lark and L.S. Lohmander, 1994. Cartilage metabolism in in the injured and uninjured knee of the same patient. Ann Rheum Dis 53: 823-827.

Daniel, D.M., M.L. Stone, B.E. Dobson, D.C. Fithian, D.J. Rossman, K.R. Kaufman, 1994. Fate of the ACL-injured patient. A prospective outcome study. Am J Sports Med. 22: 632-644.

Englund, M., E.M. Roos and L.S. Lohmander, 2003. Impact of type of meniscal tear on radiographic and symptomatic knee osteoarthritis: a sixteen-year followup of meniscectomy with matched controls. Arthritis Rheum 48: 2178–2187.

Ettinger, W.H. Jr., R. Burns, S.P. Messier, W. Applegate, W.J. Rejeski, T Morgan, S. Shumaker, M.J. Berry, M. O'Toole, J. Monu and T. Craven, 1997. A randomized trial comparing aerobic exercise and resistance exercise with a health education program in older adults with knee osteoarthritis. The Fitness Arthritis and Seniors Trial (FAST). JAMA. 277: 25-31.

Fithian, D.C., L.W. Paxton and D.H. Goltz, 2002. Fate of the anterior cruciate ligament-injured knee. Orthop Clin North Am. 33: 621-636.

Friden, T., T. Erlandsson, R. Zatterstrom, A. Lindstrand and U. Moritz, 1995. Compression or distraction of the anterior cruciate injured knee. Variations in injury pattern in contact sports and downhill skiing. Knee Surg Sports Traumatol Arthrosc. 3: 144-147.

Frobell, R., S.L. Lohmander and H. Roos, 2006. Acute traumatic hemarthrosis of the knee – poor agreement between clinical assessment and MRI findings. Scan J Med Sci Sports, (in press).

Hart, A.J., J. Buscombe, A. Malone and G.S. Dowd, 2005. Assessment of osteoarthritis after reconstruction of the anterior cruciate ligament: a study using single-photon emission computed tomography at ten years. J Bone Joint Surg Br. 87: 1483-1487.

Holm, I., M.A. Fosdahl, A. Friis, M.A. Risberg, G. Myklebust and H. Steen, 2004. Effect of neuromuscular training on proprioception, balance, muscle strength, and lower limb function in female team handball players. Clin J Sport Med. 14: 88-94.

Galois, L., S. Etienne, L. Grossin *et al.*, 2003. Moderate-impact exercise is associated with decreased severity of experimental osteoarthritis in rats. Rheumatology (Oxford) 42: 692–693.

Gelber, A.C., M.C. Hochberg, L.A. Mead *et al.*, 2000. Joint injury in young adults and risk for subsequent knee and hip osteoarthritis. Ann Intern Med 133: 321–328.

Grontvedt, T., L. Engebretsen, P. Benum, O. Fasting, A. Molsterand T. Strand, 1996. A prospective, randomized study of three operations for acute rupture of the anterior cruciate ligament. Five-year follow-up of one hundred and thirty-one patients. J Bone Joint Surg Am. 78: 159-168.

Lindberg, H., H. Roos and P. Gärdsell, 1992. The prevalence of coxarthrosis among former soccer players. Acta Ortop Scand 64: 165-167.

Lohmander, L.S., A. Östenberg, M. Englund and H.P. Roos, 2004. High prevalence of knee OA and functional limitations in female soccer players with ACL injury. Arthritis Rheum. 50: 3145-3152.

Magyar, G., T.L. Ahl, P. Vibe, S. Toksvig-Larsen and A. Lindstrand, 1999. Open-wedge osteotomy by hemicallotasis or the closed-wedge technique for osteoarthritis of the knee. A randomised study of 50 operations. J Bone Joint Surg Br. 81: 444-448.

Manninen, P., H. Riihimaki, M. Heliovaara *et al.*, 2001. Physical exercise and risk of severe knee osteoarthritis requiring arthroplasty. Rheumatology (Oxford) 40: 432-437.

Management of lameness causes in sport horses

Moseley, J.B., K. O'Malley, N.J. Petersen, T.J. Menke, B.A. Brody, D.H. Kuykendall, J.C. Hollingsworth, C.M. Ashton and N.P. Wray, 2002. A controlled trial of arthroscopic surgery for osteoarthritis of the knee. N Engl J Med. 347: 81-88.

Myklebust, G., I. Holm, S. Maehlum, L. Engebretsen and R. Bahr, 2003. Clinical, functional, and radiologic outcome in team handball players 6 to 11 years after anterior cruciate ligament injury: a follow-up study. Am J Sports Med. 31: 981-989.

Neuman, P., M. Englund, H. Roos and L. Dahlberg, 2005. Coexistent meniscal injury is a strong risk factor for radiographic OA 16 years after a total ACL rupture. Abstract Swedish Orthopaedic Society, annual meeting, 2005.

Otterness, I.G., J.D. Eskra, M.L. Bliven et al., 1998. Exercise protects against articular cartilage degeneration in the hamster. Arthritis Rheum 41: 2068–2076.

Roos, E.M., 2005. Joint injury causes knee osteoarthritis in young adults. Curr Opin Rheumatol. 17: 195-200.

Roos, E.M. and L. Dahlberg, 2005. Positive effects of moderate exercise on glycosaminoglycan content in knee cartilage: a four-month, randomized, controlled trial in patients at risk ofosteoarthritis. Arthritis Rheum. 52: 3507-3514.

Roos, H., H. Lindberg, P. Gärdsell, L.S. Lohmander and H. Wingstrand, 1994. The prevalence of gonarthrosis in former soccer players and its relation to meniscectomy. Am J Sports Med 22: 219-222.

Roos, H., M. Ornell, P. Gärdsell, L.S. Lohmander and A. Lindstrand, 1995. Soccer after anterior cruciate injury – an incompatible combination? A national survey of incidence and risk factors and a 7-year follow-up. Acta Orthop Scand 66: 107-112.

Segawa, H., G. Omori and Y. Koga, 2001. Long-term results of non-operative treatment of anterior cruciate ligament.Injury. Knee. 8: 5-11.

Tiderius, C.J., L.E. Olsson, F. Nyquist and L. Dahlberg, 2005.Cartilage glycosaminoglycan loss in the acute phase after an anterior cruciate ligament injury: delayed gadolinium-enhanced magnetic resonance imaging of cartilage and synovial fluid analysis. Arthritis Rheum. 52: 120-127.

Von Porat, A., E.M. Roos and H. Roos, 2004. High prevalence of osteoarthritis 14 years after an anterior cruciate ligament tear in male soccer players – A study of radiographic and patient-relevant outcomes. Ann Rheum Dis. 63: 269-273.

Zatterstrom, R., T. Friden, A. Lindstrand and U. Moritz, 2000. Rehabilitation following acute anterior cruciate ligament injuries--a 12-month follow-up of a randomized clinical trial. Scand J Med Sci Sports. 10: 156-163.

Physiotherapeutic options for the prevention and management of skeletal disorder

Amanda Sutton
Harestock Stud Physiotherapy Centre, Kennel Lane, SO 22 6PT Littleton, Nr. Winchester, Hampshire, United Kingdom

Take home message

The mainstay of physiotherapy intervention is to normalise afferent information into the central nervous system, which then provides material for a normal effector response. This may take many different forms and include a combination of sensory, cognitive and effective intervention in other words a multifaceted treatment plan.

Introduction

Physiotherapy is the practice of maintenance of optimum function by means of evaluation, treatment and rehabilitation. Physiotherapy treatment and management is concerned with reversing various physical conditions associated with injury or dysfunction and rehabilitating the patient.

When devising a rehabilitation plan the response of the tissues to the physiological events of trauma have to be considered and the time frame of events. The effectiveness of rehabilitation in the recovery period usually determines the degree and success of future athletic function. The two main goals are: 1) Reverse or deter the adverse effects resulting from immobility or disuse. 2) Facilitate tissue healing and avoid excessive stress on immature tissue.

The overall plan is to initiate pain relief, decrease effusion, oedema and return to a full active and pain free range of motion. The end result should be a return of full muscular strength, power and endurance. There should be a full reprogramming of neuromotor pathways and a return to full asymptomatic functional activities at preinjury level.

The initial evaluation will consist of a detailed history and movement examination. Observations in both static and dynamic positions including the effects of different surfaces and inclines are invaluable. Specific balance reactions and subtle movement tests will be performed. The use of sedation to evaluate spinal and cervical mobility may be utilised, allowing passive mobility and joint restrictions to be cross-referenced with active and active assisted movements. The use of functional exercise testing is necessary in more subtle performance problems. It is important to accurately appreciate the nature of the problem and to observe its influence. The use of videoanalysis will allow more accurate data to be collected. Repeated examination over several days, before and after exercise can help identify the significance and functional importance of the presenting problem.

As chartered physiotherapists we are employed to treat a range of conditions. Acute inflammatory responses to joints, wounds, tendons, ligaments and periosteal reactions are seen in the competitive athlete, both on the course and at home. Immediate control of the oedema and joint effusion is critical. Both serve to increase pain on sensory nerve endings and raise intraarticular pressure. The resultant afferent activity leads to muscle inhibition. In humans a small increase in joint fluid (10 ml) can produce a 50% decrease in maximal voluntary contraction of the quadriceps (Fahere *et al.*, 1988). Muscle physiotherapy modalities help control and reduce these responses allowing the athlete to begin early range of motion and strength exercises, when combined with therapeutic exercises.

Electrotherapy

Electrotherapy used at the right place, and right time, for the right reason, has the ability to assist repair (Watson, 2005). All electrotherapy modalities involve the introduction of some physical energy into the system. This energy brings about one or more physiological changes, which are used for therapeutic benefit. The effects appear to be dose dependant and so it is important to deliver the appropriate dose (Watson, 2005). There are numerous examples of research papers that have demonstrated a significant effect at one dose but nothing at another.

Electrical activity of the body has been used for a long time for diagnostic and monitoring purposes, examples are ECG, EMG, EEG. Tissues that have not been recorded as excitable but that have demonstrated endogenous electrical activity have been detected. Research has been conducted on this activity and its relationship to healing and injury. Treatment using electrotherapy modalities is therefore directed at enhancing this endogenous electrical activity and thereby the growth and healing process. This is created using an exogenous stimulation which in the form of low energy, produces membrane excitement and this results in cellular excitement (Watson, 1996).

Therapeutic ultrasound

Therapeutic ultrasound is best utilised when treating tendon, ligament, fascia or bone, this is because it is best absorbed in dense collagenous tissue. Sparrow (2005) utilised it to good effect in the treatment of the medial collateral ligament in a rabbit model. The results showed that the ligaments were larger in area, achieved a greater load before failure and had greater energy absorption capacity. Importantly the relative proportion of type I to type III collagen was greater.

In the human field there have been some papers on the increasing use of ultrasound in fracture healing (Fujioka *et al.*, 2004; Busse and Bhandari, 2004). An excellent metaanalysis on fracture healing has also been done by Busse and colleagues (2002).

The use of ultrasound for tendon healing has been demonstrated (Ng *et al.*, 2003). The ultimate tensile strength of low and high dose groups ultrasound was significantly greater than in controls. Ng *et al.* (2003) compared the outcome of two different ultrasound doses, running and swimming on achilles tendon repair in rats. The higher intensity ultrasound group and running group did best. The management of degenerative joint disease in humans and equines presents a challenge. Reduced mobility from disuse atrophy, pain and poor joint stability all affect proprioceptive input. Hilary (2005) looked at the effect of ultrasound as a means to increase the effectiveness of isokinetic exercise with patients with osteoarthritis knee. The trial consisted of 120 patients and the combination with ultrasound did significantly better.

Neuromuscular electrical stimulation

The transcutaneous application of neuromuscular electrical stimulation (NMES) has been used by physiotherapists in a rehabilitation setting to reduce the detrimental effects of immobilisation and to strengthen weakened muscles (Bromiley, 1999; Johnson *et al.*, 1997). There are many parameters for the delivery of NMES from the stimulus shape to the pulse duration rate, and intensity interval and frequency. There are no papers published on the use of this modality in equines but on rats, dogs and humans (Vinge *et al.*, 1996). Demir *et al.* (2004) looked at the use of electrical stimulation and laser on wound healing. Both had beneficial effects during the inflammatory, proliferation, and maturation phases of a wound. The electrical stimulation had more beneficial effects during the inflammatory phase than the laser, but this could have been related to the dosage parameter.

A growing area of NMES treatment is the use of microcurrent therapies. It appears to have significant potential and is currently probably somewhat underused in the clinical field. Its application has been cited in the treatment of equine tendon injuries and was used in the Demir *et al.* (2004) paper.

In NMES the recruitment order of muscle fibres is reversed to that of a voluntary contraction although some debate exists over this. Therefore type II muscle fibres are preferentially activated over type I fibres (Delitto and Synder-Machler, 1990). In chronic diseases, type II fibres are predominantly affected and therefore the use of NMES is applicable (Martin *et al.*, 1991). Evidence exists to suggest the NMES increases muscular blood flow and oxygen metabolism more than voluntary exercise of the same intensity (McKeeken, 1994; Grimmer, 1992; Tracey *et al.*, 1988). It has been shown to reduce the detrimental effects of immobilisation and may be more effective at strengthening weakened or inhibited muscle than voluntary exercise alone. NMES strength gains appear to be proportioned to the intensity of training and to involve neural mechanism (Trimble and Enoka, 1991).

Interferential therapy

Interferential therapy is a modality used for joint pain in the presence of oedema and pain in another paper by Defrin *et al.* (2005). He showed significantly decreased pain levels, morning stiffness reduction and improved range of motion with noxious stimulation levels. This in equine practice can be difficult to apply as a modality because of the sensory stimulation. It has been used particularly with chronic sacroiliac dysfunction and degenerative joint disease in practice.

Laser therapy

Pain relief is administered using low intensity laser therapy. Vinck *et al.* (2005) provide useful evidence with regards the effect of laser on nerve conduction capacity. It was originally postulated that laser's effects on inflammatory events and stimulation of tissue repair produced pain relief. For several years it was reasoned that the laser was having a direct effect on nerve conduction. Vinck *et al.* (2005) showed that the sural nerve conduction characteristics in 64 healthy human volunteers were changed on an immediate and localised level. Suggested applications for laser are acute injuries, including fractures, autoimmune diseases, calcifications and vertebrogenic radiculopathies.

Transcutaneous electrical nerve stimulation

In 1965 Melzack and Walls 'paingate theory' lead to the development of transcutaneous electrical nerve stimulations (TENS) used for pain relief. It involves the application of electrical currents to the skin to stimulate afferent nerve fibres and thereby reduces pain (Walsh *et al.*, 1997). TENS tends to be used primarily for chronic pain *e.g.* lower back pain and arthritis (Grimmer, 1992; Marchand *et al.*, 1993) but also can be used to treat acute pain (Forster *et al.*, 1994; Harrison *et al.*, 1987). Its application in equines is used to treat conservatively managed dorsal spine impingement and lumbar degenerative joint disease. Both animal and human models have been used to investigate the peripheral neurophysiological effects. Work by Walsh *et al.* (1998) has demonstrated significant neurophysiological and hypoalgesic effects of different combinations of TENS parameters.

Manual therapies

Manual therapies are employed to treat altered joint position sense as a result of incongruent joint surfaces and reflex muscle inhibition (Maitland, 1982). The result is localised muscle spasm and decreased passive and active articular movement. The application of graded mobilisations and manipulation to restore mobility are used as part of the therapeutic exercise regime. These can be applied locally or distally to the restricted site utilising fascial and muscular continuums. These techniques are part of the treatment regime of skeletal problems and allow normalisation of afferent information and therefore joint position sense leading to normal neuromotor movement patterns.

Exercise

Regardless of the mechanisms of injury any damage to muscle spindles, golgi tendon organs and joint receptors has a significant impact on function and dynamic joint stabilisation. Damage to capsuloligamentous structures results in decreased proprioception and joint instability. This dysfunction results in faulty movement patterns resulting in changes in neuromuscular control patterns. Age and injury all affect proprioception due to inadequate activation of mechanoreceptors that results in delayed muscle reaction latencies (Ellenbecker and Mattalino, 1997).

If exercised inappropriately in the rehabilitation phase by inducing fatigue from inappropriate surfaces and regimes then laxity will be increased in these already damaged structures (Barrey *et al.*, 1991). Posture and its maintenance via the use of schooling appliances should be carefully considered. Incorrect sensory stimuli initiating abnormal reflexive placement of limbs serves only to reinforce incorrect movement patterns. The use of restraint to secure the self carriage of the cervical spine has been shown to affect spinal movement and hind limb propulsion (Rhodin *et al.*, 2005). In many cases the equine musculature and skeletal frame does not allow the execution of the task and only serves to encourage poor postural control. Impaired joint position sense is often overlooked and is a major risk factor for recurrent injury. A carefully graduated exercise plan is therefore essential. This involves avoiding excessive, repeated movements on poor grip surfaces. Stability has been observed to improve by switching surfaces to prevent too much movement and to encourage stabilisation of the distal limb (Back *et al.*, 1995).

The use of proprioceptive adhesive and non-adherent materials to increase sensory awareness and to posturally re-educate movement patterns both statically and dynamically are utilised. The use of nonhabitual movement patterns such as those based on feldenkrais (Scholz, 1990) and circuit training all increase neuromotor programming by corrective posture and repetitive movements, reprogramming and re-establishing normal.

Factors central to successful physiotherapy intervention include understanding of the various tissue responses to stress and strain. Secondly, the adaptive and maladaptive changes to sensitivity of healing tissue and finally knowledge of normal functional movement and the use of efficient, optimum movement strategies. Biomechanics and adaptive strategies give us a baseline to identify dysfunction.

References

Back, W., H.C. Schamhardt, W. Hartman and Barneveld, 1995. Repetitive loading and oscillations in the distal fore and hind limb as predisposing factors for equine lameness. Am J Vet Res 56: 1522-1528.

Barrey, E., B. Landjerit and R. Wotter, 1991. Shock and vibration during hoof impact on different track surfaces. In: Equine Exer Physiol 3. S.G.B. Persson, A. Lindholm and L.B. Jeffcolt (1991), ICEEP Publications, Davis, California pp. 97–106.

Bromiley, M.W., 1999. Physical therapy for the equine back, Veterinary Clinics of North America: Equine Practice 15: 223–246.

Busse, J.W, M. Bhandari, A.V. Kulkami and E. Tunks, 2002. The effect of low – intensity pulsed ultrasound therapy on time to fracture healing: a Meta – analysis. CMAJ 166: 437–441.

Busse, J.W. and M. Bhandari, 2004. Therapeutic ultrasound and fracture healing: A survey of beliefs and practices. Arch Phys Med Rehabil 85: 1653–1656.

Defrin, R., E. Ariel and C. Peretz, 2005. Segmental noxious Versus innoculous electrical stimulation for chronic pain relief and the effect of fading sensation during treatment. Pain 115: 152-160.

Delitto, A. and L. Synder–Machler, 1990. Two theories of muscle strength augmentation using percutaneous electrical stimulation. Physical therapy 70: 158–164.

Demir, H. et al., 2004. A comparative study of the effects of electrical stimulation and laser treatment on experimental wound healing in rats. J Rehabil Res Dev 41: 147–154.

Ellenbecker, T.S. and A.J. Mattalino, 1997. Concentric isokinetic shoulder internal and external rotation strength in professional baseball pitchers. J. Orthop Sports Phys Therap 25: 323–328.

Fahere, H., H.U. Rentsch and N.J. Gerber, 1988. Knee effusion and reflex inhibition of the quadriceps. J Bone Joint Surg 70: 635–638.

Forster E.L, J.F. Krammer, S.D. Lucy, R.A. Saidds and R.J. Novick, 1994. Effect of TENS on pain medications and pulmonary function following coronary artery bypass graft surgery. Chest 106: 1343–1348.

Fujioka, H. et al., 2004. Ultrasound treatment of non union of the hook of the hamate in sports activities. Knee surg Sports Traumatol Arthrosc 12: 162–164.

Grimmer, K., 1992. A controlled double blind study comparing the effects of strong burst mode TENS and high rate TENS on painful osteoarthritic knees. Aust J Physiotherapy 38: 49–56.

Harrison, R.F., M. Shore, T. Woods, G. Mathews, J. Gardiner and A. Unwin, 1987. A comparative study of transcutaneous electrical nerve stimulation (TENS), entonox, pethidine and promazine and lumbar epidural for pain relief in labour. Acta Obstet Gynaecol Scan 66: 9–14.

Hilary et al., 2005. Use of ultrasound to increase effectiveness of isokinetic exercise for knee osteoarthritis. Archives Physical Medicine and Rehabilitation 86: 1545–1551.

Johnson, J.M., A.L. Johnson, G.J. Pijanowski, S.K. Kneller, D.J. Schaeffer, J.A. Eurell, C.W. Smith and K.S. Swan, 1997. Rehabilitation of dogs with surgically treated cranial cruciate ligament – deficient stifles by use of electrical stimulation of muscles. American Journal Veterinary Research 58: 1473–1478.

McKeeken, J., 1994. Tissue Temperature and blood flow: a research based overview of electrophysical modalities. The Australian Journal of physiotherapy 40 (spec.155): 49–57.

Maitland, G.D., 1982. Examination of the cervical spine. Australian Journal of Physiotherapy 28: 6.

Marchand, S., J. Charest, J.-R. Chenard, B. Larigrolle and L. Laurencelle, 1993. Is TENS purely a placebo effect? A controlled study on chronic low back pain. Pain 54: 99–106.

Martin, T.P, L.A. Gunderson, F.T. Blevins and R.D. Coutts, 1991. The influence of functional electrical stimulation on the properties of vastus lateralis fibres following total knee arthroplasty. Scand J Rehab Med 23: 207–210.

Melzack, R. and P.D. Wall, 1965. Pain mechanisms: a new theory. Science 150: 971–979.

Ng, C.O., G.Y. Ng, E.K. See and M.C. Leung, 2003. Therapeutic ultrasound improves strength of Achilles tendon repair in rats ultrasound. Med Bio 29: 1501–1506.

Rhodin, M., C. Johnston, K. Roethlisberger-Holm, J. Wennerstrand and S. Drevemo, 2005. The influence of head and neck position kinematics of the back in riding horses at the walk and trot. Equine Veterinary Journal 37: 7–11.

Scholz, P., 1990. Dynamic pattern theory – some implications for therapeutics. Phys Ther 70: 827–843.

Sparrow et al., 2005. The effects of low-intensity ultrasound on medial collateral ligament healing in the rabbit model. American Journal of Sports Medicine 33: 1048–1056.

Tracey, J.E., D.P. Currier and A.J. Threlkeld, 1988. Comparison of selected pulse frequencies from two different electrical stimulators on blood flow in healthy subjects. Physical Therapy 68: 1526–1532.

Trimble, M.H. and R.M. Enoka, 1991. Mechanisms underlying the training effects associated with neuromuscular electrical stimulation. Physical Therapy 71: 273–280.

Management of lameness causes in sport horses

Vinck, E, P. Coorevits, B. Cagnie, M. De Muynck, G. Vanderstraeten and D. Cambier, 2005. Evidence of changes in sural nerve conduction mediated by light emitting diode irradiation. Lasers in Medical Science 20: 35–40.

Vinge, O., L. Edrardsen, F.G. Jensen, J. Wernerman and H. Kehlet, 1996. Effect of transcutaneous electrical muscle stimulation on post operative muscle mass and protein synthesis. British Journal of Surgery 83: 360–363.

Walsh, D.M., A.S. Lowe, J.C. McCormack-Willer, G.D. Baxter and J.M. Allen, 1998. Effects of transcutaneous electrical nerve stimulation (TENS) upon peripheral nerve conduction, mechanical pain threshold and tactile threshold in humans. Arch Phys Med Rehab 79: 1051–1058.

Watson, T., 1996. Electrical stimulation for wound healing. Physical Therapy Reviews 1: 89–103.

Watson, T., 2005. Electrotherapy research: in context. In Touch Winter 2005 (113): 20–26.

Expanded abstracts

Influence of diet and sex differences on plasma serotonin and tryptophan of trained Thoroughbreds

D. Alberghina[1], G. Bruschetta[1], G.M. Campo[3], S. Campo[3], P. Medica[2] and A.M. Ferlazzo[1]
[1]Department of Morphology, Biochemistry, Physiology and Animal Production, Unit of Biochemistry, University of Messina, Italy
[2]Department of Morphology, Biochemistry, Physiology and Animal Production, Unit of Physiology; University of Messina, Italy
[3]Department of Biochemical, Physiological and Nutritional Science, University of Messina, Italy

Take home message

Different diets can influence slightly the plasma serotonin (5-HT) concentration in horses. Lower 5-HT levels are measured when horses receive a low fibre diet compared to a high fibre diet. An abnormal behaviour was observed horses when fed the low fibre diet only. Horses have a sexual dimorphism for 5-HT and tryptophan levels.

Introduction

Concentration of plasma serotonin (5-HT) represents an equilibrium state between synthesis by enterochromaffin cells of the gut and processes that inactive free circulating 5-HT (monoamino oxidase activity in liver and lung, platelet uptake mechanism). A relationship between plasma 5-HT and central 5-HT has been reported (Sarrias *et al.*, 1990). Human plasma 5-HT has been measured in physiological (Kumar *et al.*, 1998) and pathological conditions (Lee *et al.*, 2000).

Horse plasma 5-HT levels (Lebelt *et al.*, 1998; Bailey and Elliot, 1998; Alberghina *et al.*, 2004) are higher than human plasma 5-HT (Ortiz *et al.*, 1988; Baguley *et al.*, 1997). Uptake of 5-HT into platelets is an important mechanism to maintain low plasma concentrations, and platelet activation may therefore result in a significant release of this vasoconstrictor. The increase of plasma 5-HT, measured after ingestion of endotoxins and dietary amines could be related to acute laminitis (Bailey *et al.*, 2000). Cribbing horses showed plasma 5-HT levels lower than control group horses (Lebelt *et al.*, 1998) and this stereotypic behaviour significantly increased during and after feeding concentrates (Gillham *et al.*, 1994). It is well known that diets with different content of protein and carbohydrates influences plasma tryptophan levels and, likely, central tryptophan, precursor of 5-HT. Moreover, horses fed a low fibre diet have a greater susceptibility to develop stereotypic behaviour and stomach ulcers than horses fed with high fibre diet (Ellis and Visser, 2003). On this basis, the present study has been carried out in order to measure plasma 5-HT and its precursor tryptophan in two groups of trained horses fed a high fibre or a low fibre diet.

Material and methods

18 Dutch Warmblood horses (10 mares and 8 geldings, 3 years old, 510 to 590 Kg body weight) were used. Horses belongued to the Research Institute for Animal Husbandry of Lelystad, Netherlands. The protocol used for the research was the same reported by Ellis and Visser (2003). Horses were accustomed to individual housing, trainingmill and treadmill during a period of 4 months, reaching a light fitness level; then they were divided into a high fibre diet (HF) group (ratio concentrate: silage = 1:4) and a low fibre diet (LF) group (ratio concentrate: silage = 4:1). The diets were isoenergetic.

Two months after feeding the different diets blood was taken from the jugular vein of the horses. Venous blood was collected into a K_3-EDTA tube. The tubes were centrifuged at 4° C (2,500 g for 10 minutes) to obtain platelet-low plasma that was kept at –20° C until the analysis.

An isocratic HPLC (Waters 1525 binary HPLC pump) method was developed for the separation and the quantification of serotonin (5-HT) and tryptophan. The mobile phase used was: water solution of Na_2HPO_4 0.0493 M and citric acid 0.0382 M (pH = 3.8) - methanol (85:15, v/v). The flow rate was 1.2 ml/min. The detection system was an electrochemical detector (Coulochem ESA, mod. 5100 A). 100 µl of sample were added to 100 µl of an internal standard (N-Methylserotonin, Chromsystems) and 100 µl of precipitation reagent (Chromsystems), vortex-mixed for 30 s, incubated for 10 min at 4° C and centrifuged. Then 20 µl of supernatant was injected.

T-Test and Pearson correlation coefficients were calculated. Data are expressed as mean ± SEM.

Results

Results are shown in Table 1. Plasma 5-HT levels were higher in horses fed with HF diet than horses fed with LF diet, but difference of levels was not significant (P=0.09). Tryptophan levels are slightly higher in the HF group than in the LF group (P=0.5). Irrespective of the diet, females had higher 5-HT and tryptophan levels than geldings. (P<0.05).

Conclusions

The different diets influence slightly plasma 5-HT concentrations in horses. The lower levels of plasma 5-HT measured in the LF group compared to HF group could be a reflection of the increase of abnormal behaviour patterns observed (Ellis and Visser, 2003): coprophagy, eating of bedding material, and greater excitability. Further studies are needed to clarify this preliminary data. In humans, cortisol induces an increase in the expression of the gene coding for the serotonin transporter, associated with an increase of the uptake of serotonin (Tafet *et al.*, 2001). In foals, separation from the dam significantly decreases plasma serotonin and increases cortisol concentration (Alberghina *et al.*,

Table 1. Mean (± SEM) plasma 5-HT and Tryptophan in horses (in brackets the number of horses).

	LF (9)		HF (9)	
5-HT (ng/ml)	24.56 ± 2.85		31.61 ± 2.75	
Tryptophan (µg/ml)	14.11 ± 1.25		15.50 ± 0.95	
	Females (4)	Geldings (5)	Females (6)	Geldings (3)
5-HT (ng/ml)	26.25 ± 2.46	23.20 ± 4.96	33.75 ± 2.56	27.33 ± 6.67
Tryptophan (µg/ml)	16.25 ± 1.77	13.00 ± 1.39	16.33 ± 1.10	13.83 ± 1.67

2005). In this study tryptophan levels were not affected by the diet. Our data suggest the existence of sex differences. Females showed levels of 5-HT and tryptophan higher than geldings. Many studies, carried out in animal and human species, have confirmed sexual dimorphism for serotonin (Maes and Meltzer, 1995). Plasma 5-HT is higher in women than in men (Ortiz et al., 1988), in female than in castrated male pigs (Henry et al., 1996). Furthermore, prolactin response to tryptophan increases in women but not in men (Anderson et al., 1990), suggesting a different function of brain 5-HT in women, since prolactin response to tryptophan is mediated via brain 5-HT pathways (Cowen et al., 1992). In horses, significant sex differences were found in prolactin levels (lower in geldings than in females and in stallions; Thompson et al., 1994). These results could suggest a relationship, in the horse, between 5-HT and plasma prolactin, like it is reported, in women, between platelet 5-HT and plasma prolactin (Muck-Seler et al., 2004). In further studies it should be examined whether mares are more prone to develop behavioural abnormalities (Dodman et al., 1994).

Acknowledgements

Horses were kindly supplied by the Research Institute for Animal Science, Lelystad, Netherlands.

References

Alberghina, D., S. Campo, G.M. Campo, G. Bruschetta and A.M. Ferlazzo, 2004. Atti Soc. It. Sci. Vet. 58: 6.

Alberghina, D., S. Campo, G.M. Campo, G. Bruschetta, F. Di Giovanni and A.M. Ferlazzo, 2005. Atti Soc. It. Sci. Vet. 59: 91-92.

Anderson, J.M., M. Parry-Billings, E.A. Newsholme, C.G. Fairburn and P.J. Cowen, 1990. Psycol Med. 20: 785-791.

Baguley, B.C., L. Zhuang and P. Kestell, 1997. Oncol Res. 9: 55-60.

Bailey, S.R., F.M. Cunningham and J. Elliott, 2000. Equine Vet J. 32: 497-504.

Bailey, S.R. and J. Elliott, 1998. Equine Vet J. 30: 124-130.

Cowen P.J., J.M. Anderson and C.G. Fairburn, 1992. Academic Press, San Diego, CA, pp. 269-284.

Dodman N.H., J.A. Normile, L. Shuster and W. Rand, 1994. J Am. Vet. Assoc. 204: 1219-1223.

Ellis A.D. and E.K. Visser, 2003. Proc. 54th Annual Meeting EAAP Vol.9, pp.416.

Gillham S.B., N.H. Dodman, L. Shuster, R. Kream and W. Rand, 1994. Appl.Anim.Behav. Sci. 41: 147-153.

Henry, Y., B. Seve, A. Mounier and P. Ganier, 1996. J Anim Sci. 74: 2700-2710.

Kumar, A.M., S. Weiss, J.B. Fernandez, D. Cruess and C. Eisdorfer, 1998. Gerontolog, 44: 211-216.

Lebelt, D., A.J. Zanella and J. Unshelm, 1998. Equine Vet. J., Suppl. 27: 21-27.

Lee, M.S., F.C. Cheng, H.Z. Yeh, T.Y. Liou and J.H. Liu, 2000. Clin Chem. 46: 422-423.

Maes, M. and H.Y. Meltzer, 1995. In: F.E. Bloom and D.J. Kupfer (Eds.) Psychopharmacology: The fourth generation of progress New York: Raven Press. pp. 933-944.

Muck-Seler, D, N. Pivac, M. Mustapic, Z. Crncevic, M. Jakovljevic and M. Sagud, 2004. Psychiatry Res. 127: 217-226.

Ortiz, J., F. Artigas and E. Gelpi, 1988. Life Sci. 43: 983-990.

Sarrias, M.J., P. Cabré, E. Martinez and F. Artigas, 1990. J. of Neurochemistry 54: 783-786.

Tafet, G.E., V.P. Idoyaga-Vargas, D.P. Abulafia, J.M. Calandria, S.S. Roffman, A. Chiovetta and M. Shinitzky, 2001. Cogn Affect Behav Neurosci.1: 388-393.

Thompson, D.L. Jr., C.L. DePew, A. Ortiz, L.S. Sticker and M.S. Rahmanian, 1994. J Anim Sci. 72: 2911-2918.

Management of lameness causes in sport horses

Intratendinous administration of Tendotrophin™ (Insulin-Like Growth Factor I) injection following induced tendonitis leads to superior tendon healing

Andrea Britton[1], Simon Humphrys[2] and Robyn Woodward[3]
[1]*Primegro Limited PO Box 10065 BC Adelaide SA 5000, Australia*
[2]*PO Box 1024, McLaren Flat SA 5171, Australia*
[3]*Equivet Australia Pty Ltd, m/s 465 Cambooya QLD 4358, Australia*

Take home message

The study provides evidence for accelerated tendon repair and increased type I collagen in Tendotrophin™ injection[1] treated horses compared to untreated controls.

Introduction

Suboptimal healing, prolonged rehabilitation time and a high incidence of recurrence make tendon injuries difficult to treat and manage. New tendonitis treatments are focusing on the internal repair process, especially during the early stages of healing. Insulin-like Growth Factor I (IGF-I), a natural protein found in animals that is responsible for tissue growth and repair, has proven therapeutic effects in injured tendons (Murphy and Nixon, 1997; Dahlgren *et al.*, 2002). A direct physiological function of IGF-I is to induce cellular activity, leading to new extracellular matrix synthesis by stimulating tenocyte migration and proliferation (Abrahamsson, 1997; Abrahamson and Lohmander, 1996). IGF-I also minimises the local inflammatory effect and protects tenocytes from apoptosis, thereby leaving a greater viable population of tenocytes to initiate tendon healing. These physiological effects of IGF-I have targeted it as a potential therapeutic for treating connective tissue (muscle, bone, ligament and tendon) injury in humans and veterinary medicine. This study tested this hypothesis by investigating the intrinsic equine tendon repair effects of IGF-I (two doses of 250 ug) administered intralesionally to increase the quality and rate of tendon repair.

Materials and methods

The study design was a randomised, blinded, placebo control clinical study, conducted over a three-month period using 6 treated and 6 untreated (control) horses with collagenase induced tendonitis. Key parameters measured were plasma IGF-I concentrations (ng/ml), lameness scores (0-5: not lame to severely lame), rate of change in tendon echogenicity over time (measured by mean grey scale analysis of core lesions),

---

[1] Tendotrophin™ Injection is a registered treatment for tendon injury with the Australian Pesticides and Veterinary Medicines Authority (www.apvma.gov.au).

hydroxyproline and proline content and their ratio (provides indication of total collagen content), along with the proportion of type I and type III collagen and tenocyte numbers. These key parameters provide information on the rate of tendon healing and the type of structural repair, which are the main outcomes of concern in relation to intrinsic tendonitis treatments.

Following random allocation into treatment or placebo control groups, all twelve standardbred horses used for the study had mid-metacarpal superficial digital flexor tendon lesions induced in the left foreleg with 3000 units of collagenase. At days seven and fourteen following collagenase injections, tendon core lesions were treated with an intratendinous injection of 0.1 mL (250 ug) of IGF-I (treated: n=6) or equivalent volume of 10 mM phosphate buffered saline excipient (control: n=6). Blood samples were collected prior to and following intralesional treatment with IGF-I to concurrently monitor systemic plasma IGF-I concentrations. Horses were recorded every two weeks following the collagenase-induced injury for lameness. Sequential ultrasonographic monitoring of the superficial digital flexor and deep digital flexor tendons was performed for both forelegs (*i.e.* the collagenase treated left foreleg and the untreated right foreleg) immediately prior to IGF-I treatment injections and every two weeks for the duration of the study period (14 weeks).

Mean plasma IGF-I concentrations (measured using Active® Non-Extraction IGF-I ELISA) for treatment and control groups were analysed using a repeated measures ANOVA (1 pre-treatment sample and 3 samples taken until 72 hours post IGF-I injection). Treatments were compared using a two-tailed t-test. The 72 hours time period was chosen as the half life of bound IGF-I in circulation is very short, approximately 4-8 hours. The lameness scores were compiled for each horse over the monitoring period and linear regression was used to estimate the change in lameness over time. The hypothesis that IGF-I treatment increases the rate of repair and consequently returns a horse to soundness, as characterised by a more rapid decrease in lameness, was subsequently assessed using an unpaired one-tailed t-test.

The ultrasonographic images (cross sectional and longitudinal) were used to identify the maximal injury zone. Echogenicity was measured using a mean grey scale expressed as a ratio to the echogenicity of the deep digital flexor tendon within the same leg. Normalised (corrected for the contralateral tendon echogenicity) maximal injury zone echogenicity over the 12 weeks was analysed using linear regression from which the slopes equated to the rates of lesion resolution. Slopes for lesion resolution were compared using a t-test that assessed the hypothesis that IGF-I treatment increased the rate of tendon repair.

Following euthanasia the superficial digital flexor tendons were removed from both forelimbs and longitudinal sections were used for biochemical and histological analysis, with tissue excised from the central part of the lesion. For biochemical analysis tissue was dried and ground to a fine powder. The ground powder was processed and collagenous proteins were assayed for hydroxyproline/proline concentration calculated from amino acid standards and expressed as millimoles/gram of dry tissue. These results were also normalised to the contralateral tendon and compared using a paired two-tailed t-test.

The type I and type III collagen proteins in the injured and contralateral uninjured tendons were resolved using high performance liquid chromatography. The protein types were confirmed by collecting fractions corresponding to chromatographic peaks and comparing these to type I and type III standard reference proteins (Sigma Chemical Co, St Louis, MO, USA) using SDS-PAGE. Relative collagen proportions were compared using a paired one-tailed t-test.

Tissue samples were dehydrated in increasing concentrations of ethanol followed by infiltration with paraffin wax. Samples were sectioned (8um sections), mounted and stained using haematoxylin to highlight tenocyte nuclei. Computer software (Image Pro Plus) was used to calculate the number of tenocytes present in 10 distinct microscope fields from the injured tendon. The increased cellularity hypothesis was tested by comparing the mean cell counts of IGF-I treated and control horses using a one-tailed t-test.

Results and discussion

Mean circulating plasma IGF-I concentrations were not significantly different (P=0.12) between treated and control groups. Means and standard errors from the analysis of average circulating plasma IGF-I concentration were 150 ± 17.8 ng/ml vs 187 ± 12.5 ng/ml for the treated and control groups. The decline in lameness over time between IGF-I treated and control groups was not statistically different, but did indicate a tendency towards more rapid reduction in lameness with IGF-I treatment (treated *vs.* control: -0.98 ± 0.04 vs -0.74 ± 0.04; P=0.09). The normalised rate of echogenic change over the study period was significantly (P=0.03) improved in the IGF-I treatment group over the control group (8.28 ± 1.4 vs 1.49 ± 2.2).

The biochemical analysis of core lesion hydroxyproline and proline content, and their ratio, showed that there was no significant difference between the control and IGF-I treated tendons, normalised against the contralateral tendon (ratio of 1.78 ± 0.08 *vs.* 1.84 ± 0.10; P=0.72), and without normalisation. Thus, total collagen content of the tendons for treated and control horses were similar. In contrast, the proportion of type I collagen in IGF-I treated horses was significantly greater than for the saline control group (mean type I collagen, 68.4 ± 3.6% *vs.* 52.4 ± 2.4%, treated vs control). The higher proportion of type I collagen compared to type III (mean type III, 31.7 ± 3.6% *vs.* 47.6 ± 2.4%, treated vs control, P=0.004) in the repairing core lesions has the potential to lead to superior tendon healing as type I collagen forms fibrils with larger diameters and increased mechanical strength. Histology of the core lesions showed a tendency towards increased cellularity in the IGF-I treated group compared to the placebo controls (mean cell count 292 ± 15 *vs.* 221 ± 40, treated vs control groups, P=0.06).

Recent studies by Dahlgren *et al.* (2005) assessed the temporal expression of IGF-I in healing tendon lesions. In their study it was found that the levels of tendon IGF-I become low during the early stages of tendon tissue repair. Therefore administering exogenous IGF-I into the tendon lesion during the early stages of healing seeks to boost the low tendon tissue levels and enhance the metabolic response of tenocytes, leading to a superior repair. The three month study period was chosen for this study as it is during this time period that IGF-I has its major effects. However, to assess the clinical outcome of this treatment a longer controlled study would be required with stringent criteria relating to controlled exercise rehabilitation (Dyson, 2004). This intervention study and a subsequent study (n=24, unpublished) along with Dahlgren *et al.* (2002) have all shown that early treatment of tendonitis with IGF-I improves the rate and quality of early tendon healing prior to the horse increasing controlled exercise. The treated tendon is sonographically similar to its original form and has better collagen composition to withstand the controlled exercise that is critical for a superior clinical result.

Conclusions

The intratendinous administration of two doses of IGF-I does not affect the systemic concentrations of IGF-I. Therefore the exogenous IGF-I remains and acts locally within the injured tendon. The treatment course using IGF-I increased the rate of echogenic sonographic healing, promoted the synthesis of type I collagen in preference to type III collagen and showed a tendency of stimulated tendon cellularity during the early phase of tendon repair. The relatively short study period meant that it was not possible to establish whether the IGF-I treatment improved the ability of treated horses to withstand increased levels of exercise. Nevertheless, there was good evidence for improved rates and quality of tendon healing in IGF-I treated horses.

Acknowledgements

Funding for this study conducted by the Animal Science Department of The University of Adelaide was from the Cooperative Research Centre for Tissue Growth and Repair. The authors would like to thank Aloka, Australia Pty Ltd for their generous loan of ultrasound equipment and Kerry Nyland and Frank Thomas from CSIRO Division of Health Sciences for histological and statistical analysis.

References

Abrahamsson, S.O., 1997. Similar effects of recombinant human insulin-like growth factor-I and II on cellular activities in flexor tendons of young rabbits: experimental studies *in vitro*. J. Orthop. Res. 15: 256-262.

Abrahamsson, S.O. and S. Lohmander, (1996. Differential effects of insulin-like growth factor-I on matrix and DNA synthesis in various regions and types of rabbit tendons. J. Orthop. Res. 14: 370-376.

Dahlgren, L.A., H.O. Mohammed and A.J. Nixon, 2005. Temporal expression of growth factors and matrix molecules in healing tendon lesions. J. Orthop. Res. 23: 84-92

Dahlgren, L.A., M.C. van der Meulen, J.E. Bertram, G.S. Starrak and A.J. Nixon, 2002. Insulin-like growth factor-I improves cellular and molecular aspects of healing in a collagenase-induced model of flexor tendinitis. J. Orthop. Res. 20: 910-919.

Dyson, S.J., 2004. Medical management of superficial digital flexor tendonitis: a comparative study in 219 horses (1992-2000). Equine Vet J. 36 (5) 415-419.

Murphy, D.J. and A.J. Nixon, 1997. Biochemical and site-specific effects of insulin-like growth factor I on intrinsic tenocyte activity in equine flexor tendons. AJVR. 58: 103-109.

Influence of a trimming that restores latero-medial balance of the distal limb on the distribution of forces under the foot during movement

I. Caudron, J.P. Lejeune, L. Vander Heyden, D. Votion, B. Deliege, D. Serteyn
Centre Européen du Cheval, Mont-Le-Soie 1, 6690 Vielsalm, Belgium
Faculty of Veterinary Medicine, University of Liege, B41, 4000 Liege, Belgium

Take home message

A trimming that restores latero-medial symmetry of inter-phalangeal joint space induces a more central location of the center of force on the weight bearing foot and a more balanced latero-medial distribution of forces applied on solar surface during movement.

Introduction

It is a widely accepted fact that asymmetrical bearing of weight due to abnormal conformation of a horse or inadequate trimming of hooves will cause pulling on ligaments, abnormal rotational movement of phalanges and unbalanced compressive forces in joints that predispose to articular, ligamentar and tendinous pathologies (Moyer and Anderson, 1975; Stashak, 1987; Balch *et al.*, 1991; Turner, 1996). This is especially true on thoracic limb of intensive sport horses (Denoix, 1993). Literature describes contradictory methods to obtain optimal trimming of a hoof (Watrin, 1887; Liénaux, 1912; Moyer, 1980; Russel, 1988; Pollit, 1995). Our previous work described a radiographical procedure to assess asymmetrical articular compression of the inter-phalangeal joints (Caudron *et al.*, 1996, 1997). This method enables to objectivize the effect of trimming and to restore the medio-lateral balance of inter-phalangeal joints according to individual conformation of each horse. The current study shows the effect of a trimming that cancel articular pinching in the distal limb on location of the centre of force under the weight bearing foot and on latero-medial repartition of forces under solar surface during movement.

Material and methods

Four clinically sound barefoot warmblood horses were equiped for this experiment. Four reflective markers were glued on each front limb. Two on the lateral aspect of forearm give cranio-caudal inclination of the limb: lateral tuberosity of the radius and ulnar styloid process. Two on the dorsal aspect of canon-bone give latero-medial inclination of the limb: dorso-medial metacarpal tuberosity and sagittal ridge of third metacarpal bone. Three-dimensional trajectory of these markers were followed by the cinematic Elite® system. An in-foot shoe force sensor (4 sensors/cm^2) was trimmed to the tall of front hoof and sandwiched between two thin PVC protective plates to avoid impairment of sensing locations. The assembling was inserted in an Equi boot®. Two front limbs of each horse were equipped with instrumented Equi boot® (Figure 1) and connected to a computer loaded with the F-scan® software that enabled to follow the distribution of vertical forces under equine foot in motion. The systems were calibrated. Horses were put on a treadmill, warmed up and accustomed to their accessories at walk and trot. Information provided by the in-shoe foot sensors and the Elite® system were recorded at trot (4m/s) when the gait was stabilized. A sequence of 800 frames was recorded at a frequency of 100 frames/sec. This corresponded to storage of data during about twelve trot strides.

Two data sets were analyzed from Fscan® system. First were coordinates (X and Y) of the centre of force (COF) under the foot at mid stance phase. This moment was determined on a "force versus time" graphic that displayed the sum of forces sensed on a frame-by-frame basis. The mid stance phase corresponded to the moment when the sum of forces sensed was maximal. For this frame, coordinates of the centre of force (X and Y) were automatically calculated by the computer. The COF was visualized on a two-dimensional display on which the theoretical location of the palmar centre of figure (perpendicular to distal inter-phalangeal joint center) could also be represented.

The second data set was the total of forces sensed under the lateral part of foot (LTF) and the total forces sensed under the medial part of foot (MTF) during one stride. On the two-dimensional view, the window was separated in two similar focus zones, a lateral

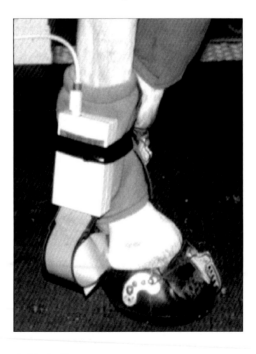

Figure 1. A foot equipped with the F-scan system.

and a medial one. A graph "force versus time" was obtained for each zone. The area under the curve of their graphic corresponded to the integrated forces during one stride. Lateral and medial total forces (LTF/MTF) were calculated by computer to obtain the rapport LTF/MTF.

The Elite® system measures the inclination of the canon bone (angulation between the vector formed by markers of the dorsal part of the canon-bone and a reference vertical line) at mid stance (when the vector formed by the markers of the lateral part of forearm is vertical).

All of these data were recorded before and after trimming according to a specific radiographical procedure called "angles method" that quantifies articular pinching or asymmetrical joint compression due to inadequate hoof trimming regarding to the individual conformation of the horse. Before the specific radiological evaluation, the foot was cleaned so that the white line was visible. The exact position of the toe was determined either by reference to a triangular, dark coloured fault in the white line that corresponded to the indentation of the third phalanx, or by tracing a straight line between the centre of the central cleft, the apex of the frog and the white line. A rigid metal wire was stuck to the front of the hoof wall from this point, aligned parallel to the hoof horn tubules. To mimic the situation of the weight bearing foot during movement when loads were maximum on the distal limb, the horse was made to stand on one foot on a rotating support so that it could take its most natural position. Furthermore the horse was positioned so as the inclination of its canon-bone corresponded to the value measured by the Elite® system in movement. A dorso-palmar X-ray was taken, centred on the coronary band with radiation beam parallel to the sagittal plane of the foot. The radiograph was valid if projection of the metal marker, placed on the toe, passed through the frog's central cleft confirming that the RX beam was parallel to the sagittal plane of foot. Two angles were measured on each radiograph: P1g was the angle between the perpendicular line to the tangent to the articular surface of the proximal phalanx and the ground. P3g was the angle between the perpendicular line to the tangent to the articular surface of the distal phalanx and the ground. The difference between P1g and P3g quantifies latero-medial inter-phalangeal pinching (Figure 2). The feet were trimmed to take off the excessive horn on the side of the articular pinching to cancel the possible joint asymmetrical compression.

After corrective trimming, the radiographical procedure was carried out again to confirm that latero-medial balance of the interphalangeal joints was obtained. When P1g equalled P3g the distal articular surface of the proximal phalanx and the articular surface of the distal phalanx were parallel, inter-phalangeal pinching was nil and latero-medial balance was obtained (Figure 3). If it was not the case the trimming continued and a new radiographical control completed. This was repeated so that inter-phalangeal pinching was cancelled. The experience of our farrier enabled us to reduce the number of attempts. In some cases the expected result can not be achieved due to insufficient horn material.

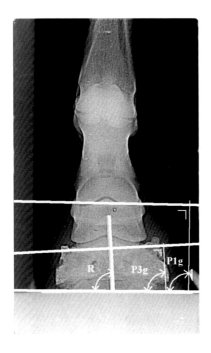 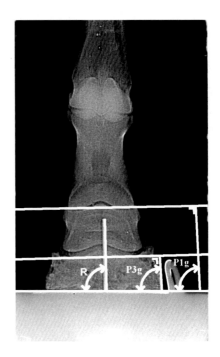

Figure 2. Angles Method before trimming. P1g-P3g = 3° = lateral inter-phalangeal pinching.

Figure 3. Angles Method after lateral corrective trimming. P1g-P3g = 0 = inter-phalangeal balance.

A new set of Elite® and Fscan® data were taken on treadmill after the final corrective trimming.

Results and conclusions

Data from eight front limbs were analyzed. Before trimming we observed a medial canon-bone inclination at mid stance phase (mean value 4.32° +/- 1,98) a lateral inter-phalangeal compression on all limbs (mean value 3,13° +/- 1,48), a COF at mid stance phase located laterally from the palmar centre of figure (mean value 1,07 cm +/- 1.2) and more lateral distribution of forces under the foot during a stride (LTF/MTF mean value 1,98 +/- 0.64) (Table 1).

After corrective trimming the canon-bone inclination was not significantly modified (mean value 4.29° +/- 1.60), the lateral interphalangeal compression was diminished (mean value 1,31° +/- 1.46), a COF at mid stance phase located closer to the palmar centre of figure (mean value 0.29 cm +/- 0.7) and a more balanced distribution of force under the foot during a stride (LTF/MTF mean value 1,29+/-0.52) (Figure 4).

Table 1. Results.

	Before trimming	After trimming
Canon-bone inclination	4.32° +/- 1.98	4.29° +/- 1.60
Articular pinching	3.13° +/- 1.48	1.31° +/- 1.46
COF position	1.07 cm +/- 1.20	0.29 cm +/- 0.7 0
LTF/MTF	1.98 +/- 0.64	1.29 +/- 0.52

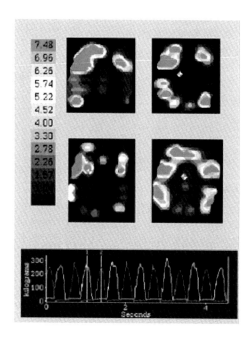

Figure 4. Distribution of forces under the foot at mid stance phase provided by the F-scan system. Left side of the picture before trimming: lateral surcharge of the foot and lateral position of the COF. Right side of the picture after lateral corrective trimming: more balanced distribution of forces and central position of the COF.

During the radiographical procedure we also noticed that the canon-bone inclination in unipodal situation before trimming does not correspond naturally to the inclination measured by the Elite® system at mid stance phase. After corrective trimming these two angulations tended to equalize themselves.

Despite that these results have to be confirmed on a larger sample, this study showed the corrective trimming diminished lateral inter-phalangeal compressions and does not seem to alter the sagittal inclination of the limb at mid stance phase. On the other hand it made the COF at mid stance phase move towards the palmar centre of figure that is located straight below the distal inter-phalangeal joint centre and improved latero-medial balance of forces under the foot during movement. These could have a beneficial impact on joint mechanics of the distal limb resulting in more comfortable sport horses. It could also delay the onset and development of osteo-articular pathologies.

References

Balch, O., K. White and D. Butler, 1991. Factors involved in the balancing of equine hooves. J. Am. Vet. Med. Assoc. 198: 1980-1989.

Caudron, I., M. Miesen, S. Grulke, P. Vanschepdael and D. Serteyn, 1996. Evaluation radiologique de l'équilibre biomécanique du pied dans les plans frontal et sagittal. Prat. Vét. Equine 28: 41-46.

Caudron, I., M. Miesen, S. Grulke, P. Vanschepdael and D. Serteyn, 1997. Clinical and radiological assessment of corrective trimming in lame horses. J. Equine Vet. Sc. 17: 375-379.

Denoix, J.-M., 1993. Biomécanique inter-phalangienne dans les plans sagittal et frontal, in Proceedings Swiss Vet. 11-S: 44-49.

Lienaud, E., 1912. Précis du cours de maréchalerie (Ed. Bothy, Bruxelles).

Moyer, W. and J.P. Anderson, 1975. Diagonal imbalance of the equine foot: a cause of lameness. In: Proceedings 38th Ann. Conv. Am. Assoc. Equine Practn., pp. 413-418.

Moyer, W., 1980. Corrective Shoeing. The Veterinary Clinics of North America, Saunders CY, London, Toronto.

Pollit, C., 1995. Color Atlas of the horse's foot. Times Mirror International.

Russel, W., 1988. Scientific Horseshoeing. Reprinted 10th ed. (1903), Loose Change publications, California.

Stashak, T.S., 1987. Adam's Lameness in Horses. 4th ed., Lea & Febiger, Philadelphia.

Turner, T., 1996. Lameness of the distal interphalangeal joint. Equine Pract. 18: 15-19.

Watrin, A., 1887. Le pied du cheval et sa ferrure. (Eds Théolier St-Etienne, France.

Adrenocorticotropin and cortisol response to competitive and not competitive races in Thoroughbreds of different age

C. Cravana, P. Medica, E. Fazio, F. Di Giovanni and A. Ferlazzo
Department of Morphology, Biochemistry, Physiology and Animal Production, Unit of Physiology, Faculty of Veterinary Medicine, University of Messina, Italy

Take home message

ACTH and cortisol levels increased after gallop during both competitive and not competitive races. Sampling time influences hormone concentrations. Age does not have an effect on ACTH and cortisol concentration changes after galloping.

Introduction

The hypotalamic-pituitary-adrenal (HPA) axis is a neuroendocrine system highly involved in the coping response to metabolic and stressful challenges. Physical exercise is a physiological challenge that induces threshold- and intensity-dependent HPA response. This has been well documented in horses by significant increases in plasma ACTH (Fazio *et al.*, 1999; Marc *et al.*, 2000) and serum cortisol concentrations (Linden *et al.*, 1991; Rose and Hodgson, 1994; Ferlazzo and Fazio, 1997; Alberghina *et al.*, 2000; Lindner *et al.*, 2000, 2002; Green *et al.*, 2002; Medica *et al.*, 2004; Ferlazzo *et al.*, 2005). ACTH responses were significantly correlated to treadmill velocity (Kurosawa *et al.*, 1998). The intensity of exercise had a larger influence than the duration of exercise in racehorses during standardized exercise test (SET) on treadmill (Nagata *et al.*, 1999). Serum cortisol response appeared to be related to the type (Ferlazzo and Fazio, 1997), duration and intensity of exercise (Raidal *et al.* 2000; 2001). Furthermore, emotional stress seemed to influence adrenocortical activity during competitive events (Ferlazzo *et al.*, 1998; Fazio *et al.*, 2000). On this basis, the aim of this study was to examine the effects of exercise on hypophysis-adrenocortical response of Thoroughbreds of different age to competitive and not competitive races.

Materials and methods

The research was carried out on 10 healthy Thoroughbreds (n= 6 males and n= 4 females), weighing 452 ± 15 kg, and divided in two groups: Group I, 2 year old horses (n = 4); Group II, >3 year old horses (n = 6). All horses were already accustomed to be trained for competition and at the end of a training period of 3 months were submitted to two different exercise conditions on a 1,600 m turf track: not competitive (Race 1) and competitive (Race 2) race.

During Race 1 each horse galloped over 1600 m at a velocity of 12-14 m/s for the first 1,000 m and of 14-16 m/s for the last 600 m. After 3 days, all racehorses were submitted to a competition over 1,600 m (Race 2). During Race 2 the velocity was maintained at 16-18 m/s in the first 1,000 m and at 18 m/s in the last 600 m.

Blood samples were collected from jugular vein prior to exercise (08.00 - 09.00 a. m.) and at 5 and 30 minutes post exercise.

Plasma ACTH concentrations were analysed in duplicate by RIA (ELSA–ACTH, CIS Diagnostics). Serum cortisol concentrations were analysed in duplicate by immunoenzymatic assay (RADIM).

Data are presented as mean ± standard deviation (SD). To determine the effects of race type and age, a two-way analysis of variance with repeated measures (RM ANOVA) was applied. When the F statistic was significant, differences between individual means were assessed with a post hoc test (Bonferroni). The comparison between races was done with the paired t-test. The level of significance was set at <0.05. Percentage differences (Δ%) between values recorded in basal condition and at different post exercise times were calculated.

Results

There was a significant interaction between time and race type on ACTH levels both in Group I (F = 10.5; $p < 0.002$) and in Group II (F = 21.0; $p < 0.0001$). In addition, time had a significant effect on ACTH levels both in Group I (F = 74.7; $p < 0.0001$) and in Group II (F = 161; $p < 0.0001$). Finally, race type had a significant effect in both groups (Group I: F = 62.9; $p < 0.0002$; Group II: F= 78.2; $p < 0.0001$).

After Race 1, plasma ACTH concentrations (Table 1) showed a significant increase at 5 min (+ 343%; $p < 0.001$) in Group I and at 5 min (+ 542%; $p < 0.001$) in Group II.

After Race 2, plasma ACTH levels were significantly increased at 5 (+ 487%; $p < 0.001$) and 30 min (+ 206%; $p < 0.001$) in Group I and at 5 min (+ 691%; $p < 0.001$) and 30 min (+ 210%; $p < 0.001$) in Group II.

The two-way RM ANOVA showed a significant interaction between time and race type on cortisol levels in both groups (Group I: F = 19.3; $p < 0.0002$; Group II: F = 43.1; $p < 0.0001$). In addition, time had a significant effect on cortisol levels both in Group I (F = 44.7; $p < 0.0001$) and in Group II (F = 88.8; $p < 0.0001$). Finally, race type was significant both in Group I (F = 49.3; $p < 0.0004$) and in Group II (F= 70.0; $p < 0.0001$).

Data obtained (Table 2) showed a significant increase of circulating cortisol concentrations 30 min (+ 39.5%; $p < 0.05$) after Race 1 in Group II only.

Table 1. Plasma ACTH levels (Mean ± SD) of Thoroughbreds during not competitive (Race 1) and competitive (Race 2) races.

Plasma ACTH (pmol/l)	Race 1		Race 2	
	Group I (n=4) 2 years	Group II (n=6) >3 years	Group I (n=4) 2 years	Group II (n=6) >3 years
Basal	3.57 ± 1.00	2.59 ± 0.98	5.50 ± 1.79[A]	4.50 ± 2.43
5 minutes	15.8 ± 3.36[a]	16.6 ± 1.99[a]	32.3 ± 6.27[aA]	35.6 ± 7.05[aB]
30 minutes	4.59 ± 1.78	3.55 ± 0.69	16.8 ± 2.11[aB]	13.9 ± 2.36[aC]

vs. basal: a= $P<0.001$.
vs. race 1: A= $P<0.05$; B= $P<0.01$; C= $P<0.001$.

Table 2. Serum cortisol levels (Mean ± SD) of Thoroughbreds during not competitive (Race 1) and competitive (Race 2) races.

Serum Cortisol (nmol/l)	Race 1		Race 2	
	Group I (n=4) 2 years	Group II (n=6) >3 years	Group I (n=4) 2 years	Group II (n=6) >3 years
Basal	170 ± 7.17	176 ± 14.8	175 ± 8.55	162 ± 12.6
5 minutes	257 ± 51.5	224 ± 25.3	455 ± 96.0[bA]	425 ± 7.7[bA]
30 minutes	260 ± 71.7	246 ± 16.8[a]	632 ± 79.1[bA]	552 ± 8.0[bB]

vs. basal: a= $P<0.05$; b= $P<0.001$.
vs. race 1: A= $P<0.01$; B= $P<0.001$.

After Race 2, serum cortisol levels were significantly increased at 5 min (+ 171%; p<0.001) and 30 min (+ 261%; p<0.001) in Group I and at 5 min (+ 163%; p<0.001) and 30 min (+ 242%; p<0.001) in Group II.

The two-way RM ANOVA showed that both the age and the interaction between age and time were not significant for all parameters.

Considerations

The results showed that gallop influences the HPA axis response, as already described in literature (Ferlazzo and Fazio, 1997; Lindner *et al.*, 2000; Marc *et al.*, 2000; Green *et al.*, 2002), showing that competitive and not competitive races induced ACTH and cortisol responses at 5 and 30 minutes after racing. Higher increases were recorded after competitive racing as compared to not competitive racing. The highest hormone levels were recorded when the horses were submitted to competition racing and this could be result of the high intensity of exercise and the psychological competition stimuli. The age-time interaction did not have an effect on ACTH and cortisol concentration modifications after gallop. However, the significantly higher ACTH basal levels, recorded in 2-yr-old horses during competitive racing as compared to the basal values of the same horses before the not competitive racing, may indicate the major sensitivity of their HPA axis, due to the greater emotional impact in inexperienced horses. Moreover, the lower ACTH and cortisol levels recorded 30 minutes after both race types in over 3-yrs-old horses, as compared to younger horses, could be related to a better recovery ability as result of training.

References

Alberghina, D., P. Medica, V. Aronica, A. Lindner and A. Ferlazzo, 2000. Atti Soc it Sci vet 54: 89-90.

Fazio, E., P. Medica, A. Lindner and A. Ferlazzo, 1999. Atti So F I Vet 3: 55-59.

Fazio, E., D. Alberghina, V. Aronica, P. Medica and A. Ferlazzo, 2000. In: The Elite Show Jumper. A. Lindner (ed), Dr Arno Lindner Science Consult, Jülich, Germany, pp. 113-115.

Ferlazzo, A. and E. Fazio, 1997. In: Performance diagnosis of horses. Lindner A (ed), Wageningen Pers, Wageningen, pp. 30-43

Ferlazzo, A., E. Fazio, V. Aronica, R. Di Majo, P. Medica and L. Grasso, 1998. In: Proc Conf on Equine Sports Med and Sci, A. Lindner (ed), Wageningen Pers,Wageningen, pp. 53-56,

Ferlazzo, A., P. Medica and E. Fazio, 2005. Chapter 11. In: Training del Caballo de deporte. Respuesta y Adaptación, F. Boffi (ed), Editorial Intermedica Saici, in press.

Green, H.M., E.A. Cogger, T.L. Miltenberger, A.k. Koch, R.E. Bray and S.J. Wickler, 2002. Equine Vet J Suppl 30: 545-550.

Kurosawa, M., S. Nagata, F. Takeda, K. Mima, A. Hiraga, M. Kai and K. Taya, 1998. J Equine Sci 9: 9-18.

Linden, A., T. Art, H. Amory, D. Desmecht and P. Lekeux, 1991. In: Equine Exercise Physiology 3. S.G.B. Persson, A. Lindholm and L.B. Jeffcott (eds), ICEEP Publications Davis, California, pp 391-396.

Lindner, A., E. Fazio, A.M. Ferlazzo, P. Medica and A. Ferlazzo, 2000. Pferdeilkunde 16: 502-510.

Lindner, A., E. Fazio, P. Medica and A. Ferlazzo, 2002. Pferdeilkunde 18: 51-56.

Marc, M., N. Parvizi, F. Ellendorff, E. Kallweit and F. Elsaesser, 2000. J Anim Sci 78: 1936-1946.

Medica, P., C. Cravana, D. Alberghina, E. Fazio and A. Ferlazzo, 2004. In: The Elite Race and Endurance Horse. A. Lindner (ed), pp 196-200, Dr Arno Lindner Science Consult, Essen (Germany)

Nagata, S., F. Takeda, M. Kurosawa, K. Mima, A. Hiraga, M. Kai and K. Taya, 1999. Equine Vet J Suppl 30: 570-574.

Raidal, S.L., D.N. Love, G.D. Bailey and R.J. Rose, 2000. Res Vet Sci 68: 246-253.

Raidal, S.L., R.J. Rose and D.N. Love, 2001. Equine Vet J 33: 238-243.

Rose, R.J. and D.R. Hodgson, 1994. In: The Athletic Horse: Principles and Practice of Equine Sports Medicine. D.R. Hodgson and R.J. Rose (eds), WB Saunders Comp, Philadelphia, pp. 63-78.

Bone marrow mononucleated cells (BMMNCs) are able to synthesize type I collagen similar to cultured bone marrow stromal cells (cBMSC) in an equine model of collagenase-induced tendonitis: A preliminary study

A. Crovace[1], L. Lacitignola[2], R. De Siena[1], G. Rossi[3] and E. Francioso[1]
[1]*Dipartimento dell' Emergenza e dei Trapianti di Organi (D.E.T.O.), Sezione di Chirurgia Veterinaria, Facoltà di Medicina Veterinaria, Università degli Studi di Bari, Italy*
[2] *Dipartimento dell' Scienze Cliniche Veterinarie, Sezione di Chirurgia Veterinaria, Facoltà di Medicina Veterinaria, Università degli Studi di Teramo, Italy*
[3]*Dipartimento dell' Scienze Cliniche Veterinarie, Università degli Studi di Camerino, Macerata, Italy*

Take home message

Both bone marrow mononucleated cells (BMMNCs) and cultured bone marrow stromal cells (cBMSCs) regenerate experimental tendon injury in the horse.

Introduction

In both horses and humans tendon injuries have a considerable impact on athletic performance. Tissue damage to tendons produces lameness that lasts several months, and is so severe that a return to the previous level of sportive activity is compromised despite what is considered appropriate orthopaedic care (Sharma and Maffuli, 2005; Smith and Webbon, 2005). Traditional therapies are often palliative at best and do not lead to complete regeneration of tendon tissue, which has important consequences for the athlete, human and horse alike, in terms of impaired performance and a substantial risk of re-injury (Sharma and Maffuli, 2005; Smith, 2004). New methods of modulating tendon repair, aimed at improving the quality and speed of tissue healing, have been investigated. Numerous studies in experimental animals have shown that transplantation of mesenchymal stem cells (MSCs) into injured musculo-skeletal tissues promote healing, most notably in skeletal and cardiac muscle (Smith, 2004; Fortier, 2005; Smith *et al.*, 2003). Smith *et al.* proposed the use of autologous BM-derived MSCs in spontaneous tendon lesions in horses (Smith, 2004; Smith and Webbon, 2005; Smith *et al.*, 2003) which produced optimal regeneration of injured tendon tissue. Despite these very promising results, the previously reported techniques carry some disadvantages that may prevent their widespread use in clinical equine practice due to the necessary in-vitro cell culturing of harvested BM cells.

Bone marrow mononucleated cells (BMMNCs) could be an alternative cell source for obtaining MSCs. Their use has been reported in the treatment of myocardial infarct lesions, bone defect reconstruction, and ischemia-reperfusion injury in muscle (Blatt *et al.*, 2005; Cho *et al.*, 2005; Crovace *et al.*, 2004a, b; Hisatome *et al.*, 2005; Ryu *et al.*, 2005; Tateishi-Yuyama *et al.*, 2002; Tse *et al.*, 2003). The idea of using BMMNC autografts is based on the assumption that MSCs among the mononucleated cells, which are present in only small numbers in BM aspirates, can be easily separated ex-vivo from the rest of the harvested cells, concentrated in small volume, and then immediately implanted into the patient's injured tissue, where the microenvironment will trigger their replication and differentiation into specialized cells. This method does not require cell culturing, and lacks any risk of immune reactions as the grafts are autologous in nature. Thus, the aim of this study was to compare tendon healing following transplantation of cBMSCs, BMMNCs, and placebo in an equine model of collagenase-induced tendonitis.

Materials and methods

The study was performed at the School of Veterinary Medicine, University of Bari, after having obtained approval from the Ministery of Health, Rome, Italy. Three male Standardbred horses, 4 years old, were used in this investigation. In each horse, in three limbs (left front, right front, and right hind) 4000 IU of *Cl. histolyticum* Type 1A collagenase were injected in each superficial digital flexor tendon (SDFT) under ultrasonographic guidance in zone 2B. The left hindlimb was not injected and used as sham control. After 3 weeks the lesions were evaluated clinically and ultrasonographically.

For BM aspiration horses were sedated with IV detomidine (20 µg/kg) and butorphanol (10 µg/kg). Following aseptic skin preparation and subcutaneous infiltration of 40 mL 2% lidocaine, BM was harvested twice from the horses' ileal crest, an average 35 mL per day of collagenase injection for production of cBMSCs; an average 46 mL on day T_0 (day 21 after collagenase injection) for processing of BMMNCs. The BM aspirate was immediately transported to the on-site laboratory. Preparations of both cBMSCs and BMMNCs for later transplantation into the lesions of the tendons were then obtained employing procedures previously described by our group (Crovace *et al.*, 2004a, b; Lacitignola *et al.*, 2005). The first passage of cBMSCs that was obtained after 3 weeks of cultivation contained on average 5.5×10^6 cells, which were suspended in a mean of 3.13 ± 1.93 mL of fibrinogen solution for transplantation into the tendon. The number of BMMNCs that were prepared in the laboratory for tendon injection was $122.3 \pm 23.1 \times 10^6$, with cells being suspended in a mean volume of 3.13 ± 1.93 mL of fibrinogen solution.

On the day of transplantation, horses were sedated as described before and under local anaesthesia with lidocaine 2% a 21-ga needle was inserted into the tendon lesion using ultrasonographic guidance. Subsequently, either cBMSC or BMMNC suspension or placebo (= saline; 1 mL) was injected to fill the defect in the tendon. Immediately after injection into the lesion a small amount of thrombin was added to clot the suspension.

Ultrasound (US) examinations were performed with a 7.5 MHz linear probe prior to collagenase injection (T_{-3}) and 0 (day of treatment), 1, 3, 6, 8, 12, 16, 18, and 21 weeks ($T_0 - T_{21}$) following tendon treatment. The following parameters were determined to quantify the degree and time-related changes of the SDFT lesion: type lesion echo score (TLS), fibre pattern score (FPS) and the percentage of cross-sectional area of the lesion (% CSA-l) assessed in the zone of maximum injury (MIZ).

At T_{21} animals were euthanized and SDFTs of all four limbs were harvested and processed for microscopic tissue examination. Quantitative data are reported as mean ± s.d.. Statistical analysis included a 2-way analysis of variance (ANOVA) for repeated measures with the confidence level set at $P < 0.05$.

Results

Three weeks following collagenase injection (T_0) US examination revealed significant SDFT lesions in all 3 legs without significant differences between limbs. The experimentally induced lesions were on average 36.5 ± 8.2 mm wide, with a ratio of lesion CSA to tendon CSA at the MIZ of 30.5 ± 13.8%. At T_0 Type lesion score were -2.8 ± 0.4 and FPS were 2.8 ± 0.4.

The number of culture dish-adhered BM stem cells that can form a colony was quantified as colony forming units of fibroblasts (CFU-f). Prior to Ficoll gradient centrifugation the original BM aspirate consisted of a mean of 428 ± 223 CFU-f per mL (pre-Ficoll) while post centrifugation (post-Ficoll) the number rose to 1697 ± 785 CFU-f per mL.

At T_8, US determination of% CSA-l revealed no statistical difference between tendons treated with cBMSC or BMMNCs, while% CSA-1 was significantly larger in placebo (saline)- injected SDFTs ($P < 0.05$). At this time point FPS and TLS were still below baseline (T_{-3}) values, but had substantially improved when compared to previous examinations. From T_{16} on and consistently until T_{21},% CSA-l, FPS and TLS were significantly different among SDFTs undergoing the three different treatments.

In cBMSC- and BMMNC-treated SDFTs microscopic examination at T_{21} revealed longitudinal orientation of newly formed collagen fibrils. In Herovici stain the presence of Methyl blue -stained (blue) fibrils mixed with acid fuchsin-stained (red) fibrils indicated still somewhat incomplete collagen maturation at this time point following treatment. In BMMNC-treated SDFTs also large numbers of mononucleated cells were present in the interfascicular zone. In placebo-injected SDFTs the tissue architecture was completely disrupted with collagen fibrils being randomly oriented.

Immunohistochemistry stains for type I and III collagen, COMP revealed a high expression of type I collagen and COMP in cBMSC- and BMMNCs-injected tendons, but very low expression of type III collagen. In contrast, in all three placebo-treated SDFTs the location of the lesion was readily identified as an area that was highly positive for type III collagen with very low expression of type I collagen and COMP and showed in some zones evidence for mineralization.

Discussion

Our study demonstrates that cultivation of BM stem cells without prior gradient centrifugation of the native BM aspirate (pre-Ficoll) yields a significantly lower number of CFU-f as compared to cultivation following gradient separation of the same BM sample. This finding also proves that BMSCs, when undergoing gradient centrifugation procedure, maintain not only viability but also their ability to clone and differentiate into fibroblastoid cells. In our experiments we studied for the first time simultaneously, *i.e.* in the same animal, the effects of cBMSCs, BMMNCs and placebo (saline) injection on tendon healing following an experimentally (collagenase-) induced tissue injury and compared the results with a sham control (intact tendon).

Our preliminary results provide evidence that in the horse regeneration of injured tendon tissue can be achieved with injection of both cBMSCs and BMMNCs into the lesion while injection of placebo (saline) leads to a repair of the lesion with scar tissue. Extracellular matrix characteristics were equally well restored in both cell graft groups with type I collagen fibrils greatly dominating over type III collagen fibres, and type I collagen fibrils being longitudinally oriented with high expression of COMP. In contrast, in placebo-treated lesions type III collagen formation predominated while type I collagen and COMP was only minimally expressed and fibrils were also randomly oriented. With respect to the presence of some immature collagen in both cBMSC- and BMMNC-treated groups, we may only speculate that the finding was due to the minimal mechanical loading due to prolonged stall rest in this group of animals.

In conclusion this study is the first one to describe the efficacy of BMMNC injection in an experimental tendonitis model in the horse. Use of BMMNCs offers significant advantages in terms of progress and quality of tendon healing when compared to native BM implantation. Although both cBMSC and BMMNC injection produced similarly good regeneration of tendon tissue in terms of quality of extracellular matrix produced, the use of BMMNCs is a more simple and cost-effective method than the use of cultured BMSCs, and thus its introduction into equine clinical practice is expected to have a great impact on tendon injury treatment in the future.

References

Blatt, A., G. Cotter, M. Leitman, R. Krakover, E. Kaluski, O. Milo-Cotter *et al.*, 2005. Intracoronary administration of autologous bone marrow mononuclear cells after induction of short ischemia is safe and may improve hibernation and ischemia in patients with ischemic cardiomyopathy. Am Heart J 150: 986.

Cho, S.W., H.J. Park, J.H. Ryu, S.H. Kim, Y.H. Kim, C.Y. Choi *et al.*, 2005. Vascular patches tissue-engineered with autologous bone marrow-derived cells and decellularized tissue matrices. Biomaterials 26: 1915-1924.

Crovace, A., E. Francioso, J. Hendry and R. Quarto, 2004a. Use of autologous bone marrow stromal cells (BMSC) and resorbable bone graft substitute in dogs with orthopedic lesions. Vet Surg 33: 435-E25.

Crovace, A., E. Francioso, J. Hendry and R. Quarto, 2004b. Use of autogenous bone marrow stromal cells (BMSC) and resorbable scaffolds in dogs with bone loss. VCOT 18: A27 (16).

Fortier, L.A., 2005. Stem cells: classifications, controversies, and clinical applications. Vet Surg 34: 415-423.

Hisatome, T., Y. Yasunaga, S. Yanada, Y. Tabata, Y. Ikada and M. Ochi, 2005. Neovascularization and bone regeneration by implantation of autologous bone marrow mononuclear cells. Biomaterials 26: 4550-4556.

Lacitignola, L., G. Ferlan, R. De Siena, E. Francioso and A. Crovace, 2005. Trapianto autologo di cellule mononucleate di midollo (BMMNCs) nelle lesioni tendinee nel cavallo. In: Proceedings of XII Congresso Nazionale SICV, Pisa, pp. 85-87.

Ryu, J.H., I.K. Kim, S.W. Cho, M.C. Cho, K.k. Hwang, H. Piao et al., 2005. Implantation of bone marrow mononuclear cells using injectable fibrin matrix enhances neovascularization in infarcted myocardium. Biomaterials 26: 319-326.

Sharma, P. and N. Maffulli, 2005. Tendon injury and tendinopathy: healing and repair. J Bone Joint Surg Am 87: 187-202.

Smith, R.K., 2004. Autogenous stem cell implantation. Vet Surg 33: 199-201 E.

Smith, R.K. and P.M. Webbon, 2005. Harnessing the stem cell for the treatment of tendon injuries: heralding a new dawn? Br J Sports Med 39: 582-584.

Smith, R.K., M. Korda, G.W. Blunn and A.E. Goodship, 2003. Isolation and implantation of autologous equine mesenchymal stem cells from bone marrow into the superficial digital flexor tendon as a potential novel treatment. Equine Vet J 35: 99-102.

Tateishi-Yuyama, E., H. Matsubara, T. Murohara, U. Ikeda, S. Shintani, H. Masaki et al., 2002. Therapeutic angiogenesis for patients with limb ischaemia by autologous transplantation of bone-marrow cells: a pilot study and a randomised controlled trial. Lancet 360: 427-435.

Tse, H.F., Y.L. Kwong, J.K. Chan, G. Lo, C.L. Ho and C.P. Lau, 2003. Angiogenesis in ischaemic myocardium by intramyocardial autologous bone marrow mononuclear cell implantation. Lancet 361: 47-49.

Serum cortisol levels of Quarter Horses: Circadian variations and effects of training and western riding events

E. Fazio, G. Calabrò, P. Medica, C. Messineo and A. Ferlazzo
Department of Morphology, Biochemistry, Physiology and Animal Production. Unit of Physiology, Faculty of Veterinary Medicine, University of Messina, Italy

Take home message

Sedentary Quarter Horses do not exhibit a clear cortisol circadian pattern. Six weeks of western type training induce increased basal cortisol levels. Barrel Racing and Pole Bending events increase post exercise cortisol levels.

Introduction

Western riding events require both anaerobic and aerobic components during contraction of skeletal muscle. Previous studies in Quarter Horses examined the circadian variations of β-endorphin (Calabrò *et al.*, 2003) and the effects of training on total and free iodothyronines and estradiol-17β levels (Fazio *et al.*, 2004, 2005; Medica *et al.*, 2005 a, b). The relationship between adrenocortical function and physical exercise of athletic horses have been often examined (Rose and Hodgson, 1994; Ferlazzo and Fazio, 1997; McKeever, 2002; Ferlazzo *et al.*, 2005), but not in horses used for western riding events.

The aim of this study was to evaluate the circadian variations of serum cortisol of sedentary Quarter Horses and the effects of training and different western riding events.

Materials and methods

10 healthy Quarter Horses (3-20 years old; 3 anoestrus mares, 3 stallions and 4 geldings) were studied. To examine the circadian variation blood samples were collected every four hours, from 5.30 a.m. to 5.30 a.m. of the day after, in sedentary conditions. To examine the effects of training, horses were then submitted to a conventional 6 weeks training for western riding. Blood samples were collected from the jugular vein at the different weeks, at 09.00 a.m., in basal conditions.

In order to examine the effects of exercise, horses were submitted to Reining, Cutting, Barrel Racing and Pole Bending events and blood samples collected before and 5, 30 min and 24 hours post exercise.

Serum cortisol concentrations were analysed in duplicate by immunoenzymatic assay (RADIM).

Data are presented as mean ± standard deviation (SD). To determine the effect of time, training and exercise an analysis of variance for repeated measures was applied. A paired t-test to compare data obtained at the different sampling times during a day, at the different weeks of training and at the different post exercise times with respect to basal levels was applied. The level of significance was set at <0.05. Percentage differences (Δ%) were also calculated.

Results

An increase of cortisol levels (Figure 1) from 5.30 a.m. to 5.30 p.m. and a successive decrease from 5.30 p.m. to 5.30 a.m. was observed (F = 2.55; $p<0.05$). No statistical differences between the different times and the different ages were obtained. Stallions and geldings showed significant higher cortisol levels than mares at 5.30 a.m. ($p<0.005$; $p<0.01$).

Training (Table 1) induced serum cortisol increase at the 2nd (+61.1%), 3rd (+93.0%; $p<0.02$), 4th (+47.2%) and 5th (+64.1%) week, and a decrease at the 6th (-34.5%; $p<0.05$) week. A significant effect of training (F=10.61; $p<0.001$) was shown.

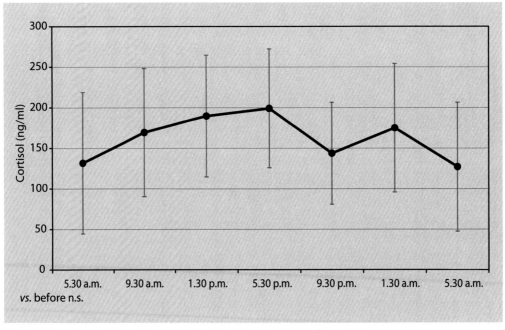

Figure 1. Circadian variations of serum cortisol levels (means ± S.D.) of Quarter Horses.

Table 1: Serum cortisol levels (mean ± SD) of Quarter Horses during 6 weeks of training.

Serum Cortisol (ng/ml)	
1st	69.9 ± 28.0
2nd	113 ± 64.0
3rd	135 ± 59.6*
4th	103 ± 62.5
5th	115 ± 55.7
6th	45.8 ± 15.1**
ANOVA	F=10.6 p<0.001

vs. 1st week: * p<0.02; ** p<0.05.

Cortisol levels showed (Table 2) a progressive decrease at 5 min (-5.2%), 30 min (-15.5%) and 24 h (-20.8%) after Reining; an increase at 5 min (+19.5%) and a decrease at 30 min (-5.3%) and 24 h (-5.4%) after Cutting; an increase at 5 min (+40.3%; p<0.02), 30 min (+20.5%) and 24 h (+10.9%) after Barrel Racing; and an increase at 5 min (+39.6%), 30 min (+72.1%; p<0.005) and 24 h (+102%; p<0.001) after Pole Bending. Significant effects of Barrel Racing (F=5.25; p<0.006) and Pole Bending (F=11.23; p<0.001) events were recorded.

Horses with an age of 7 to 20 yrs had higher cortisol levels 5 and 30 min as well as 24 hours after exercise than horses of 3 to 6 yrs (p<0.05).

Gender did not have an effect on serum cortisol concentration during the training period and the changes after exercise.

Table 2. Serum cortisol levels (means ± SD) of Quarter Horses before and after western riding events.

Exercise	Serum Cortisol (ng/ml)				ANOVA	
	Basal	5 min	30 min	24 h	F	P
Reining	113 ± 64	107 ± 41.7	95.0 ± 38.1	89.2 ± 19.9	1.04	n.s.
Cutting	135 ± 60	161 ± 65.7	128 ± 43.2	128 ± 44.8	1.21	n.s.
Barrel Racing	103 ± 63	144 ± 74.2***	124 ± 65.8	114 ± 55.3	5.25	<0.006
Pole Bending	45.8 ± 15	63.9 ± 23.5	78.8 ± 22.8*	92.4 ± 34.4**	11.2	<0.001

vs. Basal levels: * p<0.005; ** p<0.001; *** p<0.02.

Conclusions

Studies carried out in horses reported a circadian glucocorticoid rhythm, exhibiting a peak between 6.00 and 9.00 a.m. and a nadir between 7.00 and 11.00 p.m. (James et al., 1970; Toutain et al., 1988); however, circadian changes only occasionally are present (Sojka et al., 1993), because the rhythm is fragile and could be obliterated by experimental conditions (Irvine and Alexander, 1994). In this study, no clear circadian cortisol variations were recorded. Thus it would be worthwhile to understand if Quarter Horses do not exhibit a true circadian pattern of cortisol levels or if the sampling experimental protocol adopted masked the physiological daily pattern.

Training had a significant effect on serum cortisol concentration. This has been shown in other studies too (Freestone et al., 1991; Ferlazzo and Fazio, 1997; Marc et al., 2000; Ferlazzo et al., 2005). Cortisol concentration was higher in trained (in 2nd, 3rd, 5th week) than in untrained horses (in 1st week). The decrease of cortisol levels in the 6th week could be the cause of overtraining (Golland et al., 1996; Hamlin et al., 2002). The similar values detected from the 2nd to the 5th week could be the expression of an equal workload imposed during training, independently of training state. Serum cortisol levels seem not to be related to aerobic (during the 1st and 4th week) or anaerobic type of exercise (during the 2nd, 3rd, 5th and 6th week).

The significant effects of Barrel Racing and Pole Bending events on cortisol concentration show its involvement during western riding exercise, as already reported after different sport activities (McKenna et al., 1993; Ferlazzo and Fazio, 1997; Nesse et al., 2002; Ferlazzo et al., 2005). The different pattern of cortisol modifications after western riding events could be the expression of its differentiated utilization. It is known that in Barrel Racing and Pole Bending events the horse must show the best degree of motor ability; then, cortisol increase could confirm results obtained in sport horses after exercises with the highest emotional involvement (de Vries et al., 2000; Hada et al., 2003). Finally, the higher cortisol levels of older horses after Pole Bending confirm data obtained in Standardbreds during exercise (Lindner et al., 2002).

References

Calabrò, G., E. Fazio, V. Aronica, L. Grasso and A. Ferlazzo, 2003. Atti Soc It Sci Vet 57: 55-56.

de Vries, W.R., N.T. Bernards, M.H. de Rooij and H.P. Koppeschaar, 2000. Psychosom Med 62: 866-872.

Fazio, E., G. Calabrò, A. Alberghina, P. Medica and A. Ferlazzo, 2004. In: The Elite Race and Endurance Horse, A. Lindner (ed), Dr Arno Lindner, Essen, Germany, pp. 167-171.

Fazio, E., G. Calabrò, P. Medica, C. Messineo and A. Ferlazzo, 2005. Atti Congr Naz SO. F. I. Vet. VI: 46-49.

Ferlazzo, A. and E. Fazio, 1997. In: Performance diagnosis of horses. A. Lindner (ed), Wageningen Pers, Wageningen, pp. 30-43.

Ferlazzo, A., P. Medica and E. Fazio, 2005. Chapter 11. In: Training del Caballo de deporte. Respuesta y Adaptation, F. Boffi (ed), Editorial Intermedica Saici, in press.

Freestone, J.F., K.J. Wolfsheimer, S.G. Kamerling, G. Church, J. Hamra and C. Bagwell, 1991. Equine vet J 23: 219-223.

Golland, L.C., D.L. Evans, G.M. Stone, C.M. Tyler, R.J. Rose and D.R. Hodgson, 1996. Pferdeheilkunde 12: 531-533.

Hada, T., T. Onaka, T. Takahashi, A. Hiraga and K. Yagi, 2003. J Neuroendocrinol 15: 638-648.

Hamlin, M.J., J.P. Shearman and W.G. Hopkins, 2002. Equine vet J 34: 383-388.

Irvine, C.H.G. and S.L. Alexander, 1994. Dom Anim Endocrinol 11: 227-236.

James, V.H.R., M.W. Corner, M.S. Moss and A.E. Rippon, 1970. J Endocrinol 48: 319-335.

Lindner, A., E. Fazio, P. Medica and A. Ferlazzo, 2002. Pferdeheilkunde 18: 51-56.

Marc, M., N. Parvizi, F. Ellendorff, E. Kallweit and F. Elsaesser, 2000. J Anim Sci 78: 1936-1946.

McKeever, K.H., 2002. In: Veterinary Clinics of North America: Equine Practice. J.M. MacLeay (ed), Saunders WB, Philadelphia, pp. 469-502.

McKenna, B., M. Lambert and J.A. Evans, 1993. In: Proc 12th Meeting Assoc Equine Sports Medicine, Veterinary Practice Publ Comp, Santa Barbara, California, pp. 39-43.

Medica, P., V. Aronica, G. Calabrò, E. Fazio, F. Di Giovanni and A. Ferlazzo, 2005a. Atti 7° Convegno "Nuove acquisizioni in materia di Ippologia", pp. 264-269.

Medica, P., G. Calabrò, E. Fazio, C. Cravana and A. Ferlazzo, 2005b. Atti 7° Convegno "Nuove acquisizioni in materia di Ippologia", pp. 284-285.

Nesse, L.L., G.I. Johansen and A.K. Blom, 2002. Am J Vet Res 63: 528-530.

Rose, R.J. and D.R. Hodgson, 1994. In: The Athletic Horse: Principles and Practice of Equine Sports Medicine. D.R. Hodgson and R.J. Rose (eds), WB Saunders Comp, Philadelphia, pp. 63-78.

Sojka, J.E., M.A. Johnson and G.D. Bottoms, 1993. Domest Anim Endocrinol 10: 1-5.

Toutain, P.L., M. Oukessou, A. Autefage and M. Alvinerie, 1988. Domest Anim Endocrinol 5: 55-59.

The effect of induced front limb lameness on back kinematics

C. B. Gómez Álvarez[1], M.F. Bobbert[2], L. Lamers[2], J. Wennerstrand[3], C. Johnston[3] and P.R. Van Weeren[1]

[1]Department of Equine Sciences, Utrecht University, The Netherlands
[2]Institute for Fundamental and Clinical Human Movement Sciences, Vrije Universiteit, Amsterdam, The Netherlands
[3]Department of Anatomy and Physiology, Swedish University of Agricultural Sciences, Uppsala, Sweden

Take home message

It is not very probable that acute sub-clinical lameness causes back problems.

Introduction

Back problems in horses, and especially the interaction between back problems and lameness, are poorly understood. It is known that back problems can be secondary to lameness (Landman *et al.*, 2004), but so far the exact nature of the relationship between back kinematics and limbs kinematics has not been studied in depth. This is mainly because the discrimination between primary back problems and back problems secondary to lameness can be difficult under clinical conditions.

It has been documented that front limbs lameness provokes biomechanical changes on horses in the head, neck, trunk and limbs (Buchner *et al.*, 1995, 1996a, b; Galisteo *et al.*, 1997; Keegan *et al.*, 2000; Uhlir *et al.*, 1997; Vorstenbosch *et al.*, 1997; Weishaupt *et al.*, 2006). But few studies have been done about the impact of lameness over back kinematics. Landman *et al.* (2004) reported a concurrence of back problems (defined as repeatable pain on palpation) and lameness in 26% of a population of patients presented for orthopedic ailments. Back kinematics has been studied by Pourcelot *et al.* (1998). In their work a small influence of induced lameness on dorsoventral mobility was shown, but no more detail was provided because only 4 markers were used to analyze back mobility.

The aim of the present study was to improve the understanding of the interaction between kinematics of the limb and the back. For this purpose, we determined the kinematics of the vertebral column in horses before and after the induction of fully reversible, subtle forelimb lameness at walk and trot on a treadmill.

Material and methods

Kinematics of the back was measured using the infrared-based Proreflex® automated gait analysis system (Qualysis Medical AB, Gothenburg, Sweden), operating at 240 Hz, and spherical infrared light reflective 19 mm diameter markers glued to the skin in different locations of the vertebral column (T6, T10, T13, T17, L1, L3, L5, S3, coxal tuberosities and the lateral sides of the hooves) in six, sound Dutch Warmblood horses while they were walking (1.6 m/s) and trotting (4.0 m/s) on a treadmill.

Qualisys Track Manager Software (Qualisys Medical AB, Gothenburg, Sweden) was used to capture and process the data. The range of motion (ROM) of the flexion-extension and lateral bending angles of the vertebral column, and axial rotation of the sacral bone were calculated using Matlab® (The MathWorks, Inc.) and Backkin® (Qualisys Medical AB, Gothenburg, Sweden). The back angles were defined as the angle between three adjacent marked vertebrae (*e.g.* the T10 angle is the angle between the line from T10 to T6 and that from T10 to T13). Lameness was induced in the left front limb with help of a modified shoe provoking reversible pain on the hoof sole (Merkens and Schamhardt, 1988). The lameness was grade 2 according to the AAEP's guidelines for grading lameness (Stashak, 1987). In order to quantify the lameness in biomechanical terms, the changes in the vertical acceleration of the head and the length of the distal limbs were calculated. For this purpose, extra markers were located on the head for the calculation of the acceleration, and the vertical distance between markers on each limb was measured.

Data were tested for normality and analysed by paired t-test if normally distributed. If data were not normally distributed a Wilcoxon signed rank test was used. The level of significance was set at $p<0.05$.

Results

The length of the lame distal limb remained unchanged during the loading phase of the stride while the sound distal limbs normally decreased their length during this phase. Besides, there was a significant asymmetry in the peak vertical acceleration of the head as previously reported (Buchner *et al.*, 1996a). Both findings confirmed the lameness. Despite of this, there were no significant changes in the linear and temporal stride parameters.

There were no significant changes in the individual back angles or in any of the variables during walking. However, at trot, the induced lameness produced a significant increase in the flexion-extension range of motion of T13 ($P<0.05$), a significant decrease in the lateral bending range of motion of T10 ($P<0.05$) and a significant decrease of the axial rotation range of motion of the sacral bone (S3) ($P<0.01$) (Table 1).

Table 1. Range of motion (ROM) values (mean ± SD) in degrees at walk and trot in horses with induced forelimb lameness.

Motion		Walk		Trot	
		sound	lame	sound	lame
Flexion extension	T10	5.1 ± 1.0	4.8 ± 0.9	3.4 ± 0.6	4.0 ± 0.8
	T13	6.3 ± 0.6	6.1 ± 0.9	2.3 ± 0.7 *	2.9 ± 0.6 *
	T17	6.8 ± 1.0	6.6 ± 1.4	2.3 ± 0.4	2.6 ± 0.4
	L1	6.6 ± 1.4	6.4 ± 1.7	2.8 ± 1.0	2.9 ± 0.7
	L3	6.4 ± 2.0	6.1 ± 2.0	2.9 ± 0.7	3.0 ± 0.7
	L5	5.9 ± 2.0	5.7 ± 2.1	2.9 ± 0.7	2.9 ± 0.9
Lateral bending	T10	8.9 ± 1.9	8.9 ± 2.0	7.2 ± 1.2 *	6.7 ± 1.6 *
	T13	5.0 ± 1.0	4.6 ± 1.2	4.3 ± 1.3	4.1 ± 1.3
	T17	3.2 ± 0.9	3.1 ± 1.0	3.3 ± 0.9	3.4 ± 0.9
	L1	4.0 ± 1.4	4.4 ± 0.7	3.1 ± 0.9	3.1 ± 0.8
	L3	5.3 ± 1.6	6.0 ± 1.6	3.9 ± 1.1	3.9 ± 0.9
	L5	6.7 ± 1.9	7.3 ± 1.7	4.7 ± 0.9	4.6 ± 0.9
Axial rotation	S3	9.6 ± 1.3	9.4 ± 1.7	6.2 ± 0.7 **	5.6 ± 0.9 **

Significant differences between sound and lame condition $P<0.05$, ** $P<0.01$.

Discussion

The subtle induced lameness in the front limb did not influence significantly the stride variables, but became manifest through an asymmetry in the peak vertical acceleration of the head and a constant length of the lame limb; demonstrating that the lameness induction had been effective. The asymmetry in the peak vertical acceleration of the head is in agreement with earlier studies of induced lameness (Buchner et al., 1995, 1996a). During supporting limb lameness the horse tries to reduce the load of the painful limb (Buchner et al., 1996b). A way to predict the loading of the limbs is knowing the length of the distal limb because there is an inverse relationship between the length and the force of the limb (McGuigan and Wilson, 2003). In this study, the length of the lame distal limb remained constant compared with the sound limbs in order to decrease the force applied over the ground.

At trot, but not at walk, this subtle front lameness affected the pelvic rotation and the range of motion of two angles of the thoracic segment; one in the sagittal plane and one in the medio-lateral plane. These changes in back movement are not extensive, but it should be emphasised that they were provoked by an intentionally very subtle lameness that was hardly perceptible to the eye. This observation makes sub-clinical lameness as a cause for back problems not very probable, but it should be kept in mind, however, that we only looked at acute effects. If a horse suffers from a chronic ailment of the limb, which will be almost invariably the case in the clinical setting, long-term adaptation processes may perhaps ultimately lead to chronic back problems.

References

Buchner, H.H.F., H.H.C.M. Savelberg, H.C. Schamhardt and A. Barneveld, 1995. Temporal stride patterns in horses with experimentally induced fore or hind limb lameness. Equine Vet J. Suppl. 18: 161-165.

Buchner, H.H.F., H.H.C.M. Savelberg, H.C. Schamhardt and A. Barneveld, 1996a. Head and trunk movement adaptations in horses with experimentally induced fore- or hind limb lameness. Equine Vet J 28: 71-6.

H.H.F., H.H.C.M. Savelberg, H.C. Schamhardt and A. Barneveld, 1996b. Limb movement adaptations in horses with experimentally induced fore- or hindlimb lameness. Equine Vet J 28: 63-70.

Galisteo, A.M., M.R. Cano, J.L. Morales, F. Miro, J. Vivo and E. Aguera, 1997. Kinematics in horses at the trot before and after an induced forelimb supporting lameness. Equine Vet J. Suppl. 23: 97-101.

Keegan, K.G., D.A. Wilson, B.K. Smith and D.J. Wilson, 2000. Changes in kinematic variables observed during pressure-induced forelimb lameness in adult horses trotting on a treadmill. Am J Vet Res 61: 612-619.

Landman, M.A.A.M., J.A. De Blaauw, P.R. van Weeren and L.J. Hofland, 2004. Field study of the prevalence of lameness in horses with back problems. Vet Rec 155: 165-168.

McGuigan, M.P. and A.M. Wilson, 2003. The effect of gait and digital flexor muscle activation on limb compliance in the forelimb of the horse *Equus caballus*. J Exp Biol 206: 1325-1336.

Merkens, H.W. and H.C. Schamhardt, 1988. Evaluation of equine locomotion during different degrees of experimentally induced lameness: Distribution of ground reaction force patterns of the concurrently loaded limbs. Equine Vet J. Suppl. 6: 107-112.

Pourcelot, P., F. Audigie, C. Degueurce, J.M. Denoix and D. Geiger, 1998. Kinematics of the equine back: a method to study the thoracolumbar flexion-extension movements at the trot. Vet Res 29: 519-525.

Stashak, T.S., 1987. Examination for Lameness. In: Adam's Lameness in Horses, S. Stashak (ed.), 5th edn., Lippincott Williams & Wilkins, Philadelphia, pp. 113-183.

Uhlir, C., T. Licka, P. Kubber, C. Peham, M. Scheidl and D. Girtler, 1997. Compensatory movements of horses with a stance phase lameness. Equine Vet J. Suppl. 23: 102-105.

Vorstenbosch, M.A., H.H. Buchner, H.H. Savelberg, H.C. Schamhardt and A. Barneveld, 1997. Modeling study of compensatory head movements in lame horses. Am J Vet Res 58: 713-718.

Weishaupt, M.A., T. Wiestner, H.P. Hogg, P. Jordan and J.A. Auer, 2006. Compensatory load redistribution of horses with induced weight-bearing forelimb lameness trotting on a treadmill. Vet J 171: 135-146.

Musculoskeletal injuries of Arabian horses during endurance training

L.M.W Gomide, M.A.G. Silva, C.B. Martins, R.M. Albernaz, C.A.G. Orozco and J.C. Lacerda-Neto
Depto de Clínica e Cirurgia, FCAV/UNESP, Jaboticabal, SP, Brazil

Take home message

During endurance training heels, suspensory ligament of forelimbs, superficial digital flexor tendon of hindlimbs, neck and lumbar muscles must be under constant evaluation.

Introduction

The aim of a training program is to increase stamina, speed, muscular strength, improve biomechanical skill and reduce the risk of musculoskeletal injuries (Marlin and Nankervis, 2002). Comparing different training protocols, Gansen *et al.* (1999) showed that low intensity exercise sessions, 45 minutes each one, were more effective to improve endurance parameters than higher intensities in shorter durations.

Musculoskeletal problems of equine athletes can cause behaviour change, reduction of performance and lameness (Dyson, 2003), being the major international clinical issue in the management of the equine athlete (Smith *et al.*, 2000). In endurance horses, the main cause of lameness is suspensory ligament desmitis, but superficial digital flexor tendinitis, paravertebral and gluteal mialgia, lumbosacral and sacroiliac pain and sore feet are also important (Misheff, 2003; Foss and Wickler, 2004).

Clinical evaluation requires good knowledge of the horses normal movements and differences between breeds and types. Then, periodically physical examination helps to recognize subtle changes in movement (Dyson, 2003). This is a fundamental acknowledgement, since mild forelimb lameness can affect performance (Parente *et al.*, 2002).

The purpose of this study was to determine the most demanded musculoskeletal structures during endurance track training.

Material and methods

Horses

Twelve healthy Arabian horses, mares and geldings, age 4-11 years, weighing 339-422 kg were used. Before the beginning of training the horses were kept on pasture under similar environmental conditions during four months with no specific training.

Physical exam

The musculoskeletal structures were evaluated before the beginning of the training and after this each 10 days until the end. It was made an inspection at rest, to identify lesions, scars or volume increases. Later, animals were trotted to evaluate movement quality. Lameness was classified in five degrees (AAEP). Neck, paravertebral, gluteus and limb muscles were palpated; hoof sensibility was tested; structures of fetlock, cannon and knee, hock and digital flexor tendon were inspected and palpated (Taylor and Hillyer, 1997). Sensitivity was classified in four degrees: 0 no sensitivity; 1 low (described by animal reaction to strong compression); 2 moderate (reaction to a medium compression) and 3 intense (reaction to a mild stimulus) (Marxen, 2001).

Training

Horses were ridden three times a week for 90 days aiming endurance conditioning. Forty two exercise sessions of 45 minutes each were done. During the first 45 days average speed was 13 km/h and the next 45 days the intensity increased to 15 km/h. Before each session the animals were submitted to a 10 minutes warm-up.

Statistical analysis

Data are presented as intervals. To determine the effect of period a Scott-Knott test was applied (SAS). The significance level was set at $P<0.05$ and $P<0.01$.

Results

The intervals of the structures sensitivity and lameness degrees presented during the training period are shown in Table 1.

Neck and lumbar muscles, heels and suspensory ligament (SL) of forelimbs, heels and superficial digital flexor tendon (SDFT) of hindlimbs presented a higher sensitivity during the training, followed by gluteus, sacral region and semitendineous / semimembraneous muscles. In hindlimbs, SDFT demonstrated more sensitivity than SL. The other structures presented less distinct increase during training.

Discussion and conclusions

Musculoskeletal, metabolic and correct mental stimulations are necessary to reach proper conditioning (Ridgway, 1994). Metabolic and thermoregulatory adaptations of training occur in a few weeks and are associated with the spirit during exercise. However, the musculoskeletal structures need longer periods to develop strength (Hodgson and Rose, 1994; Ridgway, 1994). Musculoskeletal injuries can happen in all athletic horse (Ridgway, 1994) even when the intensity of the exercise is under aerobic capacity (Couroucé, 1998). The horses in this study exercised enthusiastically during the whole training period but musculoskeletal injuries induced lameness.

Table 1. Intervals of evaluated variables in Arabian horses during endurance training period. Jaboticabal, 2005.

Variables		Day									
		0	10	20	30	40	50	60	70	80	90
Lameness degree		0^a	$0\text{-}1^a$	$0\text{-}1^a$	0^a	$0\text{-}1^a$	$0\text{-}1^a$	0^a	0^a	0^a	0^a
Muscle sensitivity	Neck	0^b	$0\text{-}1^a$	$0\text{-}1^a$	$0\text{-}1^b$	$0\text{-}1^a$	$1\text{-}2^a$	$0\text{-}1^a$	$1\text{-}2^a$	$0\text{-}1^a$	$0\text{-}1^a$
	Lumbar region	0^b	$0\text{-}1^b$	1^a	$0\text{-}1^b$	$0\text{-}1^a$	$1\text{-}2^a$	$0\text{-}1^a$	1^a	$0\text{-}1^a$	$0\text{-}1^b$
	Gluteus*	0^b	$0\text{-}1^b$	$0\text{-}1^a$	0^b	0^b	$0\text{-}1^a$	$0\text{-}1^b$	$0\text{-}1^a$	$0\text{-}1^a$	$0\text{-}1^b$
	Sacral region*	0^b	0^b	0^b	$0\text{-}1^a$	$0\text{-}1^a$	$0\text{-}1^a$	$0\text{-}1^a$	$0\text{-}1^a$	$0\text{-}1^b$	$0\text{-}1^b$
	Semitendineous/Semimembranous*	0^b	$0\text{-}1^a$	$0\text{-}1^a$	0^b	0^b	$0\text{-}1^a$	0^b	$0\text{-}1^a$	$0\text{-}1^b$	0^b
Forelimbs sensitivity	Heel	0^c	$0\text{-}1^c$	$0\text{-}1^a$	0^c	0^c	0^c	$0\text{-}1^b$	0^c	0^c	0^c
	SDFT[1]	0^a	$0\text{-}1^a$	$0\text{-}1^a$	$0\text{-}1^a$	$0\text{-}1^a$	$0\text{-}1^a$	$0\text{-}1^a$	$0\text{-}1^a$	$0\text{-}1^a$	$0\text{-}1^a$
	SL[2]	0^d	$1\text{-}2^a$	$1\text{-}2^a$	$0\text{-}1^c$	$1\text{-}2^b$	$1\text{-}2^b$	$2\text{-}3^a$	$1\text{-}2^a$	$1\text{-}2^a$	$1\text{-}2^b$
Hindlimbs sensitivity	Heel	0^b	$0\text{-}1^b$	$1\text{-}2^a$	0^b	0^b	0^b	$0\text{-}1^b$	0^b	0^b	0^b
	SDFT[1]	0^c	$0\text{-}1^c$	$0\text{-}1^c$	$0\text{-}1^c$	$0\text{-}1^b$	$0\text{-}1^c$	$0\text{-}1^c$	$1\text{-}2^a$	$0\text{-}1^c$	$0\text{-}1^c$
	SL[2]	0^a	$0\text{-}1^a$	$0\text{-}1^a$	0^a	$0\text{-}1^a$	$0\text{-}1^a$	$0\text{-}1^a$	$0\text{-}1^a$	$0\text{-}1^a$	$0\text{-}1^a$

Different characters in the same line differ in Scott-Knott test (P<0.01).
*P<0.05.
[1] Superficial Digital Flexor Tendon.
[2] Suspensory Ligament.

After skeletal maturity, tendon presents limited capacity of adaptation to exercise. This weakness can be increased by the speed of the exercise and the rider's weight, causing cumulative micro damage and increasing the risk for tendinitis (Smith et al., 2000). Forelimb suspensory ligament sensitivity was mild to moderate and disappeared within 24 hours after exercise, according to Misheff (2003). Dyson (2000) relates higher incidence of bilateral injuries with persistent lameness even with box rest (Dyson, 2000). Although Misheff (2003) and Foss and Wickler (2004) showed that SDFT of forelimb was the most often injured structure after SL, in this study the SDFT of the hindlimb was more sensitive than in the thoracic members, suggesting that the higher prevalence of tendinitis in the hindlimbs during endurance races is because these members are more stressed.

In most cases increases in the structures sensitivity were not associated with lameness. Affected horses were kept under box rest for two days returning to training thereafter. Lame horses received a single dose of phenylbutazone, local cold therapy twice a day and box rest until lameness disappeared. Associated with the early diagnosis this treatment regime demonstrated to be effective.

During endurance training musculoskeletal structures should be constantly evaluated, to reduce the incidence of severe injuries or even athletic disability. A careful physical examination done every 10 days is a useful tool to follow the adaptations of horses to endurance type of exercise.

Acknowledgments

We thank Fundação de Amparo à Pesquisa do Estado de São Paulo (FAPESP) for financial support.

References

Couroucé, A., 1998. Endurance and sprint training. Conference on Equine Sports Medicine and Science. Proceedings, pp. 190-202.

Dyson, S., 2003. Poor performance and lameness. In: Ross, M.W.; Dyson, S. (ed,) Diagnosis and management of lameness in the horse. Missouri: Saunders, pp. 828-832.

Dyson, S., 2000. Lameness and poor performance in the sports horse: dressage, show jumping and horse trials (eventing). 46th Annual Convention of the American Association of Equine Practitioners, Proceedings, pp. 308-315.

Foss, M.A. and S.J. Wickler, 2004. Veterinary aspects of endurance riding. In: Hinchcliff, K.W.; Kaneps, A.J. and Geor, R.J. (eds.) Equine sports medicine and surgery: basic and clinical sciences of the equine athlete. Saundners, pp. 1105-1117.

Gansen, S., A. Lindner, S. Marx, H. Mosen and H.-P. Sallmann, 1999. Effects of conditioning horses with lactate-guided exercise on muscle glycogen content. Equine Vet. J., Supl. 30: 329-331.

Hodgson, D.R. and D.J. Rose, 1994. The athletic horse: principles and practice of equine sports medicine. 497 pp.

Marlin, D. and K. Nankervis, 2002. Equine exercise physiology. Oxford: Blackwell. 296 pp.

Marxen, S., 2001. Análise da eficácia do polissulfato de glicosaminoglicanas no tratamento intratendíneo de tendinite induzida enzimaticamente pela colagenase m eqüinos. Dissertação. Universidade Estadual Paulista, Campus de Jaboticabal. 76 pp.

Misheff, M.M., 2003. Lameness in endurance horses. In: Ross, M.W.; Dyson, S. (eds.) Diagnosis and management of lameness in the horse. Missouri: Saunders, pp. 996-1002.

Parente, E.J.; A.L. Russau and E.K. Birks, 2002. Effects of mild forelimb lameness on exercise performance. Equine Veterinary Journal, suppl. 34: 252-256.

Ridgway, K.J., 1994. Training endurance horses. In: Hodgson, D.R.; Rose, R.J. (eds.) The athletic horse: principles and practice of equine sports medicine. Philadelphia: Saunders, pp. 409-417.

Smith, R.K.W.; H.L. Birch, J. Patterson-Kane, S. Goodman, E.R. Cauvin and A.E. Goodship, 2000. A review of the etiopathogenesis, and current proposed strategies for prevention, of superficial digital flexor tendinitis in the horse. 46th Annual Convention of the American Association of Equine Practitioners, Proceedings, pp. 54-58.

Taylor, F.G.R. and M.H. Hillyer, 1997. Diagnostic techniques in equine medicine. London: WB Saunders. 348 pp.

Retrospective evaluation of prepurchase examinations in Purebred Spanish Horses: 2004-2005

E.M. Hernández[1,3], P.J. Ginel[1], J.L. López-Rivero[2] and M. Novales[1]
[1]Departamento de Medicina y Cirugía Animal, Spain
[2]Departamento de Anatomía y A. Patológica Comparadas, Spain
[3]Clínica Equina Vet-express. Facultad de Veterinaria; Universidad de Córdoba; Campus de Rabanales, 14014 Córdoba, Spain

Take home message

If you perform a prepurchase examination to Purebred Spanish Horse (PSH), remember that anatomical regions of higher risk are the foot, fetlocks, and the hocks. Regions of lower risk in this breed are the carpus and the stifle.

Introduction

The sales of PSH outside Spain have increased considerably along the last decade in some countries of South America, Central Europe and the Unites States. The aim of this work was to review the clinical and radiological findings detected at prepurchase examinations performed in the last two years in order to determine their prevalence and clinical relevance. This information can be useful to equine practitioners from countries where this breed is less known. The study focuses mainly on the locomotor apparatus, which is the most common cause of rejection.

Material and methods

The study population comprised a total of 148 prepurchase examinations (120 males and 28 mares) performed along 2004 and 2005. Examinations were carried out at the Radiology service of the Veterinary Hospital of the Veterinary Faculty of Córdoba (Spain), or under field conditions but following identical pre-established criteria.

Age range of examined horses varied from 2 to 13 years with a mean age of 4.72 years. The most represented age group was 4 to 5 years (n=61; 41.2%).

With respect to physical activity, at the time of examination most horses were having a light to moderate physical activity as corresponds to pleasure horses, (n=78; 52.7%), and in lesser extent to dressage horses (n=17; 11.5%). The rest of animals were free at pasture (n=24; 16.2%), being trained (n=12; 8.11%), or were used as broodmares (n=17; 11.5%).

The prepurchase examination comprised a general physical exam following the criteria recommended by the British Equine Veterinary Association (Dyson, 1998), and a radiological study of the horses not excluded during the physical examination. The radiological protocols proposed to the purchasers were based on the authors' previous experience about the more common pathologies found in this breed, also taking into account the economic value of each individual animal and the future use intended by the purchaser.

Protocol I. (12 views)

Left and right forelimb foot: LM, DPr-PaDiO.
Left and right metacarpophalangeal joint: LM
Left and right metatarsophalangeal joint: LM
Left and right hock: DL-PlMO, DM-PlLO.

Protocol II. (24 views)

All included in protocol I plus:
Left and right forelimb foot: PaPr-PaDiO
Left and right metacarpophalangeal joint: DL-PaMO, DM-PaLO
Left and right metatarsophalangeal joint: DL-PlMO, DM-PlLO
Left and right stifle: LM.

Protocol III.

Joints studied and the number of radiographical projections varied depending on the first clinical suspicion. With independence of the radiological protocol performed, additional radiological views were included in certain cases to assess specific anatomical locations where pain or deformations were suspected. Specific ecographical evaluations were made in some horses as well, detecting proximal desmitis of MIO3 in 5 horses (3.38%).

All radiological studies were made using a fixed X-ray machine (Odel Program™) or a portable X-ray machine (Porta 1030™), regular green-line films, intensifying screens and automatic developing equipment.

Results and discussion

Of the 148 horses studied 31 (21.0%) were rejected after the preliminary physical examination (Table 1).

The most frequently detected clinical anomaly was a light ataxia. The majority of affected horses (n=10, 6.75%) were able to maintain a relatively normal activity with mild locomotor deficits, more marked on the right hindlimb which showed ataxia of grade I and II (Hahn *et al.*, 1999). Only 3 of these horses were evaluated by non-contrast cervical radiographies which detected signs of vertebral desituation at C3-C4 in 2 horses and C4-C5 in one horse. All ataxic animals were rejected for purchasing due to the risk they entail for the rider.

Table 1. Horses rejected (excluding abnormalities of the locomotor apparatus; n=148).

Eyes	Cataracts	1 (0.68%)
Cardiovascular system	Cardiac arrhythmia	1 (0.68%)
	Cardiac murmur	1 (0.68%)
Urogenital system	Cryptorchid (3 cases)	3 (2.02%)
Respiratory apparatus	Laryngeal hemiplegia grade II (3 cases) grade III (1 case)	2 (1.35%)
Nervous system	Ataxia	10 (6.75%)
Other defects	Nucal crest deviation	5 (3.37%)
	Hip asymmetry and ilium fracture	2 (1.35%)

As for the nucal crest deviation, it represents a major aesthetic defect with a hereditary basis specific of this breed and affected horses should always be rejected. The low prevalence found in our study was expected since the defect is widely known and easily detected by the purchasers.

Conformation defects

We found 35 horses (23.7%) with conformation defects more pronounced than the normal standard for this breed (Souza, 2000; Hernández, 2003), especially camped under and toe in the forelimbs, stands under, sickle hocks and cow hocked in the hindlimbs. These defects deserve especial consideration when the horse is purchased for any activity that requires intense exercise (Souza *et al.*, 2004).

Locomotor system

Fifty eight (39.2%) of the studied horses showed lameness when exercised, 32 (55.2%) in more than one limb. Lameness was detected more commonly in the forelimbs (n=39, 67.2%) and to a lesser extent in the hindlimbs (n=28, 48.3%). Clinical grade of the lameness was based on the AAEP (Anonymous, 1999) classification. All horses affected by lameness of moderate degree (grade 2/5) or higher were rejected. Horses with grade 1 lameness were considered acceptable if they fulfilled the three following criteria: negative response in the joint flexion test of the affected limb, lack of radiographic signs and intended future use as pleasure horse.

The tests of joint flexion elicited a positive response in the hindlimbs of 43 horses (74.1%) and in the forelimbs of 22 horses (37.9%).

Radiological examination

Most purchasers chose the radiographic protocol I. Although in other breeds such as the Thorougbred (Kane *et al.*, 2003), the number of radiographic projections is much higher, in Spain prepurchase examinations are not so demanded and there is less concern between the purchasers for this type of procedure compared with other countries. In previous studies, we have reported that in contrast with other sport breeds, in the PSH the metacarpus and metatarsus, the carpus, and the stifle do not constitute locations of higher risk (Lopez *et al.*, 2002).

Due to space limitations, the following Tables (2-5) list only the detected radiographic changes in each one of the main anatomical regions studied.

The main radiographical signs found in the digit were close to the distal interphalangeal joint, and more commonly were representative of osteoarthritis and fragmentations of the extensor process. Less common but of greater clinical relevance were those associated with laminitis.

Table 2. Prevalence of radiographic changes in fore foot of Andalusian horses (n=92).

Fragment of the extensor process P3	9 (9.78%)
Osteitis of the palmar processes P3	2 (2.71%)
Osteoarthritis distal interphalangeal joint	6 (6.52%)
Osteoarthritis proximal interphalangeal joint	9 (9.78%)
Laminitis	7 (7.61%)
Ringbone	4 (4.35%)
Fragment proximal dorsal P2	1 (1.09%)
Cyst-like lesion P2	1 (1.09%)

Table 3. Prevalence of radiographic changes in the navicular bone (n=96).

Lucent zones along the distal border	9 (9.38%)
Enthesophyte	2 (2.08%)
Fragment of distal border	2 (2.08%)
Fracture	1 (1.04%)

Table 4. Prevalence of radiographic changes in fore fetlocks (n=113) and hind fetlocks (n=103).

	Fore fetlocks	Hind fetlocks
Osteoarthritis	7 (6.19%)	4 (3.88%)
Frament proximal dorsal P1	5 (4.42%)	0 (0.00%)
Change distal sagital ridge	3 (2.65%) MC3	5 (4.85%) MT3
Fragment proximal palmar (plantar) P1	3 (2.65%)	10 (9.71%)
Sesamoiditis	1 (0.88%)	0 (0.00%)
Palmar (plantar) supracondilar lysis	1 (0.88%) MC3	1 (0.79%) MT3
Osteophyte proximal dorsal P1	14 (2.39%)	2 (1.94%)
Modelling proximal dorsal P1	12 (10.6%)	2 (1.94%)

Management of lameness causes in sport horses

Table 5. Prevalence of radiographic changes in hock (n=117) and stifles (n=27).

Concavity/fragment intermedia rigde of tibia	17 (14.5%)
Change lateral trochlear ridge of talus	4 (3.42%)
Osteoarthritis distal joints of tarsi	24 (20.5%)
Wedging of tarsal bone	12 (10.3%)
Changes lateral trochlear rigde of femur	1 (3.70%)

Although 10% of horses presented radiographic signs affecting the navicular bone, only a minor proportion of them showed lameness and were rejected. In a previous retrospective evaluation of prepurchase examinations some authors concluded that navicular radiographies can not predict future lameness in an individual horse, and thus recommended an evaluation based only on the physical examination findings (Van Hoogmoed et al., 2000).

A common finding in the fore fetlocks was the osteophytosis at the dorsal periarticular aspect, especially in horses with a camped under conformation (Souza, 2000). In most cases this lesion was not associated with lameness, an observation we have previously reported in this breed (Souza et al., 2004).

In the hind fetlocks the proximal plantar fragment is a frequent finding, in any of its two variants of osteochondrosis type I and II but usually with a low clinical significance as the physical activity is moderate in this breed. The clinical consequences of this condition in PSH are much lower than those described in Standarbreds (Philipsson, 2002).

Concerning the pathological conditions of the hock, osteoarthritis was the more predominant especially with osteophytosis of the MT3 dorsal aspect. The osteochondrosis of the tibial intermedial ridge has consequences more aesthetical than functional in the PSH as we have previously reported (Hernández, 2003; Novalez et al., 1999).

As to the final result of the prepurchase examination, of the 148 horses evaluated a favourable response was given in 72 cases (48.7%) and a negative response in the other 76 horses (51.4%). In spite of the technical assessment, some of the recommended animals were not purchased and, what is more surprising, some rejected horses were acquired under the responsibility of the purchaser.

Conclusions

On prepurchase examinations of Purebred Spanish Horses, the regions at higher risk seem to be the foot, fetlocks and hocks. The most prevalent pathological conditions are osteoarthritis and osteochondrosis which generally have a low clinical significance if we consider the physical activity of this breed. The bone changes on the dorsal aspect of P1 and MT3 are induced mainly by several conformation defects common to this breed.

References

Anonymous, 1999. Guide to veterinary services for horse shows, ed 7. Lexington, Ky, American Association of Equine Practitioners.

Dyson S., 1998. Evaluation of the musculoskeletal system II. The limbs. In: Mair T (ed.), British Equine Veterinary Association manual: the prepurchase examination. Newmarket, Equine Veterinary Journal.

Hahn CN, Mayhew IG and Mackay RJ., 1999. Examination of the Nervous System. In: Colahan PT, Mayhew IG, Merrit AM and Moore JN (eds.). Equine Medicine and Surgery. 5th ed. Vol I. Mosby Inc. St Louis (Missouri), pp. 865-883.

Hernández EM., 2003. Incidencia de las enfermedades del tarso en el caballo Pura Raza Española. PhD Thesis. Universidad de Córdoba (Spain).

Kane AJ. Park RD, McIlwraith CW, Rantanen NW, Morehead JP and Bramlage LR., 2003. Radiographic changes in Thoroughbred yearlings. Part 1: Prevalence at the time of the yearling sales. Equine Vet J 35: 354-365.

Lopez M, Romá E, Torres R, Estepa JC and Novales M., 2002. Revisión de casos de cojera estudiados en el Servicio de Radiología del Hospital Clínico Veterinario de Córdoba, en el periodo comprendido entre el 30-09-00 y el 30-09-02. III Congreso Internacional de Medicina y Cirugía Equina (SICAB 02). Noviembre 2002. Sevilla, Spain.

Novales M, Hernández EM, Souza MV, Rodriguez M and Lucena R, 1999. Incidence of osteocondrosis in the hock of Andalusian horses. 26th World Veterinary Congress. September, 1999. Lyon (France).

Philipsson J., 2002. Hereditability of osteochondrosis in Standardbreds and effects on racing performance. In: Jeffcott L, Davies ME (eds.), Osteochondrosis into the New Millenium. Equine Vet Educ 34: 51-56.

Souza MV, 2000. Correlación entre los defectos de aplomo y la cojera del caballo. PhD Thesis. Universidad de Córdoba (Spain).

Souza MV, Galisteo AM, Novales M and Miró F., 2004. Influence of camped under associated with upright pastern in front conformation in the forelimb movement of horses. J Eq Vet Sci 24: 341-346.

Van Hoogmoed LW, Zinder JR, Thomas HL and Harmon FA, 2000. Retrospective evaluation of equine prepurchase examinations performed 1991-2000.

Evaluation of short-term analgesic effect of extracorporeal shock wave therapy in horses with proximal suspensory desmitis

I. Imboden, N. Waldern, C. Lischer, T. Wiestner and M.A. Weishaupt
Equine Hospital, Vetsuisse Faculty, University of Zurich, Switzerland

Take home message

When evaluated with ground reaction force analysis, effectiveness of extracorporeal shock wave therapy can lead to a quantifiable reduction in lameness 72 hours after treatment. Neither measurement of skin sensitivity nor thermographic evaluation can be used for the detection of shock wave application.

Introduction

Over the last few years, extracorporeal shock wave therapy (ESWT) has been successfully applied in humans and horses for a variety of orthopaedic disorders. It is used for a wide range of indications including chronic tendinopathies and desmopathies as well as osseous problems ranging from osteoarthritis (bone spavin) and osteopathies (navicular disease) to stress fractures of various bones. A particularly studied indication is its use in the treatment of proximal suspensory desmitis (PSD). Lameness that can be pinpointed to the origin of the suspensory ligament is a common problem in sport horses and especially if chronic, carries a guarded prognosis for the return to full work. The use of ESWT and radial pressure wave therapy to treat cases of chronic PSD is already well documented and can lead to an improved prognosis (Crowe *et al.*,2004; Löffeld *et al.*, 2002).

Several studies evaluating the effects of ESWT in human musculo-skeletal disorders, have reported a perceived reduction in pain immediately after its application. Subjective evaluation of horses shortly after being treated with ESWT has also led clinicians to comment on an analgesic effect, expressed as a reduction in lameness. However, this effect does not equate to the healing of the affected structure. Moreover, in a study applying ESWT directly to the lateral palmar digital nerve, no analgesic effect was observed (Waldern *et al.*,2005).

The aim of this study was to evaluate and objectively quantify the analgesic effect of focussed ESWT using treadmill integrated force plate analysis on horses diagnosed with proximal suspensory desmitis and treated with a standardised ESWT protocol. Further we aimed to test methods by which the use of ESWT in horses can be recognised, as this would help the eventual enforcement of regulations imposed on its use before competition.

Materials and methods

Seven horses (bodyweight 523 ± 66 kg) with a clinical lameness score of 1-2 on a scale of 1 (slight) to 5 (non weight bearing) were evaluated. All lamenesses were in the forelimb and had been present for between 6 weeks and 1 year. The clinical lameness investigation included walking and trotting in a straight line on a hard surface and walking on a circle, as well as flexion tests and regional nerve blocks. A negative response to a high palmar and palmar metacarpal nerve block and positive response to infiltration of the origin of the suspensory ligament (OSL) with 10 ml mepivacaine was required to confirm the clinical diagnosis of PSD.

For further assessment and documentation of the affected area, as well as to exclude the possibility of other pathological processes, radiographic and ultrasonic examinations of the subcarpal region were carried out.

Gait analysis was performed on a high-speed treadmill with an integrated force measuring system (Weishaupt *et al.*, 2002). Before analysis took place, horses were accustomed to exercising on a treadmill in 3 sessions of approximately 15 minutes to allow development of a regular gait pattern. Gait analysis was carried out before (A0) and after (A1) anaesthesia of the OSL and again before application of ESWT (S0). The S0 measurement took place at least 24 hours after anaesthesia to ensure all effects had worn off. The ESWT was carried out with an electrohydraulic shock wave generator (Equitron, High Medical Technologies, Lengwil, Switzerland) using a transducer with a penetration depth of 35 mm. Two thousand pulses at an energy level of 0.15 mJ/mm^2 and a frequency of 240 Hz were applied to the subcarpal area between the lateral and the medial splint bones (MCII and MCIV). Gait analysis was repeated 6, 24, 48 and 72 hours after ESWT (S6, S24, S48, S72) and compared to S0 and the effects of anaesthesia. Mean tread-belt velocity during all trials was 3.5 m/s. At each session of gait analysis, the horses were accorded a clinical lameness score when trotting outside on a hard surface.

Stride frequency (SF) and peak vertical force (PF) normalised to the horses' bodyweights, were determined. Contralateral limb asymmetry was expressed with the asymmetry index (ASI):

$$ASI_{PF} = \frac{(PF_{affected\ limb} - PF_{sound\ limb})}{0.5\ (PF_{affected\ limb} + PF_{sound\ limb})}$$

In a fully balanced situation between contralateral limbs, ASI is zero. A PF deficit of the affected limb results in a negative ASI.

Skin sensitivity was tested by applying electrical stimuli to the palmar aspect of the metacarpus in the region where ESWT was applied. The stimulation level was increased in increments of 1 Volt. Skin sensitivity is expressed as the voltage level at which the horse showed 1 or more of the following reactions: muscular reflex, voluntary movement of the limb or turning the head to the limb, in 3 successive stimulations of the same voltage.

Thermographic evaluation of the palmar aspect of the treated and the contralateral limb was performed using an infrared camera (ThermaCAM PM695, Flir Systems, Wilsonville, OR, USA) in an enclosed examination room after 30 minutes acclimatisation. The mean surface temperatures (°C) in the region of interest (ROI) over the ESWT treated area and in a reference region (RR) over the proximal sesamoid bones were determined.

Both tests were carried out before (S0) and after ESWT, in the same interval as gait analysis. Measurements at the different times were statistically compared by use of 1-way repeated measures ANOVA.

Results

Two of the 7 horses showed ultrasound changes clearly associated with PSD, and 3 demonstrated radiological signs of PSD. Three horses did not have any diagnostically-visible abnormalities.

The clinical lameness scores, the results of gait analysis, skin sensitivity and skin temperatures are presented in Table 1. The clinical lameness score improved after anaesthesia, but after ESWT, the score remained unchanged (compared to A0/S0).

The mean ASI_{PF} showed a significant (P<0.05) improvement in response to anaesthesia of the OSL (Figure 1), decreasing from –6.0% (A0) to –1.2% (A1). There was no significant difference in mean ASI_{PF} between the A0 and the S0 measurements. After ESWT, the mean asymmetry declined when compared to S0 and showed a reduction of statistical significance at 72 hours after ESWT. The evaluation of stride frequency (SF) showed no significant changes either after anaesthesia or at any point after ESWT.

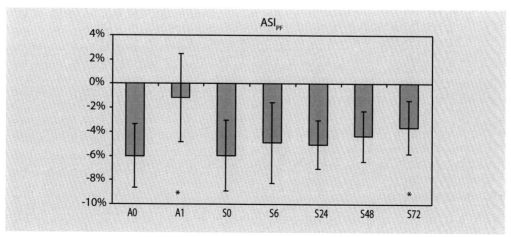

Figure 1. Asymmetry index of peak vertical force (ASI_{PF}) of the forelimbs of 7 horses measured before (A0) and after (A1) anaesthesia and before (S0) and 6 (S6), 24 (S24), 48 (S48) and 72 (S72) hours after ESWT. Values are mean ± sd. * denotes significant difference (P<0.05) to A0 and S0, respectively.

Table 1. Lameness score, selected gait analysis parameters, skin sensitivity and skin temperature of 7 horses (mean ± sd) with PSD of 1 forelimb measured before (A0) and after (A1) anaesthesia and again before (S0) and 6 (S6), 24 (S24), 48 (S48) and 72 (S72) hours after ESWT.

Parameter	unit	A0	A1	S0	S6	S24	S48	S72
Lameness								
LS		1.9 ± 0.2	0.3 ± 1.1	1.8 ± 0.4	1.9 ± 0.4	1.5 ± 0.4	1.3 ± 0.5	1.3 ± 0.7
Gait Analysis								
SF	min^{-1}	82.0 ± 5.8	80.7 ± 5.0	81.3 ± 5.9	81.5 ± 6.2	81.0 ± 5.6	81.4 ± 6.3	81.6 ± 5.8
ASI_{PF}	%	-6.0 ± 2.6^a	-1.2 ± 3.7^b	-6.0 ± 3.0^a	-4.9 ± 3.4^a	-5.0 ± 2.0^a	-4.4 ± 2.1^a	-3.6 ± 2.2^c
Skin Sensitivity								
rTV	V			4.4 ± 3.5	4.1 ± 3.6	4.6 ± 4.7	4.6 ± 4.2	4.2 ± 3.5
Skin Temperature								
ROI_{PSD}	°C			30.8 ± 4.8^a	33.8 ± 2.0^b	31.5 ± 3.1^a	31.8 ± 3.3^a	30.7 ± 3.7^a
RR_{PSD}	°C			29.2 ± 5.2	33.1 ± 1.7	30.3 ± 3.7	31.1 ± 3.4	30.1 ± 4.0
$TGRD_{PSD}$	°C			1.6 ± 1.7^z	0.7 ± 1.2	1.2 ± 1.4	0.7 ± 0.8^z	0.6 ± 0.6^z
$ROI_{Control}$	°C			29.6 ± 3.8^a	33.2 ± 1.9^b	30.2 ± 2.7^a	31.3 ± 2.4^a	30.6 ± 3.0^a
$RR_{Control}$	°C			28.4 ± 4.6^a	33.0 ± 2.0^b	29.8 ± 3.7^a	$30.7 \pm 3.0^{a,b}$	30.0 ± 3.7^a
$TGRD_{Control}$	°C			1.2 ± 1.1^z	0.2 ± 0.3	0.4 ± 1.4	0.6 ± 0.7	0.6 ± 0.9
ΔROI	°C			1.3 ± 2.1	0.6 ± 0.9	1.3 ± 1.2^z	0.5 ± 1.5	0.2 ± 1.5
ΔRR	°C			0.9 ± 1.6	0.1 ± 1.1	0.6 ± 1.5	0.4 ± 0.9	0.1 ± 1.8

a, b, c: Within a line, values with different superscript letters are significantly different (Repeated measure ANOVA; P<0.05).

z: Temperature gradient significantly greater than zero (paired t-test).

LS, lameness score; SF, stride frequency; ASI_{PF} asymmetry index of peak vertical force; RTV, reaction threshold voltage; ROI, temperature at the region of interest; RR, temperature at the reference region; PSD, PSD affected limb; Control, sound control limb; TGRD, proximodistal temperature gradient (ROI - RR), ΔROI and ΔRR: temperature difference between both limbs at the respective regions.

The skin sensitivity did not change significantly in response to ESWT. Mean ROI and RR temperatures showed a similar pattern and level over time and in both limbs. The temperature gradient between ROI and RR present at S0 disappeared in measurements S6 and S24 and reappeared at S48 and S72. Between the limbs, the mean ROI temperature only differed significantly at S24, whereas the mean RR temperature never differed at any point.

Conclusions

Proximal suspensory desmitis is a difficult problem to diagnose accurately, as a clinical diagnosis of PSD is not always confirmed by diagnostic imaging.
On average, in clinical lameness score and gait analysis, the horses did not show an improvement to the extent that they could be regarded free of lameness. Nevertheless, the ESWT led to a quantifiable improvement in gait 72 hours after its application. The improvement was smaller than that induced by local anaesthesia. This finding backs up the anecdotal reports of an analgesic effect and supports the ban of ESWT in sports horses immediately before competition.
There were no significant thermographic changes that could be conclusively linked to the ESWT. A local effect would have resulted in an increased gradient between ROI and RR and a greater difference between the limbs. Skin sensitivity did not show any changes throughout the investigation, therefore neither a skin sensitivity test nor thermography of the shockwave treated region can be considered as a suitable method for the detection of ESWT application under the conditions applied in this study.

References

Crowe, O.M., S.J. Dyson, I.M. Wright *et al.*, 2004. Treatment of chronic or recurrent proximal suspensory desmitis using radial pressure wave therapy in the horse. Equine Vet J 36: 313-316.

Löffeld, S., K.-J. Boening, K. Weitkamp *et al.*, 2002. Radiale extrakorporale Stosswellentherapie bei Pferden mit chronischer Insertionsdesmopathie am Fesselträgerursprung- ein kontrollierte Studie. Pferdeheilk 18: 147-154.

Waldern, N.M., M.A. Weishaupt, I. Imboden *et al.*, 2005. Evaluation of skin sensitivity after shock wave treatment in horses. American Journal of Veterinary Research 66: 2095-2100.

Weishaupt, M.A., H.P. Hogg, T. Wiestner *et al.*, 2002. Instrumented treadmill for measuring vertical ground reaction forces in horses. American Journal of Veterinary Research 63: 520-527.

Does warm-up in dressage horses change with level and competition type, and affect the final score?

Sarah Mann, Rachel Murray, Tim Parkin and Marcus Roberts
Animal Health Trust, Lanwades Park, Kentford, Newmarket, Suffolk, CB8 7UU, United Kingdom
Writtle College, Lordship Road, Writtle, Chelmsford, Essex, CM1 3RR, United Kingdom

Take home message

The mean warm-up time for competitors at dressage competitions was 29 min 53 s. There was no effect of rider experience, but level and type of competition affected the proportion of time spent in different paces and total time, which was increased at higher levels and championships. Increased warm-up time and specific warm-up design was positively associated with final score at Novice and Prix St George level.

Introduction

Warm-up prior to competition is considered an important component of preparation to enhance performance and potentially reduce injury risk (Safran *et al.*, 1989; Shrier, 1997; Shellock, 1985; Stewart and Sleivert, 1998; Quinn, 2005; Hournard *et al.*, 1991). Both physiological and psychological benefits have been ascribed to warm up (Gleim and McHugh, 1997; Garrett, 1996). However, there is limited knowledge of how riders or the horse-rider combination can optimise warm-up to augment performance and minimise injury. In order to improve warm-up strategies, investigation is required into the current types of warm-up strategies and how they may affect performance.

Although there has been some investigation into the effect of warm-up on horses in preparation for racing (Rokuroda, 1998; Harris *et al.*, 1995; Tyler *et al.*, 1996; Lund *et al.*, 1996; Jansson, 2005), there have been few studies into warm-up for other equestrian sports. Dressage is a sport with increasing popularity in the UK. In a previous report from Germany, it was found that dressage horses worked on average for 60 minutes on a competition day (Lindner, 2002), but there are no reports of the duration and type and of warm-up taking place at current competitions in the UK. It has been suggested that type of warm-up at a dressage competition can affect performance, however this has not previously been investigated.

This study aimed to provide baseline data on the duration and breakdown by pace, of warm-up at dressage competitions in the UK summer season, to investigate whether these were affected by level of competition, type of competition and rider experience, and to investigate whether there is an association between warm-up and final score. It was hypothesised that warm-up at higher levels of competition would be longer than at lower levels; that at championships would be longer than at local level and that increasing warm-up duration would be associated with a better result in competition.

Materials and methods

Warm up of 266 competitors at British Dressage (BD) affiliated dressage competitions was observed, including competitors at Novice (N; n=104), Medium (M; n=65), Prix St Georges (PSG; n=59) and Grand Prix (GP; n=38) levels. Competitions were classified as local (n=102), regional championship (n=54) and national championship (n=106) events. Competitions were included in the study if they were located in the BD Eastern region, except for the National championship, and both warm-up and competition tests were performed on surfaces other than grass.

All competitors at a competition that were competing at the selected level were included, but data for any horse that had already performed a test on the day was excluded from the study. Total duration of warm-up and time spent in each pace was timed using one stopwatch per pace. For each competitor, the final percentage score gained for the test was recorded. To evaluate the effect of rider experience, for N and M level, the section entered (open or restricted) was recorded.

Warm-up total duration, absolute time and proportion of time spent in each pace were compared between competitive level (N, M, PSG or GP), local, regional and national competitions, and open and restricted riders using analysis of variance and multiple comparisons of the means. At each level, Linear regression and Spearman Rank correlation were used to test for association between warm-up total time or time spent in each pace and final score. All data was analysed using a statistical software package (Analyse-It, version 1.71) with a significance level of 0.05.

Results

Total warm-up duration was 25 min 23s ± 10 min 2 (mean ± S.D.) at N level; 31 min 32 s ± 11min 32 s at M level; 32 min 53s ± 11min 19 s at PSG; and 34 min 34 s ± 10 min 10 s at GP. Mean proportion of walk, trot and canter at each level was N: walk 39.3%, trot 40.3%, canter 20.4%; M: walk 43.8%, trot 32.5%, canter 23.7%; PSG: walk 38.5%, trot 31.0%, canter 30.4%; GP: walk 38.8%, trot 33.3%, canter 28.0%.

Effect of competitive level

Overall warm-up at N level was significantly shorter than the other levels (M $p<0.001$; PSG $p<0.001$; GP $p<0.001$). Within the warm-up, there were significant variations in the proportion of walk, trot and canter between different levels. N competitors had a significantly smaller proportion of walk to M ($p = 0.046$) and a larger proportion of trot to all other levels ($p<0.001$). N and M were found to both have significantly less canter than PSG ($p<0.001$) and GP ($p=0.034$).

Management of lameness causes in sport horses

Effect of competition classification

GP warm-up time was not significantly different between competition types. Total warm-up duration at national level was significantly longer than at local level (N $p<0.001$; M $p=0.014$; PSG $p<0.001$). Within the breakdowns of the different paces N competitors at local level warmed up for a shorter total time but spent a higher percentage of it in walk than competitors warming up at regional level ($p<0.001$) and national level ($p=0.006$).

Effect of rider experience

There was no significant difference between the warm-up of open and restricted competitors at N or M level.

Association between warm up time and final score

At N and PSG level there was a significant positive association between final score and total warm-up time (N: $R^2 = 0.05$, $p=0.022$; PSG: $R^2 = 0.08$, $p=0.025$). At N level there was a positive association between final and walk percentage ($R^2 = 0.06$, $p=0.013$), time spent in trot, time spent in canter and canter percentage ($R^2 = 0.07$, $p=0.008$).

Discussion

The results of this study support the hypotheses that competitors at higher competitive levels warm-up for longer than competitors at lower levels, and that warm-up at a championship was longer than at local level. At N and PSG level, the results supported the hypothesis that increased warm-up time was associated with better performance, but this was not supported at other levels. There was no effect of rider experience at N or M level (where rider experience is classified).

Warm-up for horses begins as a generalised warm-up, in walk, trot and canter, and then becomes specific. This could provide a logical method for physiological warm-up of the body, followed by optimisation of proprioceptive pathways and specific muscles, tendons, ligaments and joints involved in the particular movements required in the competitive test. It is therefore possible that for a fit horse, increased opportunity to undertake a specific warm-up could enhance performance. However, although improved performance was associated with increased warm-up in this study, it will be important to establish whether there is a threshold past which fatigue leads to a reduction in performance. It has been shown that warm-up used in racehorses and trotters to improve VO_2 max actually led to increased muscle fatigue (Jansson, 2005). At present there is little information on how to evaluate the physiological requirements of dressage horses, but it is likely that they are subject to fatigue of specific muscle groups rather than limited by cardiopulmonary capacity, so it could be postulated that generating muscular fatigue in the warm-up could reduce performance. The results of this study, however, indicate that the warm-up duration and type used by the competitors sampled in this study was not associated with enough muscle fatigue to be limiting performance.

The mean warm-up for all competitors of approximately 30 minutes is shorter than that reported in a previous report of dressage horses at L and S level in Germany (Lindner, 2002). This may reflect a difference in practices between countries. Further information on warm-up duration and pattern between different regions would be useful to ascertain how practices differ between regions, competitors and trainers and whether these differences could influence outcome.

The difference in warm-up duration and warm-up content between N and higher levels could relate to relative rider inexperience or to a difference in the movements required at this level compared to higher levels. The increased proportion of canter performed in warm-up for PSG and GP could relate to the requirement for more canter-based movements in tests at PSG and GP level than at N and M level.

The increased warm-up duration at National level could indicate increased competitor nerves at Championships, or could be related to the competitors selected to compete. If warming up for longer is associated with enhanced performance, then it is possible that competitors have reached national level partly because they warm-up for longer and hence do better.

Conclusions

Competitors sampled in this study had a warm-up duration of approximately 30 min, consisting of varying amounts of walk, trot and canter. Warm-up duration and content was affected by competitive level, and type of competition, but not by rider experience. This is likely to provide adequate physiological warm-up of the body. However, it appears that increased warm-up duration at specific levels and increased proportion of canter at N level were associated with increased scores, which might indicate that increased opportunity for specific warm-up could lead to enhanced performance.

References

Garrett WE, 1996. American Journal of Sports Medicine: Supplement 24: 2-8.

Gleim GW and McHugh MP, 1997. Sports Medicine 24: 289-299.

Harris PA, Marlin DJ, Mills PC, Roberts CA, Scott CM, Harris RC, Orme CE, Schroter RC, Marr CM and Barrelet F., 1995. Equine Veterinary Journal Supplement 20: 78-84.

Houmard JA, Johns RA, Smith LL, Wells JM, Kobe RW and McGoogan SA, 1991. International Journal of Sports Medicine 12: 480-483.

Jansson A, 2005. Equine Comparative Exercise Physiology 2: 219-224.

Lindner A, 2002. The Elite Dressage and Three-Day Event Horse: Conference of Equine Sports Medicine and Science, Saumur, 19-21 October 2002, pp. 75-83.

Lund RJ, Gutherie AJ, Mostert HJ, Travers CW, Newton JP and Adamson DJ, 1996. Journal of Applied Physiology 80: 2190-2197.

Quinn E, 2005. http://sportsmedicine.about.com/cs/injuryprevention/a/aa071001a.htm.

Rokuroda S., 1998. M.S. Thesis. University of Kentucky.

Safran MR, Seaber AV and Garrett WE, 1989. Sports Medicine 8: 239-249.

Shellock FG and Prentice WE, 1985. Sports Medicine 2: 267-278.

Shrier I., 1997. Clinical Journal of Sports Medicine 9: 221-227.

Stewart IB and Sleivert GG, 1998. Journal of Orthopaedic Sports Physical Therapy 27: 154-161.

Tyler CM, Hodgson DR and Rose RJ., 1996. Equine Veterinary Journal 28: 117-120.

The incidence and significance of excess acupuncture channel imbalance in the equine sport horse purchase examination, 1999 - 2004[1]

William H. McCormick
Middleburg Equine Clinic, Box 1100, Middleburg, VA 20118, USA

Take home message

The TCVM channel examination is a useful component in the integrated prepurchase examination of horses.

Introduction

Prepurchase examinations are performed to provide the buyer with the medical knowledge upon which to base a decision of whether or not to buy an equine athlete. In the context of a western prepurchase examination Mitchell and Dyson cite the value of acupoint palpation (Dart *et al.*, 1992). Marks mentions acupoint palpation and provides a table of acupoints for documentation (Ramey, 1994). The objectives of the current study are 1) to relate the acupuncture channel examination to the western prepurchase examination and 2) to clarify the relationship of soundness, lameness, level channels, and unbalanced channels with respect to sale outcome. The term "level" is an adaptation of the literal translation of the term *ping mai*, or normal pulse, as opposed to *bing mai*, diseased pulse (Flaws, 1995). The word "level" is used here to depict the channel as having an absence of palpable excess muscle tension.

The prepurchase examination has come to include the possibility of a number of technical aids, such as radiography, diagnostic ultrasound, infrared thermometry, and even scintigraphy or magnetic resonance imaging. Although the use of the oriental "*si jhun*" or "four examinations" is low tech, one of the four examinations, palpation, can add valuable information to the prepurchase examination. The basic location of the TCVM acupoints used in this paper have been previously published (Van Den Bosch and Guray, 1999; Westermayer, 1993; McCormick, 2003).

Materials and methods

The medical records of all horses undergoing prepurchase examinations in a sport horse practice in Virginia (USA) from 1999-2004 were reviewed. 235 horses were examined. Geldings, mares, and stallions respectively comprised 88%, 11%, and 1% of the sample population. Thoroughbreds composed 51% (119/235) of the population followed by

---

[1] Content previously published in the Journal of Equine Veterinary Science 2006; 26 (7).

light horses of mixed ancestry, mostly Thoroughbred crosses 23% (85/235). Third most frequent were Warmbloods at 15% (35/235). Ponies, as well as Arabians and Quarter Horses were seen at low percentages. The mean age was 7 years (range 1 year to 17 years). Most horses were between 4-12 years old (85%). The horses were for sale as fox hunters (35%, 82/235), show hunters (24%, 56/235), combined training (17%, 40/235), steeplechasers (9%, 20/235), show jumpers (7%, 16/235) and others (4%, 16/235).

The physical examination included jogging on the straight away and turns, on a hard surface as well as turf, flexion tests of all four legs, and riding at a walk, trot, canter, and gallop if appropriate. Any observable lameness was recorded and categorized as lame *vs.* sound. The acupuncture channel palpation was performed after identifying the animal and examination of the ophthalmic, cardiovascular, and respiratory systems at rest, and before lameness examination. The buyer was subsequently informed of all findings. The examination procedure involved a systematic manual evaluation of a number of defined acupoints along the dorsal (*shu*) epaxial musculature of the neck, back, hindquarters, and caudal thigh as well as ventral (*mu*) acupoints. The reactivity of each acupoint was graded according to sensitivity: Gd # 1 = normal sensitivity and skin suppleness, Gd # 2 =a slightly sensitive acupoint whose reactivity fatigues easily, Gd # 3 = a painful, nonfatiguable sensitivity, Gd # 4 = a sharp, painful reaction with either an evasive maneuver or an aggressive kick or bite. Those horses with Gd # 1 or Gd # 2 acupoints were classified as having "level acupuncture channels" (CH Level). Horses with the clinically important Gd # 3 and Gd # 4 reactive acupoints were classified as having acupuncture "channel imbalance" (CH Imb). An increase in acupoint reactivity from Gd #1 or #2 to #3 or #4 coincided with a progressive increase in muscle tension.

Each case was followed up to one month after the original examination to determine if there was a subsequent sale, lease, or some other financial arrangement that would allow the horse to change hands.

A Chi-Square test (X^2) was performed to identify different distributions within the population. Significance was established as $P<0.05$.

Results

Lame horses comprised 34% (79/235) of the population. While 66% (156/235) of the horses were sound, 29% (46/156) of these sound horses had channel imbalance. However, a significantly greater 66% (52/79) of the lame horses had channel imbalance.

28% (66/235) of the total sample were not sold. Even though the horses with channel imbalance and lameness were the least apt to be sold, 6% of lame horses still managed to change custody. Therefore, 72% (169/235) of the total sample were sold. Of the unsold 18% (42/235), 12% (28/235) were lame, and 6% (14/235) were sound. Half of the lame unsold horses had channel imbalances. All of the sound horses not sold had channel imbalances. A significant 60% (102/169) of the sold horses were sound with level channels.

Management of lameness causes in sport horses

There was no statistical difference in sale outcome between lame horses with channel imbalance and lame horses with level channels. However, there was a significant difference in sale outcome between sound horses with and with out channel imbalance. Sound horses with channel imbalance had a significantly less than expected sale rate compared to sound horses with level channels.

Discussion

At issue is the integration of the palpation of acupuncture channels where an excess is signified by abnormal sensitivity at certain acupoints and a complete western physical examination within the context of the prepurchase examination of sport horses. The palpation procedure is a basic routine that can be taught to any student of veterinary medicine who has the desire and the time to learn the required manual skills. Yet the interpretation of findings has varied widely, a situation somewhat analogous to the interpretation of the flexion test.

The data show that lame horses had significantly more channel imbalance than sound horses. Secondly, the presence of channel imbalance was linked to a significant decrease in sales in sound horses. Not surprisingly lame horses did not sell as well as sound horses. There was no significant difference between the sales of lame horses with or without channel imbalance. However, there was a significant statistical increase in sales of sound horses with level channels *vs.* sound horses with unbalanced channels.

Lameness with or with out channel imbalance is a sales dampener. Buyers of sport horses, lame or sound, are averse to the gait restriction that is associated with reactive acupuncture channels. Buyers can visually perceive the asymmetric gait of the lame horse. The usually symmetrically restricted gait of the horse with channel imbalance is most easily determined by palpation. Nevertheless, a loss of extension or restricted tracking up behind can often be observed or felt by a rider. Channel imbalance is often related to lameness, and the two may occur together. However, a full 34% (27/79) of lame horses in this study had no obvious channel imbalance. Therefore, the question is what do the reactive acupoints portend for the working future of the individual in question? The vast majority of equine reactive acupoints in excess relate to joint inflammation in both spinal facets and distal extremities (McCormick, 2003). The other possibilities would be local trauma including specific muscle pain and somatovisceral pain (Smith, 1994). The origin of reactive channels referable to the distal extremities can be determined by the use of intraarticular anesthesia (mepivicaine hydrochloride) or the reactive acupoints can be rendered nonreactive by the use of intra-articular anti-inflammatory medications such as methylprednisolone acetate, triamcinalone acetonide, hyaluronate sodium or PSGAG (McCormick, 1996). The diagnostic use of intraarticular medications is governed by a neurological pathway: synovial nociceptor to sensory afferent to spinal segment to motor efferent to target epaxial muscle (McCormick, 1997). The specific joints of the distal extremities that can reliably activate such a pathway are the following: the front distal interphalangeal, the metacarpophalangeal, the carpus, the hind distal interphalangeal, metatarsophalangeal, tarsometatarsal, distal intertarsal (D. Marks, personal communication). In the stifle only the femoropatellar and medial femerotibial project reactive acupoints (McCormick, 2003). Contrary to some current texts (Cain, 1996; Fleming, 2001) extraarticular processes such as foot abscesses, splints, tendonitis and subchondral bone pathology do not activate acupoints in excess (McCormick, 2003). Often extraarticular pathologies, such as tendonitis, occur subsequent to or concurrent with joint hyperflexion. In these cases the acupuncture channels are activated because of the intra-articular component of the dual injury. In which case joint synovial nociceptors (Bowker *et al.*,1995), activated by synovial mediators of inflammation such as substance P or calcitonin gene-related peptide, are the primary neural mediators of reactive acupoints. Disease processes such as Equine Herpes (EHV 1) and Equine Protozoal Myelitis (EPM) have been postulated to have diagnostic acupuncture patterns, but neither supposition could be confirmed in western designed trials (Fenger *et al.*, 1997; Chvala *et al.*, 2004).

Although the acupuncture channel examination is low in specificity, it does have a high prevalence in working horses. In this study 42% (98/235) of the horses, which were all presented as serviceable, had channel imbalance. The increased muscle tension from unbalanced channels is a protective mechanism intended to restrict full range of joint motion under conditions of injury. The increased muscle tension need not reflect the primary injury, rather a secondary restriction of range of motion is a general precaution taken by a compromised system. The presence of reactive channels in sound horses suggests the possibility of injury despite the appearance of soundness. This is especially true in severe (Gd 4) channel reactivity, which should always signal caution to the examining veterinarian. Level channels and soundness should give the examiner a measure of optimism.

Soundness with channel imbalance should alert the examiner to the need for a change in work schedule, management, shoeing *etc.* A sore horse might require a drop in the level of competition. A less ambitious competition level would distance the individual athlete from the limit of its capabilities. For instance a Grand Prix jumper could drop to amateur owner jumper, or a Three Day Event horse could drop to Horse Trials. Channel imbalance with no change in management or a raise in competition decreases the chances for success. If the exercise work load that allows the channels to balance can be instituted, then the purchased horse would actually improve its performance.

Conclusion

The simple channel exam is appropriate for any prepurchase examination regardless of cost or use. The evaluation of channel imbalance is not a system of lameness diagnosis, but rather it is a method of assessing the response of an equine athlete to biomechanical stress. The presence of abnormal acupoints in excess indicates a lack of musculoskeletal homeostasis, frequently resulting from the inability of the individual to spontaneously recover given the current level of work and management. Therefore, channel palpation is useful in the prepurchase examination.

Acknowledgements

The author would like to thank Lydia L. Donaldson for literary criticism and statistical analysis and Cleanth B. Toledano and Dan Marks for literary criticism.

References

Bowker, R.M., Van Wulfen K.K. and Grentz D.J., 1995. Nonselectivity of Local Anesthetics Injected into the Distal Interphalangeal Joint and the Navicular Bursa. AAEP Proceedings 41: 240-242.

Cain M., 1996. Acupuncture Diagnosis and Treatment of the Equine. self published.

Chvala, S., Nowotny, N., Kotzab, E., Cain, M and van den Hoven, R., 2004. Use of the Meridian Test for the Detection of Equine Herpesvirus Type I Infection in Horses with Decreased Performance. JAVMA 225: 554.

Dart, A.J., Pascoe J.R., Snyder, J.R., Meagher, D.M., and Wilson, D.W., 1992. Prepurchase Evaluation of Horses, 134 Cases (1988-1990). Am. J. Vet. Med. 201: 1061-1067.

Fenger, C., Granstrom, D.E., Langemeier, M.S. and Stamper, S., 1997. Equine Protozoal Myeloencephalitis: Acupuncture Diagnosis. AAEP Proceedings 43: 327-329.

Flaws, B., 1995. Chinese Pulse Diagnosis. Blue Poppy Press, Boulder, CO., pp.19.

Fleming, P., 2001. Diagnostic Acupuncture Palpation Examination in the Horse. In: Shoen, A.M. (ed.), Veterinary Acupuncture, 2nd Ed., Mosby, St. Louis, pp. 436-440.

McCormick, W.H., 1996. Traditional Chinese Channel Diagnosis, Myofascial Pain Syndrome and Metacarpophalangeal Joint Trauma in the Horse. JEVS 16: 563.

McCormick, W.H., 1997. Oriental Channel Diagnosis in Foot Lameness of the Equine Forelimb. JEVS 17: 318-320.

McCormick, W.H., 2003. Understanding the Use of Acupuncture in Treating Equine Lameness and Musculoskeletal Pain in Diagnosis and Management of Lameness in the Horse. In: M.W. Ross and S.J. Dyson (eds.), Elsevier Science, St. Louis, MO., pp. 798-803.

Ramey, D.W., 1994. Navicular Bone and Future Lameness: A Retrospective Study of Prepurchase Examinations in Practice. Proc. Am. Assoc. of Equine Pract. 40: 47-48.

Smith, F.W.K. Jr., 1994. The Neurophysiologic Basis of Acupuncture. In: Shoen, A.M. (ed.), Veterinary Acupuncture, 1st Ed., American Veterinary Publications, Inc., Goleta, CA, pp. 43-44.

Van Den Bosch E and Guray J-Y, 1999. Acupuncture Points and Meridians in the Horse. Stuttgart, Germany, self-published.

Westermayer E., 1993. Lehrbuch der Veterinarakupunktur, Vol 2, Akupunktur des Pferdes. Heidelberg, KF Haug.

Treatment of tendon and ligament injuries with UBM Powder

Richard D. Mitchell
Fairfield Equine Associates, P. C., 32 Barnabas Rd., Newtown, CT 06470, USA

Take home message

This study reviews the use of an extracellular matrix material derived from swine urinary bladder for the treatment of injuries of tendons and suspensory ligaments. A review of cases 12 months or greater post treatment (107 cases) indicated an overall rate of return to soundness and the original level of performance in all treated horses to be 85.9%.

Introduction

Recent work in human and veterinary medicine using growth stimulants, bone marrow implants and stem cells have stirred interest in regenerative medicine as a technique for tissue repair. Extracellular matrix or ECM has been tested and proposed as an agent for tissue reconstruction (Badylak, 2002). ECM's have been derived from several tissues including the submucosa of pig small intestine and urinary bladder. The objective of this retrospective study was to assess the therapeutic value of Urinary Bladder Matrix Powder (UBM) for tissue regeneration and return to function in tendon and ligament injuries of the equine limb. Assessment of response was by review of lameness evaluation, physical characteristics of involved structures, and visible improvement of identified ultrasound lesions in affected structures.

Materials and methods

A total of 190 lesions of affected equine suspensory ligaments and tendons were treated during the period from April 1, 2002 to June 15, 2005. One hundred and twenty-nine proximal suspensory and suspensory body lesions were treated; 75 hind limb suspensory lesions and 54 forelimb suspensory lesions. A total of 75 suspensory lesions were treated using fasciotomy. Thirty-two suspensory branch lesions and 25 superficial digital flexor tendon lesions were treated. Additionally, two lesions of forelimb inferior check ligaments, one deep digital flexor tendon and one gastrocnemius tendon were treated.

Treated horses were initially presented for evaluation of lameness of presumed suspensory ligament or tendon origin. The origin of lameness was confirmed by a variable combination of palpation, lameness score assessment, diagnostic nerve blocks, nuclear scintigraphy, and, in all cases, diagnostic ultrasound (Denoix, 1994).

Treatment was accomplished by intra-lesional injection of 0.2-0.4 grams of UBM powder suspended in 6-10 ml of normal saline (Saline solution, 0.9%, Phoenix Pharmaceutical,

St.Joseph, MO 64503). All horses treated after August 1, 2003 received no more than 0.2 grams UBM suspended in 6 ml saline for any one specific lesion. Injection was performed after ultrasound examination determined the location of the injured tissue. Proximal suspensory lesions of the forelimb (and the two inferior check ligaments) were injected percutaneously with the exception of two cases that were performed via a proximal metacarpal fasciotomy. All proximal suspensory lesions of the hind limb were injected through a proximal metatarsal fasciotomy incision with the exception of three cases. Suspensory branch and superficial flexor lesions were treated percutaneously. The one deep digital flexor lesion was treated intra-operatively during an annular ligament desmotomy. The gastrconemius lesion was treated with ultrasound guidance. A thorough surgical prep was performed regardless of the subsequent procedure. All percutaneous injections were performed under standing sedation using detomidine (Dormosedan, Pfizer Animal Health, NY, NY 10017) and butorphanol (Torbugesic, Fort Dodge Animal Health, Fort Dodge, Iowa 50501) and a nose twitch. Regional anesthesia was used only with those horses that remained sensitive to needle puncture. All surgical cases were anesthetized with a combination of diazepam (Diazepam Injection, Abbot Laboratories, North Chicago, IL 60064), xylazine (Xyla-Ject, Phoenix Pharmaceutical, St. Joseph, MO 64503), and ketamine (Ketaset, Fort Dodge Animal Health, Fort Dodge, Iowa 50501) and maintained with halothane (Halothane, Halocarbon Laboratories, River Edge, NJ). In all proximal suspensory cases a 20 gauge, 1½ inch needle was used to distribute the suspension through the tissue. All suspensory branch lesions and all superficial digital flexor lesions were injected percutaneously with a 23 gauge, 3/4 inch needle. The one gastrocnemius tendon was injected percutaneously using ultrasound guidance with a 20 gauge, 1½ inch needle.

Proximal suspensory ligament lesions were injected via one location using a 'fanning" technique throughout the substance of the ligament in the region of injury. In the case of percutaneous injections this was accomplished from the lateral aspect of the limb just distal to the head of the fourth metacarpal/metatarsal bone. Suspensory branches and superficial digital flexor tendons were injected at multiple sites in the lesion at approximately 1 cm intervals. Approximately 1 -1.5 ml of suspension was used per injection site. While 0.2 grams UBM powder was most often used, up to 0.4 grams was used in some therapies per limb prior to Aug 1, 2003. The greater quantity was judged to be more than necessary with experience in using the product. If more than one limb was involved, routinely 0.4 grams UBM was used.

Following injection therapy, all non-surgical cases were placed in a sterile bandage for 2- 4 hours. The bandage was removed and the limb was iced for 30 minutes around the affected area. This was performed q6h for 3 days. A dry wrap was used during the day and a moist "clay" poultice under paper was applied over night for 3 consecutive days. Surgically treated horses underwent bandage changes initially every 2 days for 2 changes, then every 3 days until suture removal. Surgically treated horses were given 15 grams trimethoprim/sulfdiazine paste (Tribrissen ® 400 Oral Paste, Schering-Plough Animal Health, Union, NJ) once daily for 5 days as prophylaxis. All treated horses received an injection of 500mg flunixin meglumine (Banamine, Schering-Plough Animal Health,

Union, NJ) intravenously at the time of treatment and continued on 250 mg flunixin meglumine, q12h, orally for a total of five days.

Twice daily hand walking was begun on the day following injection. Even if the horse was uncomfortable, activity was encouraged. Hand walking continued on an increasing basis for thirty days. From August 2003 through January 2004, all cases (if available) underwent an ultrasound examination at 5 days post-treatment to assess post-injection response. Activity was normally increased after ultrasound evaluation at thirty days. More chronic lesions of the suspensory origin and body were started at walk/trot work after thirty days in most non-surgical cases. Newer injuries continued to walk another thirty days but often did so under saddle. All injection cases were walking and jogging to a limited extent after 60 days, however surgical cases were restricted to walking or a round pen for 120 days. Surgical cases were returned to work after 120 days walking/rest.

All horses receiving therapy underwent ultrasound examination prior to treatment and were then re-examined periodically to assess progress, typically at 30, 60, 90 and 120 days (Dyson, 2003). A limited number of horses were examined at five days post injection to assess injection response. Improvement in lesion grades and soundness jogging in hand were assessed at all examinations performed thirty days or greater post treatment. A review of response to therapy was performed on all horses that were deemed to be twelve months or greater post-treatment at the time of this writing.

Results

A total of 190 lesions were treated with UBM powder. Varying degrees of post injection pain and swelling were noted. Early in the use of this product, 2 horses were non-weight bearing within 24 hours of injection. This led to a modification of aftercare protocol (icing and NSAIDS). Two horses were subsequently significantly painful within 24 hours of injection (for a total of 2.1% of all treated), while 27 horses were mildly to moderately painful (14.2%). The majority of the treated horses did not demonstrate post injection pain (159 horses or 83.7%). Some mild edema was present in 169 cases 3 days post-injection. The responses of pain and swelling led to establishment of the management protocol mentioned in the previous paragraphs. Medical and physical therapy as previously described dramatically reduced side effects of pain and swelling. Surgical cases demonstrated mild local edema and generally were moderately thickened at the surgical site at thirty days. All surgical sites were very cosmetic by 90 days with the exception of one that remained thickened with some distal limb edema of unknown origin. Results of progressive soundness evaluations and client reports of horses 12 months or greater post-treatment were reviewed, and a satisfactory response was judged to be by ability to return to the previous level of work. Results were found as follows: of 77 proximal/body suspensory ligament lesions, 65 were sound and in work and 12 were still convalescing or lame (84.4% recovery); of 15 suspensory branch lesions, 13 were sound and in work and 2 were convalescing or lame (86.7%); of 14 superficial digital flexor tendon lesions, 13 were sound and in work and one was convalescing (92.9%); the one gastrconemius tendon had returned to soundness. A total of 92 of 107 cases or 85.9% of cases that were 12 months or greater post-treatment were sound and in work.

Ultrasound evaluation of post-injection lesions demonstrated significant fluid infiltrate at the 5-day and most 30 day follow-up examinations. In contrast, the 60-day examinations consistently demonstrated good fiber pattern formation and minimal edema in treated lesions. The noted fiber pattern demonstrated good linearity along the lines of stress and loading. Lameness was generally improved at the 60 day post treatment inspection.

Discussion

Equine tendon and ligament injuries are generally regarded as having a predictably prolonged convalescent period with high probability for re-injury. Healing is thought to be prolonged in part due to relatively poor blood supply to the affected tissues and opportunity for re-injury in the daily course of activity. Historically, tendon injuries have often been regarded as taking a full year for recovery often with poor healing quality (Dyson, 2003). In private practice, topical and internal blisters (coupled with prolonged rest or light exercise) have been the more traditional means of treating these injuries. Such "counterirritation" may have even been harmful with regard to future athletic function (Henninger, 1994). In recent years numerous devices have been proposed to be of benefit for tendon and ligament healing, i.e., pulsed magnetic therapy, low-level therapeutic laser, and ultrasound therapy (Henninger, 1994). Tendon splitting and superior check ligament desmotomy have gained favor for SDF injuries (Ross, 2003). Splitting has also gained some acceptance for suspensory body core lesions and suspensory branch lesions. More recently, fasciotomy and injection of bone marrow/blood has been suggested to increase the rate and quality of healing in proximal suspensory ligament injuries (Herthel, 2003). Injection of insulin growth factor (IGF-1) in conjunction with superficial check desmotomy has been promising for SDF injuries in racehorses (A.J. Nixon, personal communication). Stem cells derived from equine adipose tissue are currently commercially available for tissue repair purposes.

UBM powder is a lyophilized, acellular powder manufactured from the ECM of the urinary bladder of SPF pigs. UBM powder suspension produces a local inflammatory-like response when injected into injured tissue, as evidenced by localized heat, pain, swelling and sometimes mild redness. Histopathology in species other than the equine have indicated a profound angiogenic response developing in the first 5-7 days post treatment in studies where UBM membrane was implanted in tissue. Accompanying this response is the recruitment of bone marrow-derived cells into the treated tissue (Badylak et al., 2001, 2003). As time passes, and tissue heals, implanted UBM membrane is no longer evident histologically and scarring is not present, only normal tissue of the type that was injured (Badylak et al., 1998). It is proposed that UBM powder containing the same collagen, peptides and other substances of UBM membrane would have a similar effect.

Tendons and ligaments injected with UBM develop profound fiber pattern response by 60 days post injection. Ultrasonographic appearance of these fibers appears very similar to normal tissue. Clinical response and soundness would indicate that affected horses are able to return to moderate activity at an earlier time than with other therapies.

The encouraging results of this investigation suggest the need for a more objective, prospective and blinded investigation of this product for the treatment of ligamentous and tendon injuries in horses. Serial examination of histological samples as healing progresses may help investigators determine the nature of this regenerative process and if UBM is an appropriate therapy for tendon and ligament repair. The commercial availability of products that do not require harvesting and ex vivo expansion would be advantageous to practitioners, potentially safer for the horse, and would allow some flexibility that may not be currently available for treatments that use autogenous mesenchymal stem cells.

References

Badylak SF, 2002. The extracellular matrix as a scaffold for tissue reconstruction. Seminars in Cellular and Developmental Biology 13: 377-383.

Badylak SF, Kropp B, McPherson T, Liang H and Snyder PW, 1998. Small intestinal submucosa: a rapidly resorbed bioscaffold for augmentation cystoplasty in a dog model. Tissue Engineering Journal 4: 379-387.

Badylak SF, Park K, Peppas N, McCabe G and Yoder M, 2001. Marrow-derived cells populate scaffolds composed of xenogenetic extracellular matrix. Experimental Hematology 11: 1310-1318.

Badylak S, Obermiller J, Geddes L and Matheny, R, 2003. Extracellular matrix for myocardial repair." The Heart Surgery Forum 6: #2002-72222.

Denoix J-M, 1994. Diagnostic techniques for identification and documentation of tendon and ligament injuries. In: Tendon and Ligament Injuries I, Veterinary Clinics of North America. Equine Practice, 1994, W.B. Saunders, pp. 365-407.

Dyson SJ, 2003. Superficial flexor tendonitis in event horses, show jumpers, and dressage horses. In: Diagnosis and Management of Lameness in the Horse. W.B. Saunders, pp. 639-643.

Henninger R, 1994. Treatment of superficial flexor tendonitis. In: Tendon and Ligament Injuries I, Veterinary Clinics of North America. Equine Practice, W.B. Saunders, pp. 414-419.

Herthel D, 2003. Clinical use of stem cells and bone marrow components to stimulate suspensory ligament regeneration In: Diagnosis and Management of Lameness in the Horse. W.B. Saunders, pp. 673-674.

Ross MW, 2003. Surgical management of superficial digital flexor tendonitis. In: Diagnosis and Management of Lameness in the Horse. W.B. Saunders, pp. 635-639.

Lope kinematics of the leading fore and hind limbs as performed under 2005 Stock Horse Breed Association guidelines

M.C. Nicodemus and J.E. Booker JE
Animal & Dairy Sciences, Mississippi State University, Box 9815, Mississippi State, MS 39762, USA

Take Home Message

The Quarter Horse, a stock horse breed, is the largest breed in the United States and one of the fastest growing breeds in other countries. One of the reasons for this popularity is the breed's western pleasure gaits, the jog and the lope. In 2005, stock horse breed associations updated the western pleasure lope definition in order to discourage excessive slow, artificial-appearing loping as performed in the show arena. The kinematics described in this study will assist in objectively defining the lope as performed under current breed association guidelines in order to assist in evaluation of the western pleasure horse.

Introduction

Stock type horse breeds make up the majority of registered horses in the United States (AQHA Report, 2003; APHA Report, 2003). This popularity is rapidly growing outside of the United States borders. While stock type breeds excel in various disciplines, the most competitive and popular competition is western pleasure. The pleasurable, slow-moving gaits of the western pleasure horse make this discipline popular for novice equestrians.

Understanding of the mechanics of the western pleasure gaits can be difficult with the lack of research concerning the gaits and the current changes in breed association guidelines. While the lope is described as a slower, more collected adaptation of the canter, the demand in the show arena for an excessively slower and lower moving western pleasure horse has resulted in an artificial-looking gait (Nicodemus and Clayton, 2001). Before current rule changes, Nicodemus and Clayton (2001) found the lope performed in the show arena was a four-beat, stepping gait with a lateral footfall sequence, similar to gaits of the gaited horse breed (Nicodemus and Clayton, 2003), and periods of quadrupedal support. Stock breed associations initiated changes in their guidelines in 2003 to redefine the lope as to encourage a more natural-looking gait (AQHA Rules and Regulations, 2004; Compton and Copeland, 2003). Therefore, the objective of this study was to measure the kinematics of the lope in order to objectively define the lope that is currently being performed in the show arena.

Materials and methods

Four registered stock breed western pleasure horses were selected for this study by 1) demonstrating desirable gait qualities according to breed association guidelines; 2) proving themselves by consistently placing at the top of their respective western pleasure classes at breed recognized shows; 3) and actively competing at a national level.

Since the judge evaluates the leading limb side of the horse during competition, joint angular motion was only measured on the leading limbs of the lope. Circular retroreflective markers were placed over seven palpation points on the lateral side of both the left, leading, fore and hind limbs (Back *et al.*, 1994). Additional markers were tracked on the proximal aspect of the medial hoof wall of the right, trailing, fore and hind limbs. Markers were placed along the vertebral column at the withers, lumbosacral junction, and point of the croup. One marker placed on the temporal bone along the zygomatic process determined head position. The markers were used to calculate angles between the proximal and distal bone segments of the joints with angles measured on the flexor side.

A JVC GR-DVL 9500 VHS camcorder (US JVC Corp, Wayne, New Jersey, USA) set perpendicular to the plane of motion videotaped at 60 Hz the horse being ridden to the left at a left lead lope through the sagittal plane. A successful pass was determined by noticeable hoof contact and lift-off, consistency and correctness of gait, and complete marker attachment throughout the stride. Four successful strides of the lope for each horse (n=16) were analyzed using an Ariel Performance Analysis System (APAS) (Ariel Dynamic Inc., Trabuco Canyon, California, USA). Means and standard deviations (SD) of the joint angles and displacements were calculated. Paired t-tests were performed on the fetlock range of motion (ROM) and vertical and horizontal displacements ROM using Microsoft Excel 2000 (Microsoft Corporation, Redmond, Washington, USA). P-values less than 0.05 (P<0.05) were considered significantly different between variables.

Results

The lope had a velocity of 1.74 ± 0.13 m/s with a head vertical displacement ROM of 44.5 ± 14.2 cm. Hoof vertical displacement ROM was the greatest in the trailing fore (29.8 ± 7.85 cm) followed by the trailing hind (27.4 ± 5.55 cm), leading fore (25.4 ± 5.52 cm), and leading hindlimb (24.9 ± 7.54 cm). The vertical displacement of the hock had the greatest ROM (28.0 ± 5.46 cm) followed by the carpus (20.7 ± 3.65 cm), croup (18.2 ± 4.17 cm), loin (15.5 ± 3.78 cm), and withers (15.1 ± 2.68 cm). Significant differences were not found when comparing the ROM for vertical displacements between the withers (15.1 ± 2.68 cm) and loins (15.5 ± 3.78 cm; P=0.67); leading fore (25.4 ± 5.52 cm) and hind hooves (24.9 ± 7.54 cm; P=0.74); trailing fore (29.8 ± 7.85 cm) and hind hooves (27.4 ± 5.55 cm; P=0.24); and leading (24.9 ± 7.54 cm) and trailing (27.4 ± 5.55 cm) hind hooves (P=0.18) indicating vertical balance over the horse's topline and between ipsilateral fore and hind hooves. However, significant difference was seen between the vertical displacement ROM of leading (25.4 ± 5.52 cm) and trailing (29.8 ± 7.85 cm) fore hooves (P=0.01), and thus, distinguishes the leading limbs of the lope. Horizontal displacement ROM for the leading (203 ± 12.1 cm) and trailing (193 ± 9.34 cm) hindlimb hooves showed significant difference (P=0.0001), as did the leading forelimb (193 ± 11.8 cm) and leading hindlimb (24.9 ± 7.54cm; P=0.002) hooves.

Fore (48.8 ± 10.6°) and hind (51.1 ± 6.52°) fetlock joint ROM for the leading limbs were not significantly different (P=0.36) (Table 1). The elbow and hip had the smallest flexion angles, while both fetlocks demonstrated the largest extension angles. ROM was similar between the carpus and elbow with both exhibiting the greatest joint ROM.

Conclusions

Similar to the canter, the lope demonstrates distinguishable leading limbs, but is performed at a slower velocity. When comparing Dutch Warmbloods cantering on a treadmill (Back *et al.*, 1997), leading forelimb joints demonstrate greater ROM with greater flexion peaks for the shoulder and fetlock, which may be explained by the slower velocity of the lope. The canter of the Warmblood is performed with less ROM of the stifle, hock, and hindlimb fetlock joints. In addition, the canter has a larger flexion peak joint angle for the hindlimb fetlock. The hip has similar ROM (Back *et al.*, 1997) between gaits, which may be explained by the high degree of engagement required by both gaits. The movement of the hindquarters may explain the large ROM of the head vertical displacement during the lope as the head and neck may move to counterbalance the hindquarters.

In general, along with velocity, the ROM and flexion peaks distinguish the lope from the canter. Further changes in the breed association guidelines to encourage a more forward moving lope may find less distinction between the kinematic variables. These findings will assist in objectively evaluating the movement of the western pleasure horse according to current breed association guidelines.

Table 1. Means (SD) for peak flexion and extension joint angles (°) measured on the flexor side of the joint and Range of Motion (ROM) (°) for leading fore and hindlimbs at the lope.

Joint	Peak Flexion Angle (°)	Peak Extension Angle (°)	Joint ROM (°)
Leading Forelimb			
Shoulder	115 (1.9)	137 (3.6)	21.9 (3.9)
Elbow	97.3 (3.1)	165 (3.2)	67.4 (4.7)
Carpus	112 (6.0)	180 (0.4)	67.5 (6.0)
Fetlock	181 (1.0)	230 (10.0)	48.8 (10.0)
Leading Hindlimb			
Hip	83.5 (10)	117 (9.0)	33.8 (10.9)
Stifle	122 (9.7)	167 (7.7)	44.8 (6.7)
Hock	117 (5.2)	166 (4.7)	49.7 (6.1)
Fetlock	181 (0.7)	232 (6.6)	51.2 (6.5)

References

American Paint Horse Association, 2003. APHA 2003 Annual Report. Fort Worth, Texas.

American Quarter Horse Association, 2003. AQHA 2003 Annual Report. Amarillo, Texas.

American Quarter Horse Association, 2004. Official Handbook of Rules & Regulations. 52nd Ed, Amarillo, Texas, 201 pp.

Back, W., W. Hartman, H.C. Schamhardt, G. Bruin and A. Barneveld, 1994. Kinematic response to a 70-day training period in trotting warmbloods. Eq Vet J Supplement 18: 127.

Back, W., H.C. Schamhardt and A. Barneveld, 1997. Kinematic comparison of the leading and trailing fore- and hindlimbs at the canter. Eq Vet J Suppl 23: 80-83.

Compton, T. and S.M. Copeland, 2003. Practice pen. Horse & Rider, October, pp. 28-32.

Nicodemus, M.C. and H.M. Clayton, 2001. Temporal variables of the 4-beat stepping jog and lope. In: Proc 17th Eq Nutr Physiol Symp Lexington, Kentucky, pp. 248-253.

Nicodemus, M.C. and H.C. Clayton, 2003. Temporal variables of four-beat, stepping gaits of gaited horses. Appl Anim Scien 80: 133-142.

Risk factors for tendon injuries that result in retirement from racing at the Hong Kong Jockey Club

T. Parkin[1], K. Lam[2], C. Riggs[2] and K. Morgan[3]
[1]Centre for Preventive Medicine, Animal Health Trust, Newmarket, United Kingdom
[2]Department of Veterinary Clinical Services, Hong Kong Jockey Club, Hong Kong
[3]Epidemiology Group, Faculty of Veterinary Science, University of Liverpool, United Kingdom

Take home message

1. Tendon injury is the most commonly cited reason for retirement from racing at the Hong Kong Jockey Club.
2. The number of veterinary and ultrasound examinations can help manage tools to identify increased risk and changing the racing intensity can be used to manage the occurrence of serious tendon injury.
3. Older horses at the time of import into Hong Kong and greater racing intensity soon after import, both increase the likelihood of retirement due to tendon injury.
4. Identification of true case date is extremely difficult, but essential in order to investigate changes in training patterns that may be associated with tendon injury.

Introduction

The Hong Kong Jockey Club (HKJC), in collaboration with the University of Liverpool and the Animal Health Trust, commenced an epidemiological study of the factors affecting the performance of Thoroughbreds at the HKJC, in June 2004. The strategic aim of this study, funded by the HKJC, was to reduce the financial losses associated with the premature retirement of horses in training. This will enhance customer confidence by improving the consistency and continuity of the racehorse population. It will optimise the health and welfare of animals under the Club's care and maximise the output from the current investment in the collection and storage of health and performance related data.

Approximately 1200 racehorses are stabled at the HKJC. On average 24% of these horses retire from racing and are replaced each year. Since 1992 details of reasons for retirement from racing have been stored electronically. A total of 3,727 horses retired from racing between the 1992/93 and 2003/04 seasons. Content analysis using Simstat (Provalis Research, Quebec, Canada) was used to categorise individual reasons for retirement. A reason for retirement was given for 98% (3,634/3,727) of retired horses. Most retirements were due to a single veterinary cause (54%; 2,021/3,727). Tendon injury (25%; 512/2,021) and degenerative joint disease (16.3%, 329/2,021) were most common.

A case-control study was designed to identify risk factors for retirement from racing at the HKJC due to tendon injury. This will enable the implementation of intervention strategies that will not only reduce the risk of tendon injury but also potentially enable early identification of susceptible horses.

Materials and methods

Case definition and identification

Cases were defined as horses that were retired from racing at the HKJC, due to tendon injury, between the 1992/93 and 2003/04 seasons. Horses with tendon injury cited as the sole reason for retirement were identified using content analysis software (Provalis Research, Quebec, Canada) and exported to an Access database (Access 2000, Microsoft Corp., Redmond, Washington, USA). It was assumed that most, but not all tendon injuries occurred during fast work. In order to increase the accuracy of the date of injury, only those cases whose final exercise, prior to retirement, was at fast pace (race, barrier trial or gallop during training) were included in this study.

Control selection

Three control horses were selected at random, for each case, from all horses that raced, performed a barrier trial or galloped during training on the day defined as the last fast work date for the case. Matching on assumed date of tendon injury enabled the investigation of several training related risk factors in set time periods prior to the case date.

Conditional logistic regression

Univariable conditional logistic regression was performed with the outcome being retirement from tendon injury. Multivariable conditional logistic regression models accounting for confounding of explanatory variables were developed, using a forward stepwise procedure. All variables with a p-value of <0.25 during the univariate screening process, were available for inclusion in the final multivariable model. Variables with strong *a priori* biological reasons for inclusion were also considered for inclusion in the final model.

Statistical power

This study had more than 80% power to detect odds ratios of 2 or more for exposure variables with a prevalence of between 10% and 77% amongst the control population.

Results

A total of 175 cases of retirement due to tendon injury were included in this study based on the stated case definition.

The final multivariable conditional logistic regression model contained eight variables: The type of work on the last fast work date was associated with the outcome with cases being 12 and 9.8 times more likely to have been performing a barrier trial or racing, respectively. Cases were 10 times more likely to have had a previous positive tendon ultrasound examination and 18 times more likely to have had a previous official veterinary examination due to tendon injury. Older horses at the time of import into Hong Kong were more likely to retire due to tendon injury. For every extra year of age at import, horses were 2.6 times more likely to retire due to tendon injury. A greater distance raced in the first six months post import was associated an increased risk of retirement due to tendon injury. For every extra 1000 metres raced within the first six months the risk of being a case increased by 1.2 times. The number of episodes of fast work in both the 1-90 day and 91-180 day periods prior to the case date, was associated with the likelihood of retirement due to tendon injury. In both time periods, a reduced number of fast work events were associated with an increased likelihood of being a case (Odds ratio (O.R.) = 0.86 for 1-90 day period; O.R. = 0.92 for 91-180 day period. During univariate analysis a lower average earnings per year was associated with a greater likelihood of being a case. However, when fitting the final multivariable model a stepwise form of this variable produced the best fit: The risk of retirement due to tendon injury was unchanged up to approximately HK$1,100,000 per year, but for those horses that earned more than this per year, the risk was significantly reduced.

Conclusions

A number of risk factors associated with retirement from racing at the HKJC have been identified. Some of these factors such as previous ultrasound or official veterinary examination are examples of associations that are clearly very unlikely to causative. Although it is therefore not possible to introduce interventions based on these factors that would reduce the risk of tendon injury it will, in the future, be possible to monitor the number of examinations for individual horses that may indicate a greater degree of susceptibility to tendon injury. In addition, the reduced amount of fast work done by cases in the 1-90 and 91-180 day periods prior to last fast work date indicates that cases were most likely to be already suffering mild tendon injury, reducing the amount of exercise these horses could undertake. Therefore identification of changes in training patterns could also be used to enable closer examination of susceptible animals, potentially preventing career ending injury.

Older horses at the time of import into Hong Kong were at greater risk of retirement from tendon injury. Perkins and Reid (2005) also demonstrated that older horses were more likely to suffer tendon injuries compared to 2-year olds. The finding in the current study may be due to an increased level of tendon degeneration prior to the start of a racing career in Hong Kong. Smith *et al.* (1999) hypothesise that tendons gradually reduce in strength after maturation at a rate dependent on the amount of training undertaken.

Horses that raced a greater distance in their first 6 months after import were also at greater risk of retirement due to tendon injury. This risk factor could also be related to a greater degree of degeneration associated with increased training. It is however, interesting that although many different time periods were investigated only the first

6 months post import proved to be of significance. The reason for this is not obvious, however it does suggest that a limit on the distance raced immediately after import may reduce the likelihood of horses retiring due to tendon injury.

Case horses were more likely to be performing a barrier trial or racing, than galloping in normal training, on their last day of fast work prior to retirement. This finding may indicate that these types of exercise are more likely to result in tendon injury. However, it is likely that some case horses were already injured prior to the defined last fast work date, as indicated by the reduced level of activity for cases in the 180 days prior to this date. Further information on the motivation behind trainer decisions to enter barrier trials or races after reduced levels of fast work in training may help to explain the apparent difference in risk associated with different types of fast work. This finding does highlight the difficulty with the identification of training related risk factors for problems such as tendon injuries, some of which are likely to be chronic in nature, making identification of the true date of injury extremely difficult. Nevertheless, it was important in this study to match cases and control on time so that seasonal differences in training regimens could be accounted for. Without this matching use of set time periods prior to different dates for individual case and control horses would have potentially resulted in the identification of erroneous training related risk factors.

References

Perkins, N.R. and S.W.J. Reid, 2005. Risk factors for injury to the superficial digital flexor tendon and suspensory apparatus in Thoroughbred racehorses in New Zealand. N.Z. Vet J. 53: 184-192.

Smith, R.K., H. Birch, *et al.*, 1999. Should equine athletes commence training during skeletal development?: changes in tendon matrix associated with development, ageing, function and exercise. Equine Vet J Suppl. 30: 201-209.

Effects of intensity and duration of exercise in training on myosin transitions in Thoroughbreds

José-Luis L. Rivero[1], Antonio Ruz[1], Pablo Palencia[1], Silvia Martí-Korff[3], Escolástico Aguilera-Tejero[2] and Arno Lindner[3]

[1]Departments of Comparative Anatomy and Pathological Anatomy, University of Cordoba, Campus Rabanales, Edificio de Sanidad Animal, Crtra. Madrid-Cadiz km 396, 14014 Cordoba, Spain
[2]Faculty of Veterinary Sciences, University of Cordoba, Spain
[3]Arbeitsgruppe Pferd, D-52428 Juelich, Germany

Take home message

This study defines the relative contribution of the intensity and duration of exercise on the myosin heavy chain (MHC) response to training in Thoroughbred racehorses. Overall, training increased the fraction of MHC IIA and decreased that of MHC IIX isoform. Exercise intensity effects on fast MHCs were highly significant, whereas exercise duration only had a marginal effect on the IIA:IIX MHC ratio. Thus, exercises for up to 25 minutes per day at velocities eliciting a blood lactate concentration between 2.5 and 4 mmol/L every second day for 3 weeks improve stamina in Thoroughbreds.

Introduction

In general, the muscular response to training depends of 2 groups of factors: 1) the basal status of the muscle (determined by the breed, age, sex and level of fitness of the horse) and 2) the stimulus applied (*i.e.*, type, intensity, duration, frequency and total volume of the training exercise; Rivero and Piercy, 2004). Unfortunately, little is still known about the relative influence of most factors included into the second group. Training Thoroughbred racehorses is probably much more difficult than training endurance and other racehorses (Evans, 1994). In general, practical training of Thoroughbreds would appear to involve short distance and low-to-moderate workouts because of serious concern for muscle and tendon damage (Miyata *et al.*, 1999). But, although there is an extent literature describing muscular adaptations to particular training protocols in Thoroughbreds and other racehorses, the relative influence of relevant exercise parameters such as intensity and duration on this response remains to be precised. As a consequence, results from many of these experimental studies are of little, if any, application in practice. The present study describes the relative contribution of exercise intensity and duration on the short-term myosin heavy chain (MHC) response during the specific phase of training in 2-to-3 years-old Thoroughbreds.

Materials and methods

Six clinically healthy Thoroughbred horses (4 mares and 2 geldings) were used. Four horses were 2 years old, whereas the other 2 were 3 years old at the beginning of the study. All the exercise tests and exercise workouts were done on a treadmill[1] at 6% incline. In a cross-over study following a randomized 6x6 latin square design, horses performed 6 consecutive conditioning programmes of varying lactate-guided intensities and durations (Table 1). Horses were exercised at their individual $V_{2.5}$ or V_4 (see below) for 5, 15 or 25 minutes in each consecutive conditioning program. Each program lasted 22 days and consisted of 11 exercise sessions once a day every second day and followed by a 10 day resting period between consecutive programmes. Before and after each conditioning program, horses performed a standardized exercise test (SET) to determine their individual $V_{2.5}$ and V_4. Blood lactate analysis was done *in situ* with test-stripes BM-lactate[2] on whole blood samples. Before and after the 2-month acclimatisation period and again before and after each conditioning program, percutaneous needle biopsies were taken from the M. gluteus medius at 2 and 6 cm depth using the technique described by Lindholm and Piehl (1974). Muscle samples were always collected at rest before each SET. Samples were frozen in isopentane kept in liquid nitrogen, and stored at -80 ºC until analysed.

A total of 168 muscle biopsies [7 experimental stages (6 conditioning programmes plus the acclimatisation period) x 2 times (before and after) x 2 sampling depth (2 and 6 cm) x 6 horses] were available for electrophoretical analysis. Myosin heavy chain (MHC) electrophoresis was performed with the 8 % sodium dodecyl sulphate polyacrylamide gel electrophoresis protocol previously described and validated in horse muscle (Rivero *et al.*, 1997). Three bands of MHCs I, IIA and IIX were clearly visualised in the gels. Gels were then scanned with a videoscanning densitometric system and a quantification of each MHC isoform was obtained in relative terms for each muscle biopsy.

Table 1. *Study design with the order in which each individual horse was assigned to each conditioning program with exercises of different intensity (Int) and duration (Dur, expressed in minutes).*

	Conditioning programmes											
	1st		2nd		3rd		4th		5th		6th	
Horse	Int	Dur	Int	Dur	Int	Dur	Int	Dur	Int	Dur	Int	Dur
1	$V_{2.5}$	15	V_4	5	V_4	25	V_4	15	$V_{2.5}$	5	$V_{2.5}$	25
2	$V_{2.5}$	5	V_4	15	$V_{2.5}$	15	$V_{2.5}$	25	V_4	5	V_4	25
3	$V_{2.5}$	25	$V_{2.5}$	5	V_4	15	V_4	5	V_4	25	$V_{2.5}$	15
4	V_4	15	$V_{2.5}$	25	V_4	5	V_4	25	$V_{2.5}$	15	$V_{2.5}$	5
5	V_4	25	$V_{2.5}$	15	$V_{2.5}$	25	$V_{2.5}$	15	V_4	15	V_4	5
6	V_4	5	V_4	25	$V_{2.5}$	5	$V_{2.5}$	5	$V_{2.5}$	25	V_4	15

A 2-way ANOVA was done within each training stage (pretraining and posttraining) to investigate the fixed effects of both intensity and duration of exercise carried out in each conditioning program on MHC composition. In the presence of a significant F ratio ($P<0.05$), a one-way ANOVA for repeated measurements was done within each sampling depth among the six experimental conditioning programmes and post hoc comparisons of means were provided by Tukey's least significant difference test. Finally, paired Student's t tests were applied on a per individual basis to analyse possible effects of each conditioning program on MHC content.

Results

Overall, training status had a marginal ($0.05<P<0.1$) effect on V_4 (mean ± s.d. 7.71 ± 0.43 to 7.89 ± 0.36 m/s, before and after conditioning programmes; Figure 1). Exercise intensity fixed effect on V_4 was not significant ($P>0.05$), but the duration of the exercise had a marginal effect ($P<0.1$) on this variable with the longer the exercise duration for a particular conditioning program, the greater value of the V_4 variable. Thus, when data were analysed on a per individual basis, conditioning impact on V_4 was only significant ($P<0.05$) in horses exercised for the longest duration (25 minutes) at V_4 (Figure 1).

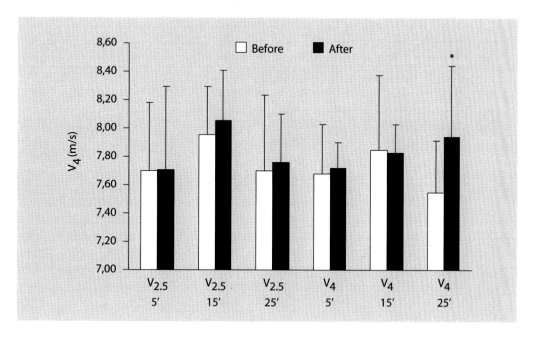

Figure 1. Mean (s.d.) V_4 of horses (n=6) before and after conditioning programmes with exercises of varying intensity ($V_{2.5}$ and V_4) and duration (5, 15 or 25 minutes). * The effect of conditioning program is significant (P<0.05).

No significant differences (P>0.05) in MHC content was observed before and after the 2-month acclimatisation period, but the IIA:IIX MHC ratio tend to be higher after this period (0.73 ± 0.12 *vs.* 0.86 ±0.13, P<0.1).

The mean MHC composition of the muscle samples before and after each conditioning program where horses exercised at different intensities and duration shown in Table 2. Overall, both training and sampling depth effects on MHC content were highly significant. Training increased the fraction of MHC IIA (41.1 ± 3.5% to 43.4 ± 4.4%, P=0.0004) and decreased that of MHC IIX isoform (from 50.2 ± 4.4% to 47.4 ± 5.6%, P=0.001), but did not affect the percentage of MHC I (P>0.05). As expected, samples from the deep sampling site of the M. gluteus medius had significantly higher percentages of both MHC I and MHC IIA and a lower percentage of MHC IIX than the superficial sampling site (P<0.001 in all comparisons).

Exercise intensity and duration fixed effects on MHC composition were not significant in the set of samples collected before conditioning programmes. After training, however, exercise intensity fixed effect on both fast MHC isoforms were highly significant (P<0.01), whereas exercise duration only had a marginal effect (P<0.1) on both the fraction of MHC IIX and the IIA:IIX MHC ratio. As a consequence, no significant differences among the 6 experimental conditioning programmes existed before training, whereas mean MHC IIA and IIA:IIX MHC ratio differed significantly after training (Table 2). Thus, in biopsies removed from the deep sampling site of the muscle, horses exercised for 25 minutes at V_4 had the greatest MHC IIA fraction and IIA:IIX MHC ratio, whereas horses exercised for only 5 minutes at $V_{2.5}$ had the lowest values for these same variables.

On a per individual basis, horses exercised for the longest duration (25 minutes) at both intensities ($V_{2.5}$ and V_4) increased significantly (P<0.05 to P<0.001) their fractions of MHC IIA and decreased that of MHC IIX (P<0.05) in the deep region of the muscle (Table 2). But the fraction of MHC IIA and the IIA:IIX MHC ratio in the superficial region of the muscle also increased after training in horses exercised for 25 minutes at V_4 (P<0.001 and P<0.01, respectively).

Discussion

The lack of significant influence of intensity of training on V_4 observed in the present study is not a new finding (Evans *et al.*, 1995; Werkmann *et al.*, 1996). Thus, our data showed that 3 weeks of training with exercises of different intensity and duration only had a discrete (but significant) impact on V_4 when horses were exercised at high intensity (V_4) for 25 minutes per day every second day. Together, duration rather than intensity of the exercise during training seems to be the main contributor to this metabolic adaptation of blood lactate concentration.

The results of the present study have demonstrated collectively that, after a 2-month basic training during the acclimatisation period, a brief period of 3 weeks of training promotes a significant increase in the IIA-to-IIX MHC isoform ratio. In racehorses,

Table 2. Mean (s.d.) myosin heavy chain (MHC) composition before and after each conditioning program (n= 6 horses).

Conditioning programmes		Superficial sampling depth (20 mm)							
		MHCI		MHCIIA		MHCIIX		MHCIIA:MCHIIX	
Intensity	Duration (min)	Before	After	Before	After	Before	After	Before	After
$V_{2.5}$	5	4.1 (2.0)	4.5 (2.3)	40.1 (3.4)	39.1 (4.1)	55.8 (4.2)	56.4 (5.4)	0.72 (0.12)	0.71 (0.15)
$V_{2.5}$	15	5.9 (1.0)	6.6 (1.8)	38.2 (2.7)	39.3 (4.8)	55.8 (3.0)	54.1 (4.2)	0.69 (0.08)	0.74 (0.15)
$V_{2.5}$	25	6.3 (2.1)	5.5 (1.5)	40.4 (3.2)	40.0 (5.9)	53.3 (3.9)	54.5 (5.3)	0.78 (0.11)	0.75 (0.18)
V_4	5	6.1 (1.1)	6.7 (3.0)	39.3 (2.1)	41.9 (4.1)	54.5 (2.0)	51.4 (3.7)	0.72 (0.06)	0.82 (0.14)
V_4	15	5.2 (2.8)	8.1 (4.4)	40.4 (3.9)	41.2 (1.8)	54.5 (1.8)	50.7 (6.0)	0.74 (0.09)	0.83 (0.14)
V_4	25	7.4 (4.5)	7.2 (2.7)	38.9 (2.9)	43.2*** (2.5)	53.7 (3.7)	49.7 (4.0)	0.73 (0.08)	0.88** (0.12)
		Deep sampling depth (60 mm)							
$V_{2.5}$	5	9.7 (3.3)	10.8 (3.1)	41.4 (4.3)	42.6[b] (4.3)	49.0 (7.0)	46.5 (6.7)	0.87 (0.23)	0.94[b] (0.21)
$V_{2.5}$	15	10.9 (2.4)	12.9 (2.2)	43.0 (4.5)	43.9[ab] (3.3)	46.1 (6.5)	43.2 (1.5)	0.96 (0.25)	1.02[ab] (0.11)
$V_{2.5}$	25	11.1 (2.7)	12.0 (3.4)	40.4 (3.0)	46.4***[ab] (3.1)	48.5 (1.6)	41.6* (5.4)	0.83 (0.08)	1.14**[ab] (0.22)
V_4	5	13.8 (3.9)	10.9 (5.3)	42.0 (3.2)	46.8[ab] (4.6)	44.1 (4.2)	42.2 (7.5)	0.96 (0.15)	1.14[ab] (0.25)
V_4	15	12.6 (3.6)	12.5 (2.3)	45.2 (3.1)	47.2[ab] (4.1)	42.2 (4.3)	40.4 (6.2)	1.08 (0.15)	1.20[ab] (0.28)
V_4	25	10.7 (3.2)	12.5 (4.4)	44.1 (3.2)	49.6*[a] (3.2)	45.3 (5.0)	37.9* (6.1)	0.99 (0.15)	1.34*[ab] (0.28)

*,**,*** P<0.05, P<0.01, P<0.001, respectively, compared with before. For each sampling depth, within a column means with different letters are statistically different (P<0.05 at least).

a comparable adaptation to training was reported after only 5 (Rivero *et al.* 2002) or 6 (Sinha *et al.*,, 1993) weeks of training. Changes in skeletal muscles similar to those reported in the present study were caused by training and not by growth in a recent study of adolescent Thoroughbreds (Yamano *et al.*, 2002).

The current results also imply that this muscular adaptation is more dependent on the intensity than the duration of exercise during training. This is not surprising since the very forceful contractions required for rapid speed result in the type IIX fibres, containing the MHC isoform with the fastest shortening velocity, being recruited (Valberg, 1996). This finding is also supported by other previous studies in young Thoroughbreds in which exercises of very high intensity were programmed during the anaerobic phase of training (Miyata *et al.*, 1999; Yamano *et al.*, 2002) and in the study by Sinha *et al.* (1993). Together, intensity of training-exercise may therefore be an important factor in determining the degree of local adaptations to training in skeletal muscles of Thoroughbred racehorses.

Nevertheless, the prevalent effect of the exercise intensity during training on MHC adaptations can be modulated by the concurrent effect of the duration of exercise sessions during training. Thus, exercises for up to 25 minutes per day at low or moderate intensity ($V_{2.5}$) can induce MHC adaptations similar or even superior than training protocols with exercises of the same duration at higher intensity (V_4; Table 2). This is also not surprising since the fastest IIX fibres are also recruited after prolonged submaximal exercises (Valberg, 1996). This observation is also in agreement with results reported by Gansen *et al.* (1999), which concluded that exercises of long duration at low speed are more effective to improve endurance of horses than faster and shorter exercises. Furthermore, an increase in the muscle aerobic capacity of Thoroughbreds can also be induced with exercises of low intensity (~55% of VO_{2max}) over long distances (60 minutes, ~13-14 km) for only 10 consecutive days (Geor *et al.*, 1999). Together, these findings have practical implications in Thoroughbreds since a reduction of training intensity is beneficial to minimise the risk of injuries in the musculoskeletal system (Miyata *et al.*, 1999).

In conclusion, the results of the present study show that the intensity of exercise during the specific phase of training in Thoroughbreds is a more important factor than exercise duration in determining the degree of IIX-to-IIA MHC fibre type transformation in skeletal muscles. But conditioning protocols with prolonged (25 minutes) exercises of moderate intensity ($V_{2.5}$) can induce MHC changes similar to those promoted by programmes with exercises of the same duration but of higher intensity (V_4). The study also implies that values for V_4 after training are not suitable indices of changes in skeletal muscles with training.

Acknowledgements

We gratefully acknowledge the assistance of J. Werkmann, M. Sobotta, A. Köster and H.H.L. Sasse during the project. The treadmill was kindly provided by the Wissenschaftliche Gesellschaft der Schwarzwald-Tierklinik e.V. (Dr. H. Lauk), and laboratory space by the Institut für Klinische Biochemie der Universität Bonn (Dr. F. Bidlingmaier). This project was possible through the financial support of Verein zur Förderung der Forschung im Pferdesport e.V., Höveler Kraftfutterwerke GmbH, Boehringer Mannheim and Horst Dieter Beyer, who provided the horses.

References

Evans, D.L., 1994. Training Thoroughbred racehorses. In: The Athletic Horse: Principles and Practice of Equine Sport Medicine, D.R. Hodgson and R. J. Rose (eds.), W.B. Saunders Company, Philadelphia,.pp. 393-397.

Evans, D.L., Rainger, J.E., Hodgson, D.R., Eaton, M.D. and Rose, R.J., 1995. The effects of intensity and duration of training on blood lactate concentrations during and after exercise. Equine vet. J. Suppl. 18: 422-425.

Gansen, S., Lindner, A., Marx, S., Mosen, H. and Sallmann, H.P., 1999. Effects of conditioning horses with lactate-guided exercise on muscle glycogen content. Equine vet. J. Suppl. 30: 329-331.

Geor, R.J., McCutcheon, L.J. and Shen, H., 1999. Muscular and metabolic responses to moderate-intensity short-term training. Equine Vet. J. Suppl. 30: 311-317.

Lindholm, A. and Piehl, K., 1974. Fibre composition, enzyme activity and concentration of metabolites and electrolytes in muscles of Standardbred horses. Acat Vet. Scand. 15: 287-309.

Miyata, H., Sugiura, T., Kai, M., Hiraga, A. and Tokuriki, M., 1999. Muscle adaptation of Thoughbred racehorses trained on a flan or sloped track. Am. J. Vet. Res. 60: 1536-1539.

Rivero, J.L.L. and Piercy, R.J., 2004. Muscle physiology: responses to exercise and training. In: Equine Sports Medicine and Surgery: Basic and Clinical Sciences of the Equine Athlete, K.W. Hinchcliff, A.J. Kaneps and J. Geor (eds.), Saunders Elsevier, Edinburgh, pp. 45-76.

Rivero, J.L.L., Sporleder, H.P., Quiroz-Rothe, E., Vervuert, I., Coenen, M. and Harmeyer, J., 2002. Oral L-carnitine combined with training promotes changes in skeletal muscle. Equine Vet. J. Suppl. 34: 269-274.

Sinha A.K., Ray, S.P. and Rose, R.J., 1993. Effect of constant load training on skeletal muscle histochemistry of Thoroughbred horses. Res. Vet. Sci. 54: 147-159.

Yamano, S., Eto, D., Sugiura, T., Kai, M., Hiraga, A., Tokuriki, M. and Miyata, H., 2002. Effect of growth and training on muscle adaptation in Thoroughbred horses. Am. J. Vet. Res. 63: 1408-1412.

Valberg, S.J., 1996. Muscular causes of exercise intolerance in horses. Vet. Clin. North Am.: Equine Pract. 12: 495-515.

Werkmann, J., Lindner. A. and Sasse, H.H.L., 1996. Conditioning effects in horses of exercise of 5, 15 or 25 minutes' duration at two blood lactate concentrations. Pferdeheilkunde 12: 474-479.

Does application of focussed shock waves to the digital palmar nerve affect skin sensitivity?[1]

N.M. Waldern, M.A. Weishaupt, I. Imboden, T. Wiestner and C.J. Lischer
Equine Hospital, Vetsuisse Faculty, University of Zurich, Switzerland

Take home message

Application of extracorporeal shock wave treatment or radial pressure wave treatment to the palmar digital nerve had no effect on cutaneous sensation distal to the treated region for at least 2 days after application. The analgesic effect of sedation on reaction to electrical stimuli is distinct but varied among horses.

Introduction

Shock waves are high-energy pressure waves characterised by a rapid rise in pressure followed by a rapid decrease in pressure and a phase of subpressure known as the tensile wave. Extracorporeal shock wave treatment [ESWT] can be focussed directly on a site within the body; while with radial pressure wave treatment [RPWT], the pressure waves are transmitted radially, decreasing in energy in proportion to the square of the distance to the surface (Schnewlin and Lischer, 2001).

A short term analgesic effect after shock wave treatment resulting in a decrease of pain has been observed in a variety of orthopaedic problems in humans. Some clinicians feel that application of 50 to 500 shock wave pulses induces an effect similar to that of local infiltrative anaesthesia or even inhibition of nerve conduction that lasts for 15 minutes to 24 hours (Dahmen *et al.*, 1993). Also in horses, clinicians claim to have observed a similar effect (Bär *et al.*, 2001).

The mechanism by which ESWT and RPWT induce an analgesic effect is unclear. Multiple theories involving the activation of endogenous nociceptive or antinociceptive systems (gate control, hyperstimulation analgesia), as well as direct effects on the nerve have been suggested (Rompe *et al.*, 1997) concerning possible mechanisms of action. However, results of studies (Haake *et al.*, 2001, 2002a, b; Takahashi *et al.*, 2003) to confirm these theories have been contradictory.

At present there are no objective data that confirm the appearance or duration of the presumed analgesic effect after ESWT or RPWT in horses. Because a post-treatment analgesic effect could mask pain caused by certain orthopaedic diseases, ESWT and RPWT are among the mechanical doping procedures prohibited by the Federation Equine International (FEI, 2002). The required withdrawal time between shock wave treatment

---

[1] Content previously published in the American Journal of Veterinary Research 2005; 66: 2095–2100.

and participation in a competition is currently 5 days at international equestrian events, an interval that was determined on the basis of subjective opinion. In contrast to the increasingly efficient detection of chemical substances, the use of ESWT or RPWT cannot be detected via routine screening tests. There is a need for reliable detection methods to guarantee animal welfare and fairness in equine competitive sports.

The objective of this study was to evaluate cutaneous nerve function by means of electrical stimulation of the skin at a site distal to a section of nerve treated with extracorporeal shock waves [ESW] or radial pressure waves [RPW]. Results were compared with the effects of an abaxial nerve block at the same site on the contralateral limb and with the effect of sedation with a combination of intravenously administered xylazine and levomethadone.

Materials and methods

Animals

Eighteen Swiss Warmbloods were used for the study. Horses were judged to be clinically sound before admission. Hair was clipped to a uniform length from above the metacarpophalangeal (*i.e.*, fetlock) joint to the coronary band in both forelimbs ≥ 24 hours before the experiment to ensure uniform testing conditions among horses for the skin sensitivity test.

Experimental protocol

Skin sensitivity was tested by means of electrical stimulation before (A0) and 10 minutes after an abaxial sesamoid nerve block (A1) on a randomly chosen forelimb. The nerve block (Stashak, 1987) was performed with 2 ml of 2% mepivacaine. On the following day, baseline measurements (T0) were made on the contralateral limb. The horse was sedated (xylazine, 0.35 mg/kg, IV, and levomethadone, 44 μg/kg, IV) and skin sensitivity was reevaluated 5 minutes later (T_{sed}). Subsequently, ESWT or RPWT was performed and the sensitivity tests were repeated 4 (T4), 24 (T24), and 48 (T48) hours after the treatment.

Shock wave treatment

Horses were randomly allocated to 3 groups and shock waves were applied to the lateral palmar digital nerve at the level of the proximal sesamoid bones on 1 forelimb. Two groups were treated with focussed shock waves delivered by an electrohydraulic shock wave generator (Equitron, High Medical Technologies, Lengwil, Switzerland) with a 5-mm transducer at a pulse rate of 240 pulses/min and an energy level of 0.15 mJ/mm². Horses in the first group (ESWT 1000) received 1000 pulses, and horses in the second group (ESWT 2000) received 2000 pulses. Horses in the third group (RPWT 2000) received 2000 pulses delivered by a pneumatic shock wave generator (Electro Medical Systems, Swiss Dolor Clast Vet, Switzerland) with a 15-mm applicator at a mean pressure of 2.5 bar and an energy level of 0.14 mJ/mm².

Skin sensitivity

The skin above the coronary band was stimulated with 2 surface electrodes which were electrically isolated and mounted on an S-shaped metal spring. The whole device was affixed to a small metal plate that was glued to the lateral hoof wall with cyanacrylate vacuum glue. Electrodes were placed in exactly the same position for repeated investigations. One stimulation consisted of a burst of 3 rectangular electrical pulses (duration, 2 milliseconds) with pulse intervals of 40 milliseconds. The stimulation was triggered manually. Four types of corporeal reactions were observed: restlessness or uneasiness, muscular reflex, conscious movement of the limb, and turning of the head. The stimulation voltage was increased in 10-V increments until the horse had at least 1 of the reaction types after each of 3 successive stimulations at the same voltage level. This level was defined as the reaction threshold.

Statistical analyses

The reaction threshold voltages at T0, T4, T24 and T48 from each horse were compared using a 1-way ANOVA on ranks to assess the differences among horses. The reaction thresholds of both forelimbs which served as baseline (T0 *vs.* A0) as well as those before and after sedation (T0 *vs.* T_{sed}) were compared with paired *t*-tests. The influence of ESWT on cutaneous sensation was tested with repeated-measures ANOVA for each treatment method in a separate test (n=6 horses) and additionally with data from all 18 horses to investigate the combined influence of method and time.

Statistical analyses were done with commercially available software (SigmaStat, SPSS Inc, Chicago, USA), and values of $P \leq 0.05$ were considered significant.

Results

Horses' mean reaction thresholds at times T0, T4, T24, and T48 ranged from 22.5 to 90.0 V and were significantly ($P<0.001$) different among horses. Mean baseline reaction thresholds (n=18) between the contralateral limbs (at T0, 60.0 ± 25.9 V; at A0, 58.9 ± 27.2 V) were not significantly ($P=0.85$) different.

After the nerve block, complete insensitivity of the skin resulted in all horses. No reactions were evoked after stimulation with voltages up to 4 times the baseline threshold voltage (defined as a negative result).

After sedation, 15 of 17 horses responded with an increase in the reaction threshold. In 4 of those horses, increasing the stimulation voltage up to 4 times the baseline voltage evoked no reaction and no threshold values were available. Excluding the 4 horses with no measurable reaction thresholds while sedated (n=13), values for T_{sed} (151.5 ± 79.1 V) were significantly ($P < 0.001$) higher than the measurements for T0 (63.1 ± 25.1 V).

There were no detectable changes in skin sensitivity after treatment with either type of shock wave (Table 1). The 2-way repeated-measures ANOVA model indicated that neither the treatment method ($P=0.95$) nor length of time after treatment ($P=0.10$) had a significant influence on mean reaction threshold voltage.

Conclusions

No cutaneous analgesia was observed at sites distal to the shock wave-treated section of the palmar digital nerve up to 48 hours after application. The response of horses to cutaneous stimulation was not influenced by the mode of treatment or the number of applied pulses. Similar to our findings, no changes in skin sensitivity were detected in a comparable study (McClure *et al.*, 2005). We conclude that application of ESWs or RPWs directly to a nerve does not interfere with nerve conductivity or affect functional integrity.

With regard to the doping issue, the absence of significant changes in skin sensitivity after direct treatment of a nerve suggests that, in a model as it was used in this study, cutaneous electrical stimulation is not a suitable method for detecting the application of ESWs or RPWs.

After sedation, the mean reaction threshold was more than twice as high as the threshold in the non-sedated state and furthermore, a high degree of interindividual variation was observed. This individually variable antinociceptive effect on the distal limb should be regarded with caution when interpolated to a clinical situation because there may be differences among horses in tolerance to different nociceptive stimuli (*i.e.*, electrical vs mechanical) (Moens *et al.*, 2003; Schatzman *et al.*, 2003).

Table 1. Threshold voltages (mean ± sd) for reaction to electric stimulation of coronary band skin after shock wave treatment of the palmar digital nerve with 1 of 3 treatment protocols. Reaction threshold voltages were determined before anaesthesia (A0) and on the contralateral limb before (T0) and at 4 (T4), 24 (T24), and 48 (T48) hours after treatment.

Shock wave treatment	n	A0	T0	T4	T24	T48	P value
ESWT 1000	6	66.7 ± 17.5	56.7 ± 25.8	58.3 ± 16.0	56.7 ± 10.3	53.3 ± 15.1	0.91
ESWT 2000	6	70.0 ± 28.3	61.7 ± 27.1	51.7 ± 26.4	50.0 ± 23.7	48.3 ± 21.4	0.18
RPWT 2000	6	50.0 ± 37.4	61.7 ± 29.3	50.0 ± 28.3	51.7 ± 27.9	48.3 ± 21.4	0.32
Total	18	58.9 ± 27.2	60.0 ± 25.9	53.3 ± 23.0	52.8 ± 20.8	50.0 ± 18.5	0.10

ESWT = extracorporeal shock wave treatment; RPWT = radial pressure wave treatment; 1000 and 2000 = number of wave pulses delivered; P value = probability of repeated measures ANOVA.

Management of lameness causes in sport horses

References

Bär K, Weiler M, Bodamer J, et al., 2001. Extrakorporale Stosswellentherapie (ESWT)- eine Möglichkeit zur Therapie der Podotrochlose. Tierarztl Prax 29: 163-167.

Dahmen GP, Nam VC and Meiss L, 1993. Extrakorporale Stosswellentherapie zur Behandlung von knochennahen Weichteilschmerzen: Indikation, Technik und vorläufige Ergebnisse In: Chaussy C, Eisenberger F, Jocham D, et al. (eds). Stosswellenlithotripsie - Aspekte und Prognosen. Tübingen: Attempto Verlag, pp. 143-148.

FEI, 2002. Alternative treatment of horses at FEI events. In: Veterinary Regulations. 9 ed. Lausanne: Fédération Equestre Internationale, pp. 35.

Haake M, Thon A and Bette M, 2001. Absence of spinal response to extracorporeal shock waves on the endogenous opioid systems in the rat. Ultrasound Med Biol 27: 279-284.

Haake M, Thon A and Bette M, 2002a. No influence of low-energy extracorporeal shock wave therapy (ESWT) on spinal nociceptive systems. J Orthop Sci 7: 97-101.

Haake M, Thon A and Bette M., 2002b Unchanged c-Fos expression after extracorporeal shock wave therapy: an experimental investigation in rats. Arch Orthop Trauma Surg 122: 518-521.

McClure SR, Sonea IM, Evans RB, et al., 2005. Evaluation of analgesia resulting from extracorporeal shock wave therapy and radial pressure wave therapy in the limbs of horses and sheep. Am J Vet Res 66: 1702-1708.

Moens Y, Lanz F, Doherr MG, et al., 2003. A comparison of the antinociceptive effects of xylazine, detomidine and romifidine on experimental pain in horses. Vet Anaesth Analg 30: 183-190.

Rompe JD, Kullmer K, Vogel J, et al., 1997. Extracorporeal shock-wave therapy. Experimental basis, clinical application. Orthopade 26: 215-228.

Schatzman U, Armbruster S, Stucki F, et al., 2001. Analgesic effect of butorphanol and levomethadone in detomidine sedated horses. J Vet Med A Physiol Pathol Clin Med 48: 337-342.

Schnewlin M and Lischer C, 2001. Extracorporal shock wave therapy in veterinary medicine. Schweiz Arch Tierheilkd 143: 227-232.

Stashak TS, 1987. Diagnosis of lameness In: Stashak TS (ed.), Adams` lameness in horses. 4. ed. Philadelphia: Lea& Febiger, pp. 134-139.

Takahashi N, Wada Y, Ohtori S, et al., 2003. Application of shock waves to rat skin decreases calcitonin gene-related peptide immunoreactivity in dorsal root ganglion neurons. Auton Neurosci 107: 81-84.

A preliminary study of comparative measurements of near foreleg third metacarpal circumference and length within selected groups of event horses

T.C. Whitaker
Centre for Equine and Animal Science, Writtle College, Chelmsford, Essex, CM1 3RR, United Kingdom

Take Home Message

Various studies have indicated a link between third metacarpal (MC3) size and performance in the equine. This study investigated four groups of mature (>4 years) event horses; a base level group, two potential achieving groups, and an achieving group of advanced event horses. MC3 circumference was observed to be significantly (P<0.01) larger within the base level group when compared to the potential achieving and achieving groups. Additionally MC3 length was significantly (P<0.01) shorter in the base level group when compared to the other groups. These observations may prove to be an aid to selection; however the effect of environment on both MC3 development and performance level attained needs careful consideration.

Introduction

The use of objective conformational measures as a method of assessment of potential performance has been undertaken previously in a variety of selection models (Saastamoinen and Barrey, 2000). However there has been limited application of objective conformational measurements within the selection of sport horses in the UK (Royal Agricultural Society of England, 1998). This study conducts a preliminary investigation and comparative analysis of near-fore measurements of the third metacarpal – MC3 (circumference and length) within four selected groups of event horses, base level, potentially achieving (two groups) and achieving.

The use of MC3 circumference and length as a means of selection in horses has been undertaken in a subjective manner for many years by assessors. Minimal soft tissue structures surrounding the MC3 make the MC3 a good site for measurement and assessment (Davies, 2002). Unsoundness associated to the third MC3 has been documented within the equine (Davies, 2002; Walter and Davies, 2001). Speirs (1994) states that the ability of bone to resist imposed loads is related to many factors – including bone geometry. Additional work (Davies, 2001) has concluded that bone strength and stiffness depend on the overall anatomical shape as well as the physical properties of the bone and loading effects. Davies (2001) states that MC3 size and shape are significantly related to strain loadings, an increase in size related to a reduction in strain. He concluded that unsoundness (shore shins) may be closely related to bone size and shape.

Materials and methods

Four groups of event horses were assessed. Base level eventing horses (n=20) were selected from pre-novice event horses under the criterion to have competed for two or more years at eventing and not have won any British Eventing (BE) points. Two groups of potential achieving horses. They were five year old novice event horses qualified for the British Eventing Breeding Championships (n=30) and four and five year old British Equestrian Federation's Young Horse Evaluation (YHE) horses (all eventers; n=22) Finally a group of achieving horses, international advanced eventers (n = 20) was selected. The base line group consisted of horses ranging in height from 157-167 cm; novice group 160-172 cm, YHE group 162-170 cm; achieving 162-172 cm. The base line group consisted of a wide variety in type/breed consisting of 11 horses of unknown breeding, 6, ½ or ¾ bred thoroughbreds, 3 horses of warmblood origin and 1 full thoroughbred. The novice group consisted of 13, ¾ bred thoroughbreds, 7, ½ bred thoroughbreds, 8 of warmblood origin, 2 unknown breeding. The YHE group consisted of 8, ¾ bred thoroughbreds, 5 horses of warmblood origin, 4, ½ bred thoroughbreds, 4 full thoroughbreds, 1 Irish Sports Horse. The elite group consisted of 7, ¾ bred thoroughbreds, 4 horses of unknown breeding, 4 horses of Irish origin, 3, ½ bred thoroughbreds, 2 horses of warmblood origin.

All measurements were collected in the field at equine competitions. Measurements were taken with accuracy to the nearest millimetre. All horses were shod when measurements were taken. All groups of horse were at least five years of age. Two measurements were taken from the near-fore MC3. Circumference was obtained from approximately 2 cm below the bottom of the fourth carpal bone. Length was obtained measuring from the bottom of the fourth carpal bone to the top of the lateral proximal sesamoid bone. To assist with accuracy and reliability all measurements were collated by the same individual. Additionally the recorded measurements for each group were collated at the same location and time.

Comparative measures of distribution between the four groups were investigated. Additionally analysis between the groups was undertaken using a one way ANOVA. Analysis where significance was observed was undertaken using appropriate *Post hoc* Bonferroni test (Zar, 1999). Further investigation of the data set for each measurement group was undertaken using product moment correlations (Zar, 1999).

Results and conclusions

Table 1 shows the distribution of all measured parameters. Table 2 presents' returns for analysis of variance for all parameters studied. Significant differences (P<0.01) in MC3 circumference are reported between the four groups studied (Figure 1). *Post hoc* analysis highlighted specific differences between the base level group and the other three selected groups. The base level group displayed a MC3 circumference +3.6 cm (P<0.05), +3.8 cm (P<0.05) and +3.7 cm (P<0.05) greater than the novice group, YHE group and advanced group respectively. A similar effect was observed in relation to MC3 length (Figure 2). *Post hoc* analysis indicated a specific difference between the base level group and other

Table 1. Descriptive statistics and measures of dispersion: MC3 Circumference and length.

Parameter measured	Group	Mean	Std. Dev	Std. Err	CV %	Skew	Kurtosis
MC3 Circum	Base Level	24.8	1.642	0.367	8.2	-1.625	4.894
	Novice	21.2	0.824	0.150	2.8	0.167	-0.212
	YHE	21.0	0.740	0.158	3.4	0.969	1.249
	Advanced	21.1	0.810	0.180	4.0	-0.445	0.512
MC3 length	Base Level	21.6	0.981	0.219	4.9	-0.124	-0.399
	Novice	26.6	1.187	0.217	4.0	0.531	0.614
	YHE	23.1	2.550	0.543	11.6	0.556	-1.380
	Advanced	27.6	1.340	0.299	6.7	0.671	0.777

Table 2. ANOVA results for all measured parameters.

Measured Dimension	Sums of Squared – within groups	Sums of Squared – between groups	F Value	Significance
MC3 circumference	94.704	212.065	65.684	0.001
MC3 length	229.410	518.642	66.316	0.001

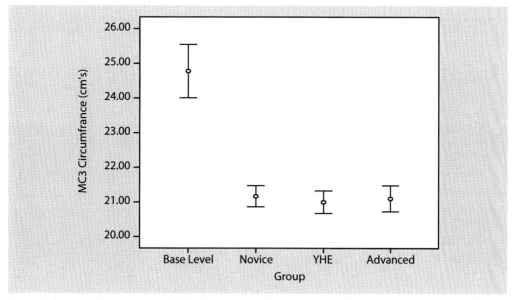

Figure 1. Comparative measures of MC3 circumference between assessed groups (error bar 95% confidence interval).

groups. The base level group was observed to have a mean MC3 length -5.0 cm (P<0.05), -1.5 cm (P<0.05) and -6.0 cm (P<0.05) smaller than the novice group, YHE group and advanced group respectively. Additionally differences were observed between the YHE group and novice and advanced groups. The YHE group displayed a MC3 length -3.5 cm (P<0.05) and -4.5 cm (P<0.05) smaller than the novice and advanced groups respectively. Product moment correlations between MC3 circumference and length were weak to moderate for the four groups (Table 3). The strongest correlation was observed within the YHE group at 0.511 (P<0.05).

The groups assessed during exhibited normality in distribution for MC3 measurements with limited variation being observed within groups. With the exception of MC3 length the base level group displayed the highest coefficients of variation. This may indicate a degree of non-uniformity within the base level sample. Further work need to be conducted to establish whether this trend is apparent in the base level population as a whole. Greater variation in distribution was also observed for the length measurement within the YHE group. This was highlighted by the divergence from the novice and achieving populations with regard to MC3 length (Figure 2).

Potential confounding factors within the study include measurement technique, breed type and base line group selection. The collection of data by a single researcher at a specific time and location for each group theoretically should mean minimum variation in recording of measurements. However the issue of reliability and repeatability of measurement techniques needs further investigations within any larger study. Additionally the influence of breed type in relation to MC3 needs investigation within a much larger population. The nature and type of horses within the base line group may include horses that are owned by amateur riders who have limited competitive aspirations. Consequently competition exposure and limited rider ambition may be a factor for non-progression of horses within this group.

The study demonstrates a clear relationship between MC3 circumference, length and group achievement. The results indicate that potential achieving horses and achieving horse have significantly smaller MC3 circumferences and greater MC3 lengths than the base level horses. This relationship requires further investigation in light of other research conducted into MC3 size and shape and potential unsoundness in the equine (Davies, 2001).

Table 3. Correlation coefficience: MC3 circumference and length.

Base Level	0.235
Novice	0.420[*]
YHE	0.511[*]
Advanced	0.215

* significant at the 0.05 level

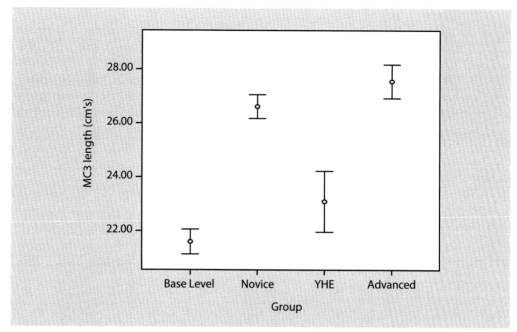

Figure 2. Comparative measures of MC3 length between assessed groups (error bar 95% confidence interval).

Both these differences in MC3 dimensions might be factors to consider in the selection of potential 'elite' event horses. However the influences of environmental management has been well documented (Speirs, 1994) and need careful consideration. Correlations indicate that only a moderate to weak relationship exists between MC3 circumference and length. It is evident that both measurements should be considered in any selection process. It should be noted that the sample sizes within this study are small and a further study involving a larger population needs to be performed before any firm conclusions or recommendations can be drawn. Further work to examine whether optimum measurements exists for elite performance needs to be undertaken.

Acknowledgements

Graham Suggett, Director of British Breeding, British Equestrian Federation, British Eventing

References

Davies, H.M.S., 2002. Monitoring soundness in sport horse. In: The Elite Dressage and Three-Day-Event Horse, A. Lindner (ed.), Arbeitsgruppe Pferd, Jülich, pp. 109-114.

Davies, H.M.S., 2001. Relationship between third metacarpal bone parameters and surface strains. Equine Veterinary Journal 33: 16-20.

Royal Agricultural Society of England, 1998. A Breeding Strategy for the British Sport Horse Industry. Kenilworth, RASE.

Saastamoinen M.T. and E. Barrey, 2000. Genetics of Conformation Locomotion and Physiological Traits. In: The Genetics of the Horse, A.T. Bowling and A. Ruvinsky (eds.), Oxford, CABI International, pp. 439-472.

Speirs, V.C., 1994. Lameness: approaches to therapy and rehabilitation. In: The Athletic Horse, Hodgson D.R. and Rose R.J (eds.), Philadelphia, W.B. Saunders Company, pp. 342-369.

Walter, L.J. and H.M.S. Davies, 2001. Analysis of a radiographic technique for the measurement of equine metacarpal bone shape. Equine Veterinary Journal, Supplement 33: 141-144.

Zar, J.H., 1999. Biostatistical Analysis. New Jersey, Prentice Hall, Inc.